Medical Radiography

PreTest®
Self-Assessment
and Review

Medical Radiography

PreTest®
Self-Assessment
and Review

Linda LeFave, M.Ed., R.T.(R)(M)
Professor and Clinical Coordinator
Radiologic Technology Program
Quinsigamond Community College
Worcester, Massachusetts

McGraw-Hill
Health Professions Division/PreTest® Series

New York   St. Louis   San Francisco   Auckland
Bogotá   Caracas   Lisbon   London   Madrid
Mexico City   Milan   Montreal   New Delhi
San Juan   Singapore   Sydney   Tokyo   Toronto

Medical Radiography PreTest® Self-Assessment and Review

Copyright © 1996 by The McGraw-Hill Companies. All rights reserved. Printed in the United States of America. Except as permitted under the Copyright Act of 1976, no part of this publication may be reproduced or distributed in any form or by any means, or stored in a data base or retrieval system, without the prior written permission of the publisher.

1 2 3 4 5 6 7 8 9 0   SEMSEM   9 9 8 7 6 5

ISBN 0-07-052078-X

The editors were Gail Gavert and Bruce MacGregor.
The production supervisor was Gyl A. Favours.
This book was set in Times Roman by V&M Graphics.
Semline was printer and binder.

The ARRT does not review, evaluate, or endorse publications. Permission to reproduce ARRT copyrighted materials within this publication should not be construed as an endorsement of the publication by the ARRT.

Library of Congress Cataloging-in-Publication Data

LeFave, Linda.
Medical radiography : PreTest self-assessment and review / Linda LeFave.
    p. cm.
  ISBN 0-07-052078-X
  1. Radiography, Medical—Examinations, questions, etc.   I. Title.
  [DNLM: 1. Radiography—examination questions.   WN 18.2 L488m   1996]
RC78.15.L44   1996
616.07′572′076—dc20
DNLM/DLC
for Library of Congress   95-14113

•   •

In Loving Memory of

William T. Carrigan
Marie B. LeFave
Holly Woodward, R.T.(R)

•   •

Contents

Preface

Medical Radiography: PreTest® Self-Assessment and Review is designed to provide a source of review questions as a means of preparation for ARRT certification and state licensing requirements. A total of 1000 board-type questions are included along with their answers and a full explanation of the answers. Specific references are also provided for each answer for further study. A bibliography of currently available texts in medical radiographic imaging and procedures concludes the book. Additionally, supplemental material is included to aid the reader in preparation and understanding of the concepts and principles involved in radiography, such as tips for reviewing and taking the exam, standard definitions used by the ARRT, and explanation and review of the mathematical principles associated with radiography.

The section on "Preparing for and Taking the ARRT Examination" provides simple suggestions for organizing study material and time, proper study techniques, and items to consider in preparation for exam day. It further offers techniques for taking the exam, as well as for handling anxiety associated with testing.

Terminology associated with radiography can be confusing and requires the reader to be fully informed to accurately interpret the questions being asked. To assist with this task, the ARRT's standard definitions for the radiography exam and for positioning and projections are also included, with permission of the ARRT.

A separate section entitled "Review of Mathematical Skills" is included to review the various mathematical concepts associated with radiography. Although modern radiographic equipment requires minimal calculations, the competent radiographer must have a thorough understanding of the relationships involved in the imaging process. This section explains the pertinent relationships, gives examples of the mathematical principles, and provides practice problems for the reader. A full listing of the answers to the practice problems follows this section.

The review questions are grouped in five categories representing the major areas of the ARRT exam. Each category contains five times the number of questions to be found on the exam for that category. The subject matter that the questions address is based on the 1995 Content Specifications for the ARRT exam. Each question is a multiple choice, board-type question with three to five distractors from which to select the one best answer. It is suggested that the reader answer a group of questions (10 to 20), then check the answers and read the explanation for further clarification. If the explanation still does not adequately explain the concept, the reader should use the references offered for further study.

It is important to note that although this text is based on the ARRT exam Content Specifications, the ARRT does not review, evaluate, or endorse publications. Permission to reproduce ARRT copyrighted materials within this publication should not be construed as an endorsement of this publication by the ARRT.

Acknowledgments

Although writing questions is a required activity of any educator, constructing questions and answers for this project was a time-consuming effort and required the support and understanding of many important groups and individuals. My thanks and sincere appreciation go to the new and future radiographers of the Quinsigamond Community College Radiologic Technology Classes of 1994, 1995, and 1996. Their pride in and support of my efforts was truly encouraging. My thanks and respect to the clinical instructors associated with the QCC Radiologic Technology program for their professional abilities, which keep problems to a minimum and thus enable me to act in an efficient manner as the program's clinical coordinator. My greatest thanks and admiration to my coworker and friend Sandra Ostresh, R.T.(R), program director, for her leadership, knowledge, and devotion to the QCC program and the profession of radiologic technology.

Of course many thanks must also go to my wonderful family for their encouragement in a project that has limited the amount of time I could spend with them. I know I am truly fortunate to have a loving mother; wonderful brothers, sisters, and brothers- and sisters-in-law; adorable nieces and nephews; and the best children and husband any woman could ever be blessed with. Each of you are in my prayers and hold a special place in my heart.

Medical Radiography

PreTest® Self-Assessment and Review

INTRODUCTION

Preparing for and Taking the ARRT Examination

The ARRT examination is the culmination of the education process for the radiologic technology student. However, it is not a "do or die" event! The importance of the exam should be kept in perspective. The added stress can be overwhelming and contribute to poor performance and ill health. Fortunately, examinees are allowed to take the exam three times. While having to repeat the exam may be disappointing and inconvenient, just remember that your future does not depend on only one chance. To be eligible to apply for the ARRT exam, the candidate must have successfully completed a radiologic technology program and have been presented with the information necessary to pass the exam. The time between completing the educational process and actually sitting for the ARRT exam should be used to reinforce your understanding and mastery of the topics studied. Using a text of practice questions, such as this one, should help to identify areas in need of further study. Memorization of questions and answers in this or any review question book is a waste of time. In the long run, the effort to thoroughly *understand* the various concepts of radiologic technology will enable successful performance. Candidates should be able to reason through test questions and answers, based on their knowledge, which will also enhance their skills as a competent radiologic technologist.

Topics and Strategies for Review

The ARRT exam is divided into five topics:

(A) Radiation Protection (30 questions). Patient protection material includes the biologic effects of radiation as well as methods for reducing patient dose. Factors affecting radiologic personnel include protection practices, NCRP guidelines, and sources of radiation exposure. Finally, topics related to the properties of radiation and methods of monitoring and measuring radiation exposure are covered.

(B) Equipment Operation and Maintenance (30 questions). This section includes topics related to the structure, function, and maintenance of the x-ray tube and exposure controls and generator systems for diagnostic, fluoroscopic, and mobile units. The structure, function, and maintenance of accessory radiographic equipment is also included, e.g., film, screens, grids, beam restrictors, and filters.

(C) Image Production and Evaluation (50 questions). This section of the exam focuses on the elements that contribute to optimum image quality: density, contrast, recorded detail, and distortion. These elements involve the exposure factors, accessory devices for imaging, patient factors, and proper use of technique charts and automatic exposure control. The components of and quality control practices for film storage, handling, and processing are also covered. Finally, this section contains questions related to evaluation of the final image to include determination of and effective remedies for poor image quality.

(D) Radiographic Procedures (60 questions). This is the longest section of the exam and consists of topics related to the anatomy and positioning of the human body to satisfy the requirements for radiographic imaging. Specific topics include understanding terminology related to anatomy, physiology, disease processes, and exam procedures. The anatomic areas referred to include the thorax, abdomen (including the GI and GU systems), upper and lower extremities, spine, pelvis, and head and neck. Specialty procedures such as tomography, arthrography, myelography, venography, and hysterosalpingography are also covered.

(E) Patient Care (30 questions). This section includes material pertaining to the legal and ethical responsibilities of the technologist in relating to patients and carrying out exam requirements. Patient safety and education before, during, and after a radiologic procedure are also included. Other questions cover such topics as monitoring of a patient's vital signs and any ancillary equipment involving the patient, as well as understanding and employing techniques for infection prevention and control. Finally, this section of the exam contains questions regarding the types of contrast media, their correct use, and possible reactions.

Getting Started. Review for the ARRT exam should be conducted over several weeks prior to the exam. This will produce more effective study periods and minimize "cramming" just before the exam. For this reason it is important to plan study time to fit realistically with other responsibilities, such as work, family, and social activities. Once you determine how much time will be available for study, divide the five topics of the exam into this time. The amount of study time needed for each topic is determined by your own weaknesses and strengths. Emphasis should be place on those topics you are least confident in; however, each area of subject matter covered by the exam should be reviewed, no matter how confident one feels. On a weekly basis, review how well you are following your plan of study and reevaluate the plan if it is not working.

Individual vs. Group Study. Effective reviewing and organizing of study material can be done as an individual. Include such activities as rereading class notes, making note cards, practicing solving mathematical problems, and reading texts as needed to reaffirm one's understanding. As the exam gets closer, encouragement and clarification can be obtained by studying in groups of five to six participants. You can quiz each other with practice questions and answers. Follow-up discussions will enhance your understanding of the concepts raised during the quiz period.

Whether working in groups or individually, plan study for a time when it will be most effective. If you are hungry or tired when trying to study, you will find it harder to concentrate. Other distractions may be less easily dealt with (family or job concerns), but must be resolved, at least momentarily, if your study period is to be productive. The place where you study should offer sufficient work space to be comfortable, without being overly relaxing and promoting sleep. The area should include a desk or table to accommodate necessary books and notes, and a supportive chair to keep you alert—not an easy chair or recliner. The study area should be free of distractions such as television, loud music, recreational activities, or noisy conversation. When studying at home, make others aware of the study plan and tell them that you wish to study for a specific time period. Include family and friends when you construct your original plan to help them understand how important study time is and how you need their support. *Effective* study time can cut down on the number of study periods, freeing up time for other purposes. If a conducive environment cannot be made at home, use a library.

Set a reasonable length of time for a study period. Short study periods (2 to 3 hours) conducted frequently (three to four times a week) can be more effective than marathon sessions (all day once a week). If a long session is the only option, plan a short break every hour or two and vary the subject matter to include several topics over the course of the session.

How to Review. Start reviewing by organizing all notes, tests, quizzes, and previous reading assignments according to the content of the exam. Those who were organized note-takers during their courses probably already have their materials pretty well ordered. However, you still may need to consolidate related material from various courses. Construct outlines of the various concepts of radiography, showing relationships and influencing factors. As mentioned previously, if the principles of radiography are *learned* rather than memorized, you will be better able to analyze a question and determine the best answer by logic. If your notes are not orderly, making them so will be an important task to accomplish. Again, use the content specifications of the ARRT exam to help organize the notes and other related materials. Review textbooks for notes made in the margins or other key points listed. Use 3 × 5 cards to record specific facts, key concepts, and practice questions based on your notes and readings. Putting information on index cards can increase study time by providing an opportunity for a quick study whenever a few moments are available (e.g., during waiting times or a lunch break).

When reviewing mathematical matters, practice, practice, practice. Many math problems related to radiography are stated in the form of a word problem. Read the entire question and determine what, specifically, is being asked. Before beginning the solution, decide what the relationship between the factors is and whether or not the new value will be increased or decreased from the original. Then write out the relationship or mathematical expression to solve the problem. Finally, carry out the math using the factors stated in the problem. Most numerical values will be carried out to the first or second decimal place. Answers should be rounded to the extent suggested by the answer options. Practice converting numerical values between their various equivalent forms. Basic calculators are allowed in the examination room, but programmable types are not. Therefore, you must know the various mathematical relationships used in radiologic technology. For a review and practice of the most common math concepts, see the section "Review of Mathematical Skills" below.

Staying in Tune. When you study, read, write, and even talk, your mind will frequently drift off into some other activity. You may daydream or suddenly realize that you have read a number of pages about which you have no recall. This is normal. Simply recognize your loss of attention and refocus on the task at hand. When concentration drifts again, bring it back. Accepting the fact that concentration may need to be gently refocused is more effective than getting irritated. When you find you can no longer concentrate, take a break or quit for the day.

Preparing to Go to the Examination

A few days before the examination, begin to prepare for the actual day. If the exam site is a distance away, be sure to get specific directions and plan sufficient travel time, remembering to allow for traffic problems. It may help to drive to the test site before exam day to work out the best route and learn how long it will take. Locate parking facilities and the proper entrance. Plan to arrive early for the exam to allow time for finding the exam room and relaxing, not rushing in at the last minute.

In addition to being mentally prepared for the exam, be physically ready. During the days prior to the exam, be sure to eat balanced meals, get plenty of rest, and enjoy some recreational activities. These activities will keep stress to a minimum. Although successful completion of the exam on the first attempt is the best outcome, it is a real possibility that a second test will be necessary. However, do not start worrying about the "next time" even before taking the exam once. Maintain a positive attitude and be confident of a successful result.

Each candidate will receive an admission ticket 2 to 3 weeks prior to the exam date. This ticket and a signed photographic identification card are required to enter the testing center. All examinees are expected to bring their own pencils, erasers, watch, and calculator. Sharing of supplies between examinees is strictly prohibited. Books, notes, and scrap paper are not allowed. Any computation work may be done on the exam booklet.

Since the conditions of the exam site will be unknown beforehand, be prepared and bring or wear a sweatshirt or sweater. Just as when you are studying, it is important to be comfortable during the exam. Being too warm or cold is an unnecessary distraction.

Taking the Examination

Once the examination materials have been distributed and pertinent instructions given, the time to begin the exam will be announced. Do not break the seal of the test booklet until instructed to do so. The exam session will be for 3 hours from the announced "start" time.

Make Notations. Once the exam has commenced, it is fair to mark down a few notes or reminders that may be needed during the test. No scrap paper is allowed, but there is space within the test booklet for such notes. These notes may include math formulas or frequently confused terms or concepts.

Read Thoroughly. Be sure to read all *directions* and *questions* completely and thoroughly. Understand what you are expected to do and what the question is asking. Note key words that may provide clues or relevant data for answering the item. Define technical and medical terms by their proper meaning and application in reference to the question and answer.

Select the Answer. Once the exam item has been read, anticipate the possible answer before reading the answer options. Read each option completely. Eliminate improbable answers, thereby narrowing the selection to two or three. Select the single best answer to satisfy the exam item *as written*; do not read "into" the question. Resist the impulse to change answers, as the first choice is usually the correct one. Change answers only when there is a significant difference in your interpretation of the item or answer when you reread it.

Mark the Answer Sheet. Mark all answers by completely filling in the circle representing your selected answer. Completely erase any answer you wish to change and mark the correct answer. Each exam item has only *one* correct answer. Multiple answers for an item will be marked wrong. Be sure the item number on the answer sheet matches the exam item from the test booklet. It is a good idea to check for a numerical match on every fifth question.

Pace Yourself. The 3-hour time frame allows approximately 50 seconds to answer each of the 200 questions. Some questions will take less time while others will require more. Pace your time by checking the number of questions completed every 20 to 30 minutes.

Leave No Blanks. *Answer all questions.* Blanks are counted as wrong, so a guessed answer is better than no answer at all! If a question stumps you, answer it as best you can, then mark it to be returned to later, if time permits. When guessing an answer, narrow down the possibilities and then choose the first one. For example, if you can rule out answers A and C, which leaves answers B and D, choose B.

Control Anxiety. If feelings of panic or anxiety begin to develop during the exam, take a few moments to calm down and regain control by using the following techniques. *Recognize*—Be aware if you begin to feel frustrated or are unable to think clearly. Also note any muscle tension in your face, neck, shoulders, or thorax. *Breathe*—If symptoms should occur, stop work on the exam, and, with your eyes closed, take a few slow, deep breaths. Do so quietly, so as not to disturb other examinees. *Visualize*—While doing the relaxation breathing, imagine a calm, pleasant scene (such as a vacation, so richly deserved after this exam!). *Work the muscles*—Repeatedly tense and relax the muscles that feel tight or where discomfort is most disturbing. Allow your mind to wander and unwind for a few moments, letting the tension flow out of your body.

Review of Mathematical Skills

As with any science-based educational program, the radiologic technology curriculum has included numerous topics based on mathematical principles. A thorough understanding of many formulas is necessary to perform as a highly skilled radiographer. Although modern radiographic equipment strives to reduce the number of variables a radiographer must consider, this does not mean you can be ignorant of the basic principles of radiography. There will always be occasions in which the radiographer must determine a new set of exposure factors to accommodate suboptimum imaging conditions. Relying on the equipment to suggest correction factors can erode your ability to accurately apply all the skills you were taught. Even when automated equipment is used, the radiographer should make it a habit to check the postexposure milliampere-second readout in order to acknowledge the level of exposure delivered. The ARRT exam will contain questions that need to be solved mathematically. This section will review the most commonly used math formulas and attempt to assist the reader in understanding the relationships involved. By knowing these relationships, you can frequently set up the correct proportion for the question at hand, thereby reducing the number of actual formulas to be remembered. Practice questions are also included here; their answers can be found at the end of this section.

Numerical Prefixes. Performing calculation requires understanding the wide variety of ways to express numerical values using *prefixes*. You must be able to convert seconds to milliseconds, volts to kilovolts, and millimeters to micrometers or angstroms. A review of the commonly used prefixes is strongly encouraged. These would include the following:

Prefix	Exponential value	Decimal value
mega (M)	10^6	1,000,000
kilo (k)	10^3	1,000
deka (da)	10^1	10
centi (c)	10^{-2}	0.01
milli (m)	10^{-3}	0.001
micro (μ)	10^{-6}	0.000001
nano (n)	10^{-9}	0.000000001
angstrom (Å)	10^{-10}	0.0000000001
pico (p)	10^{-12}	0.000000000001

As the prefix unit gets smaller, the numerical value will increase (decimal point moves to right). Larger prefix values require the decimal point to move to the left. Equivalents of numerical values as stated with various prefixes are as follows:

$$15 \text{ m} = 15,000 \text{ mm} = 15,000,000 \text{ μm}$$

$$20 \text{ V} = 0.020 \text{ kV} = 0.000020 \text{ MV}$$

$$1 \text{ mm} = 1,000 \text{ μm} = 1,000,000 \text{ nm} = 10,000,000 \text{ Å}$$

For practice, convert the following values to their equivalent with the prefix indicated.

1. The wavelength of an x-ray photon measures 0.5 Å. What is the equivalent in millimeters and meters?
    _____ mm _____ m
2. The potential difference applied to an x-ray tube is 75 kV. What is the equivalent in volts and megavolts?
    _____ V _____ MV
3. The wavelength of light emission from the rare earth intensifying screens equals 540 nm. What is the equivalent in angstroms and micrometers? _____ Å _____ µm
4. A radiographer has a cumulative occupational exposure history of 580 mrem. What is the equivalent in rem (roentgen-equivalent–man) and microrem? _____ rem _____ µrem
5. A radiographic examination delivers a dose of 0.15 gray (Gy). What is the equivalent in centigrays and milligrays? _____ cGy _____ mGy

Image Production

The art of radiography requires total understanding of the wide array of variables within the imaging chain that must be correctly manipulated to produce optimum quality images. Many of these variables have an effect on the quantity of radiation that ultimately reaches the image receptor and require a change in exposure factors (milliamperage-seconds and kilovoltage). The relationship between radiographic density and technical variables can be expressed in a mathematical manner and utilized in correcting for technical variation. These useful formulas include those listed below. Practice in working through the relationships between the variables stated and the primary beam will assist the reader in implementing variations in technique .

Milliampere-second Calculations: mAs = mA × time. Milliampere-seconds are the product of milliamperes and time. Time may be expressed as a fraction, as a decimal, or in milliseconds (ms). Find the milliampere-seconds for the following milliamperage-time combinations.

1. 500 mA, 0.012 s = _____ mAs
2. 400 mA, 1/20 s   = _____ mAs
3. 200 mA, 80 ms   = _____ mAs
4. 600 mA, 0.02 s   = _____ mAs
5. 600 mA, 15 ms   = _____ mAs

Solving for Milliamperage or Time: mA = mAs/time; time = mAs/mA. If either milliamperage or time is known for a particular milliampere-second value, the unknown factor is found by dividing the milliamperage-seconds by the known factor. For example: If a technique calls for 20 mAs when using 0.2 s of exposure time, what milliamperage will be required? The solution is found by dividing the milliampere-seconds by the time: $20/0.2 = 100$ mA. Practice this concept by solving the problems below for x.

	mAs	Time	mA
1.	32	0.08 s	x
2.	12	x	500
3.	5	0.0167 s	x
4.	48	x	600
5.	18	30 ms	x

Relationship between Milliamperage and Time: $mA_o/mA_n = time_n/time_o$ or $mA_n = mA_o \times time_o/time_n$. The relationship between milliamperage and time, for the same milliampere-second value, is *indirectly proportional*. That is, as one factor increases by two (2), the other must decrease by one-half (1/2). In a proportionate relationship, the value on each side of the equal sign must be the same. For example: 200 mA at 0.1 s equals 20 mAs; if the time is doubled to 0.2 s, then milliamperage must be decreased to 100 to maintain the same milliampere-second value. In this case the proportion is equal:

$$\frac{200}{100} = \frac{0.2}{0.1}; \ 200 \times 0.1 = 100 \times 0.2; \ 20 = 20$$

Practice this concept with the following examples.

	mA_o	$Time_o$	mA_n	$Time_n$
1.	200	0.05 s	400	x
2.	300	10 ms	200	x
3.	600	0.015 s	300	x
4.	400	20 ms	x	40 ms
5.	600	0.02 s	x	0.03 s

Relationship between Milliamperage-seconds and Kilovoltage Peak in Maintaining Radiographic Density: 15 percent increase in kilovoltage peak is equal to double the milliampere-seconds in regard to image density. Radiographic density is *directly* influenced by both milliamperage-seconds and kilovoltage peak. Increasing the milliampere-seconds increases the quantity of x-rays in the primary beam and, ultimately, the amount of exposure received by the patient and image receptor. This is achieved by increased thermionic emission that makes more electrons available for interaction with the target of the x-ray tube. Increasing kilovoltage peak also increases the quantity of radiation that reaches the image receptor by the ability of kilovoltage peak to produce high-energy, more penetrating photons and a higher conversion efficiency in the x-ray tube. However, the degree of influence of milliamperage-seconds and kilovoltage peak on photon quantity is not the same. The quantity of photons produced by milliamperage-seconds follows a *directly proportional* relationship (double milliampere-seconds equals double x-ray photons). The quantity of photons produced by kilovoltage selection is equal to the square of the kilovoltage peak $(kVp_1 / kVp_2)^2$. Thus kilovoltage peak has a direct, but not proportionate effect on radiographic density. If density is the image quality factor that needs to be altered, milliamperage-seconds is the most appropriate factor to vary. However, some situations do require the kilovoltage peak to be altered. Since a change in kilovoltage peak would affect density, milliamperage-seconds must be varied *indirectly* in order to maintain density. For example, a radiographic density of 1.2_D is achieved using 25 mAs at 70 kVp. If the kilovoltage peak was increased by 15 percent to 80 kVp, the milliampere-seconds would need to be decreased to 12 in order to maintain the same density level. Solve the following examples to practice this concept.

1. 32 mAs at 60 kV would be equal to 16 mAs at _____ kVp.
2. 15 mAs at 80 kV would be equal to 7 mAs at _____ kVp.
3. 18 mAs at 92 kV would be equal to _____ mAs at 78 kVp.
4. 10 mAs at 114 kV would be equal to _____ mAs at 96 kVp.
5. 20 mAs at 70 kV would be equal to 5 mAs at _____ kVp.

Relationship between Grid Ratio and Milliamperage-seconds: mAs_o/mAs_n = grid ratio factor$_o$/grid ratio factor$_n$. Grids are used to absorb scattered radiation between the patient and the image receptor and thereby improve radiographic contrast. However, grid use will also lower radiographic density owing to the loss of scattered radiation and inadvertent absorption of some primary radiation. The amount of reduced density increases as grid ratio increases. For this reason, grid use will require an increase in milliampere-second values (*direct relationship*). The amount of increase in milliamperage-seconds is determined by conversion factors assigned to the various grid ratios found in common use. This author subscribes to the following grid conversion factors.

Grid Ratio	Conversion Factor
Nongrid	1
5:1 linear	2
6:1 linear	3
8:1 linear	4
10:1 linear	5
12:1 linear	5
16:1 linear	6

An example of finding a new milliampere-second value for a change in grid ratio is as follows: 10 mAs is used for a nongrid examination. If an 8:1 grid was substituted, what new milliampere-second value would be required? The conversion factors will be 1 for the nongrid system and 4 for the 8:1 grid. The solution would be $10/x = 1/4$; $x = 10 \times 4$; $x = 40$ mAs. Practice this concept by solving the following problems.

	mAs_o	Grid ratio$_o$	mAs_n	Grid ratio$_n$
1.	8	nongrid	x	10:1
2.	15	8:1	x	12:1
3.	24	16:1	x	5:1
4.	18	10:1	x	8:1
5.	32	12:1	x	nongrid

Relationship between Screen and Milliamperage-seconds: mAs_o/mAs_n = relative screen speed$_o$/relative screen speed$_n$. The role of the intensifying screen is to amplify the action of x-rays on film exposure. As a result, the use of screens requires less milliamperage-seconds to achieve the desired density. Since screens are available in a variety of speeds, the amount of change in milliamperage-seconds will vary also. The relationship between relative screen speed (RS) and density is *indirectly proportional*. Therefore, as screen speed doubles, milliamperage-seconds must be reduced to one-half (1/2) to achieve the same density. For example: An examination suggests exposure factors of 25 mAs with a 100 speed screen. What milliamperage-seconds would be needed if screen speed were increased to 200? Solve this as follows:

$$\frac{25}{x} = \frac{200}{100}; \ 200x = 25 \times 100; \ 200x = 2500; \ x = 12.5 \text{ mAs}$$

The speed doubled and the milliamperage-seconds was halved. Solve the following problems to practice this concept.

	mAs_o	Relative speed$_o$	mAs_n	Relative speed$_n$
1.	48	100	x	50
2.	50	100	x	400
3.	24	200	x	400
4.	5	400	x	50
5.	12	600	x	400

Inverse Square Law: $I_o/I_n = D_n^2/D_o^2$. The inverse square law (ISL) states that radiation intensity (quantity) is *inversely proportional to the square of the distance*. This means that as the source-to-image distance (SID) is doubled, radiation intensity to the patient and image receptor is one-fourth (1/4) its original value. Thus, both radiographic density and patient dose will be similarly affected. For example: If a set of exposure factors produced an exposure of 340 mR using a SID of 40 inches, what would the intensity be if SID was changed to 48 inches? Solve this problem as follows:

$$\frac{340}{x} = \frac{48^2}{40^2}; \ \frac{340}{x} = \frac{2304}{1600}; \ 2304x = 340 \times 1600; \ 2304x = 544,000; \ x = 236 \text{ mR}$$

Use the following problems to practice this concept.

	I_o	SID_o	I_n	SID_n
1.	182 mR	40″	x	56″
2.	222 mR	40″	x	60″
3.	85 mR	100 cm	x	180 cm
4.	156 mR	60 cm	x	120 cm
5.	92 mR	72″	x	50″

Relationship between SID and Milliamperage-seconds: $mAs_o/mAs_n = SID_o^2/SID_n^2$. As a result of the inverse square law, changes in SID must be accompanied by changes in milliamperage-seconds. This relationship is *directly proportional to the square of the distance*. An example of this relationship is as follows: A technique chart recommends using 15 mAs, 70 kV, and 40 inches SID for a particular examination. Due to patient limitations, only 35 inches SID is possible. What new milliamperage-seconds should be used? Solve this problem as follows:

$$\frac{15}{x} = \frac{40^2}{35^2}; \; \frac{15}{x} = \frac{1600}{1225}; \; 1600x = 15 \times 1225; \; 1600x = 18,375; \; x = 11.48 \approx 12 \text{ mAs}$$

Complete the following problems to further practice this skill.

	mAs_o	SID_o	mAs_n	SID_n
1.	22	40″	x	56″
2.	40	72″	x	40″
3.	12	40″	x	60″
4.	8	100 cm	x	140 cm
5.	28	140 cm	x	60 cm

Relationship between Kilovoltage Peak and Beam Intensity: $I_o/I_n = kVp_o^2/kVp_n^2$. The effect of kilovoltage peak on the intensity of the x-ray beam is a *proportional to the square of the change in kilovoltage*. As kilovoltage peak is increased, the penetrability of the beam as well as the quantity of photons produced increases and has a more dramatic effect on beam intensity, patient dose, and radiographic density. For example: If a technique of 10 mAs at 72 kVp produces a beam intensity of 360 mR, what would the intensity be at 82 kVp and the same 10 mAs? The solution is found as follows:

$$\frac{360}{x} = \frac{72^2}{82^2}; \; \frac{360}{x} = \frac{5184}{6724}; \; 5184x = 360 \times 6724; \; 5184x = 2,420,640; \; x = 466.94 \approx 467 \text{ mR}$$

To practice this concept, solve the following problems.

1. If 60 kV produces 214 mR, a decrease to 50 kV produces an mR of _____.
2. If 85 kV produces 440 mR, an increase to 100 kV produces an mR of _____.
3. If 110 kV produces 622 mR, a decrease to 90 kV produces an mR of _____.
4. If 72 kV produces 338 mR, a decrease to 65 kV produces an mR of _____.
5. If 68 kV produces 276 mR, an increase to 72 kV produces an mR of _____.

Magnification Factor: Source-to-image distance (SID)/Source-to-object distance (SOD). In addition to influencing radiographic density, SID *indirectly* affects magnification of images. In general, magnification is undesirable due to misrepresentation of the structure's size and to the geometric blur. Efforts should be made to keep magnification to a minimum. Magnification is controlled by maintaining an optimum relationship between SID and SOD. This means that any increase in object-to-image distance (OID) must be associated with an equal increase in SID. There will always be some degree of magnification in radiographic images. An example of how to calculate the magnification factor is as follows: An SID of 40 inches and OID of 4 inches will result in a magnification factor of 1.11. This is solved by first finding the SOD (SID − OID). The magnification factor will be 40/36 = 1.11. Practice this concept with the following problems.

1. 56″ SID and 4″ OID creates a magnification factor of _____.
2. 72″ SID and 8″ OID creates a magnification factor of _____.
3. 40″ SID and 20″ OID creates a magnification factor of _____.
4. 36″ SID and 2″ OID creates a magnification factor of _____.
5. 40″ SID and 2″ OID creates a magnification factor of _____.

Magnification Percentage: SID/SOD − 1 × 100. The magnification factor may be more relevant when expressed in terms of magnification percentage. Finding the percentage of magnification begins by calculating the magnification factor then subtracting 1 and multiplying the result by 100. For the example used in the preceding section on magnification factor, the percentage would be 40/36 = 1.11 − 1 = 0.11 × 100 = 11 percent. Practice this concept with the following problems.

1. 56″ SID and 4″ OID has a magnification percentage of _____.
2. 72″ SID and 8″ OID has a magnification percentage of _____.
3. 40″ SID and 20″ OID has a magnification percentage of _____.
4. 36″ SID and 2″ OID has a magnification percentage of _____.
5. 40″ SID and 2″ OID has a magnification percentage of _____.

Geometric Blur: Blur = OID/SOD × focal spot size. The factors that control geometric blur are focal spot size (*direct effect*), SID (*indirect effect*), and OID (*direct effect*). The effect of these factors on geometric blur can be quantified using the above formula. For example, 40 inches SID, 3 inches OID and 1.2 mm focal spot size would produce an area of blur measuring 0.097 mm or 97 µm. Complete the following problems to practice this skill.

	SID	OID	Focal spot size	Blur
1.	100 cm	6 cm	1.2 mm	x
2.	180 cm	10 cm	0.6 mm	x
3.	180 cm	10 cm	1.2 mm	x
4.	100 cm	8 cm	0.6 mm	x
5.	100 cm	10 cm	0.3 mm	x

Film Speed: 1/R. Film speed or sensitivity is defined as the reciprocal (reverse) of the amount of exposure, measured in roentgens, required to produce an optical density of 1.0 above base-plus-fog. The more sensitive a film is, the less exposure will be required, indicating a faster film. For example, if a film requires an exposure value of 32 mR to provide a density of 1.0 above base-plus-fog, its speed value would be 31.25. This is found by converting 32 mR to 0.032 R, then finding the reciprocal value: $1/0.032 = 31.25 \approx 31$. Practice finding various film speeds and rank order the films according to most sensitive to least, using the following problems.

1. Film A requires an exposure of 100 mR; its speed value is _____.
2. Film B requires an exposure of 15 mR; its speed value is _____.
3. Film C requires an exposure of 50 mR; its speed value is _____.

Average Gradient: $D_2 - D_1$ / $LRE_2 - LRE_1$. Average gradient is used to provide a numerical value for film contrast, based on the slope of the body of a film's H&D curve. The formula represents the ratio between the log relative exposure (LRE) required to produce a low density (D = 0.25) and the log relative exposure required to produce a high density (D = 2.0). Therefore, the values for D_1 and D_2 are 0.25 (plus base-plus-fog) and 2.0 (plus base-plus-fog), respectively, and their difference will always be 1.75. The LRE values are either given in a word problem format or found on an H&D curve. For example: A particular film type produces low and high densities with LRE values of 0.6 and 1.2, respectively. The average gradient of this film type is $2.0 - 0.25/1.2 - 0.6$; $1.75/0.6 = 2.9$. Practice finding average gradient values for the following problems.

1. LRE values of 0.9 and 1.6; average gradient = _____.
2. LRE values of 0.6 and 2.1; average gradient = _____.
3. LRE values of 0.55 and 1.9; average gradient = _____.
4. LRE values of 0.7 and 1.3; average gradient = _____.
5. LRE values of 0.8 and 1.7; average gradient = _____.

Radiographic Equipment

This section will present those mathematical expressions that explain the elements and characteristics of x-rays and the electrical systems of radiographic equipment. While skill in this area is not generally used as part of the day-to-day activities of radiography, understanding of these principles improves the ability to analyze components within the radiographic imaging chain and the nature of x-rays themselves.

Ohm's Law: $V = I \times R$; *or* $I = V/R$; *or* $R = V/I$. Ohm's law expresses the relationship between the components of an electrical circuit, specifically voltage, amperage (current, or intensity), and resistance. As stated in Ohm's law, voltage is the product of amperage and resistance. Therefore, for a specific voltage, current and resistance are *inversely proportional*, while for a specific current (or resistance), voltage is *directly proportional* to the given resistance (or current). Ohm's law may be applied to the circuit as a whole or to individual components of a circuit. For example: A circuit has a resistance of 24 ohms and potential difference of 12 V. What is the current? $12/24 = 0.5$ A. Practice the use of Ohm's law by solving the problems on the facing page.

	V (voltage)	I (amperage)	R (resistance in ohms)
1.	x	20 A	3 ohms
2.	6 V	x	2 ohms
3.	120 V	5 A	x
4.	x	200 mA	15 ohms
5.	15 V	500 mA	x

Transformer Law: $V_s/V_p = N_s/N_p$. The transformer law indicates the change between input and output voltage as a result of the type of transformer used (step-up or step-down). Transformers operate on the principle of mutual induction based on the ratio of the number of windings between the primary (P) and secondary (S) sides of the transformer. The relationship between the voltage and number of turns (windings) is *inversely proportional*. The step-up transformer has more windings on the secondary side than the primary and will increase the input voltage. (The opposite is true of the step-down transformer.) The transformer ratio is always stated in terms of secondary:primary sides. An example of this law is as follows: A step-up transformer with a ratio of 5:1 receives an input voltage of 220 V. What will the output voltage be? The answer is $x/220 = 5/1$; $x = 220 \times 5$; $x = 1100$ V. Complete the following problems to practice this skill.

	Transformer ratio	Input V	Output V
1.	2:1	110	x
2.	1:5	110	x
3.	100:1	220	x
4.	1:20	110	x
5.	x	110	440

Relationship between Voltage and Amperage: $V_s/V_p = I_p/I_s$. The relationship between voltage and amperage (current, or intensity) is *inversely proportional* for a specific wattage (measurement of power). This means that as voltage doubles, amperage must decrease by one-half (1/2) to yield the same power. For example: The input power to a 6:1 transformer is 220 V and 10 A. What will the output voltage and amperage be? First, find the output V: $x/220 = 6/1$; $x = 220 \times 6$; $x = 1320$ V. Second, find the output I: $1320/220 = 10/x$; $1320x = 220 \times 10$; $1320x = 2200$; $x = 1.67$ A. Solve the following problems for practice.

	Input V	Input A	Output V	Output A
1.	110 V	5 A	220 V	x
2.	220 V	25 A	1000 V	x
3.	220 V	125 A	70 kV	x
4.	220 V	500 mA	22 V	x
5.	110 V	500 A	82 kV	x

Power Ratings: $W = V \times I$. Power is defined as the rate at which energy is used or converted. The unit of measure is the *watt* (W), which is equal to 1 amp of current flowing through a potential difference of 1 V. The value for power is the product of voltage and amperage. The power rating of a radiographic unit is determined by the maximum kilovoltage and milliamperage possible as indicated by the overload protection circuit. This rating is stated in units of *kilowatts* (kW). For example, a unit capable of 600 mA at 120 kV has a power rating of 0.6 A × 120,000 V = 72,000 W (72 kW).

Due to increased ripple factor of single-phase, fully rectified units over the nearly constant voltage of three-phase units, it is recommended that one include a correction factor of 0.7 (70 percent effective voltage) when determining wattage. Using the previously stated voltage and current factors, the power rating of a single-phase unit would be equal to 0.6 A × 120,000 V × 0.7 = 50,400 W (50.4 kW). For practice with this skill, complete the following problems.

	Current	Voltage	Generator type	Power Rating (kW)
1.	1000 mA	90 kV	three-phase	x
2.	500 mA	100 kV	single-phase	x
3.	600 mA	90 kV	single-phase	x
4.	1200 mA	100 kV	three-phase	x
5.	400 mA	125 kV	single-phase	x

Heat Units: HU = mA × time × kV × C. The heat loading of an x-ray tube is calculated in terms of heat units (HU). This value is the product of the exposure factors of milliamperage-seconds and kilovoltage and a constant value (C) representing the type of generator employed. The values for C are 1.0 for single-phase, fully rectified units; 1.35 for three-phase, 6-pulse units; and 1.41 for three-phase, 12-pulse units. Heat loading can be calculated for a single exposure or a series of exposures. This action may be required as part of monitoring the tube for adequate cooling time between runs of serial imaging. The calculation of total heat load would be conducted as follows: The use of 1000 mA, 25 ms, 68 kV with a three-phase, 12-pulse generator would result in 2397 HU for a single exposure ($1000 \times 0.025 \times 68 \times 1.41$). To find the total heat loading for a series of exposures, multiply the above value by the total number of exposures. For example, a serial run of 10 images at the above exposure factors would result in 23,970 HU. Practice calculating heat unit values by completing the following problems.

	mA	Time	kV	Generator type	No. of exposures	HU
1.	600	1/60 s	70	single-phase	1	x
2.	600	8 ms	76	three-phase, 6-pulse	1	x
3.	1000	32 ms	72	three-phase, 12-pulse	5	x
4.	800	0.02 s	80	three-phase, 6-pulse	12	x
5.	400	0.033 s	80	single-phase	1	x

Wave Equation: Velocity = wavelength × frequency; $c = v\lambda$. The relationships of the characteristics of x-ray photons are expressed in the wave equation. This relationship states that the speed of an x-ray photon is the product of wavelength and frequency of the photon. Since the speed of x-rays in a vacuum is constant (equal to the speed of light, or c), it can be stated that photon wavelength and frequency are *inversely proportional*. If either wavelength or frequency of a photon is known, the wave equation may be used to determine the unknown value. For example, a photon with a wavelength of 1 Å would have a frequency of 3×10^{18} Hz. This value is found using a variation on the wave equation, **frequency = c/wavelength:**

$$x = \frac{3 \times 10^8 \text{ m/s}}{1 \times 10^{-10} \text{ m}}; \qquad x = \frac{3 \times 10^8 \text{ m}}{\text{s}} \times \frac{1}{1 \times 10^{-10} \text{ m}};$$

$$x = (3 \times 1)(10^{8+10}); \qquad x = 3 \times 10^{18} \text{ cycle/s or Hz}$$

If frequency is known and wavelength needs to be found, the wave equation is again varied: **wavelength = c/frequency**. A photon with a frequency of 1.5×10^{19} cycle/s has a wavelength of 0.45 Å (0.45×10^{-10}). This value is found as follows:

$$x = \frac{3 \times 10^8 \text{ m/s}}{1.5 \times 10^{19} \text{ cycle/s}}; \qquad x = \frac{3 \times 10^8 \text{ m}}{\text{s}} \times \frac{1}{1.5 \times 10^{19} \text{ cycle}};$$

$$x = (3 \times 1.5)(10^{8-19}); \qquad x = 4.5 \times 10^{-11} \text{ m } or \ 0.45 \times 10^{-10} \text{ m } = 0.45 \overset{\circ}{A}$$

Radiation Protection

Calculations in this section will be needed in determining radiation exposure totals, dose equivalent limits, and conversion of standard units of radiation measurement to SI units. For each piece of radiographic equipment, a chart should be constructed and posted that states the tube output per milliampere-seconds of exposure (mR/mAs) for various kilovoltage peak stations. These charts may then be referred to as needed to determine the total tube output for a particular exam. This provides the radiographer specific information when questioned as to the quantity of exposure being delivered for a particular exam. Since most radiographers in the U.S. still use the standard rad, rem, and roentgen units of measure, yet most scientific data are expressed in SI units, it is important to be able to convert these figures.

Entrance Skin Exposure—Diagnostic Exposure: Exposure is inversely proportional to the square of the SID to the SOD; $mR_1/mR_2 = SOD^2/SID^2$. This method for calculating exposure requires knowing the output of an x-ray tube, as expressed in terms of milliroentgens per milliampere-seconds. These values are found by measuring the output at each kilovoltage station and a constant source-to-detector distance. Such charts must be devised for each radiographic/fluoroscopic installation. A sample of an exposure intensity chart is included to be used to practice solving for estimated entrance skin exposure (ESE):

Sample Exposure Intensity Chart
(100 cm SID)

kVp	mR/mAs
50	1.7
60	1.9
70	2.8
80	3.8
90	4.7
100	5.7
110	7.1

For example, a radiographic examination requires 20 mAs and 70 kV. What is the total exposure? The milliroentgens per milliampere-seconds is 2.8, which multiplied by 20 mAs equals an exposure of 56 mR at a 100 cm SID. ESE will be *inversely proportional to the square of the distance* (*SID to SOD*). To estimate the ESE, set up an inverse proportion based on exposure to distance; mR_1 equals the exposure at the SID, while mR_2 is the exposure at the SOD (ESE). The SOD is found by measuring the patient and subtracting that value from the SID. For example, if the patient measured 24 cm, the data for the proportion would be $mR_1 = 56$; $mR_2 = x$ (unknown); SOD = 76 cm (100 − 24); and SID = 100 cm. The solution would be found as follows:

$$\frac{56}{x} = \frac{76^2}{100^2}; \quad \frac{56}{x} = \frac{5776}{10,000}; \quad 5776x = 56 \times 10,000; \quad 5776x = 560,000; \quad x = 96.95 \text{ mR} \approx 97 \text{ mR ESE}$$

Practice finding milliroentgen per milliampere-second values and ESE by solving the problems below.

1. What will the total exposure (tube output) be for 15 mAs at 60 kV?
2. What will the total exposure (tube output) be for 2.5 mAs at 110 kV?
3. If the exposure is 10 mR at 100 cm, what will the ESE be for a 15 cm part?
4. If the exposure is 24 mR at 100 cm, what will the ESE be for a 20 cm part?
5. Find the ESE for a 30 cm part when using a 100 SID and exposure factors of 5 mAs at 60 kV.

Entrance Skin Exposure—Fluoroscopic Exposure: Exposure rate × mA × exposure time. The calculation of ESE for fluoroscopic exposure is a little more direct, as the exposure rate is stated for the SSD (source-to-skin distance). Therefore, ESE only requires finding the product of the fluoroscopic exposure rate, milliamperage, and exposure time (in minutes). The maximum exposure rate for fluoroscopic tubes is 10 R/min and usually the rate is less than 5 R/min. Calculating fluoroscopic dose would require knowing the exposure rate and the milliamperes and minutes used. For example, a fluoroscopic procedure is performed with an exposure rate of 2.2 R/min, using 2 mA and 3 min of fluoroscopic time. The total exposure would be 2.2 × 2 × 3 = 13.2 R. Practice this skill by solving the problems listed.

	Exposure/min	mA	Exposure time	Total mR
1.	2 R/min	3	5 min	x
2.	3.75 R/min	1.5	3 min	x
3.	1.4 R/min	3	3 min	x
4.	2 R/min	4	2 min	x
5.	1.75 R/min	2.5	3.5 min	x

Dose Equivalent Limits: 1 rem × age of radiation worker (1 cSv × age). According to NCRP No. 91 and No. 116, the dose equivalent limit (previously known as *cumulative dose*) for occupational exposure is determined by multiplying the worker's age by 1 rem (1 cSv). Therefore, for a 40-year-old radiographer, the dose equivalent should not be greater than 40 rem (40 cSv).

Converting Units of Radiation Measurement

Exposure Conversions: 1 R = 2.58 × 10^{-4} C/kg. The measurement of radiation *exposure* or *intensity* provides a value for the quantity of photons in the x-ray beam, also known as *tube output*. For this reason, it is referred to as *exposure in air,* as opposed to a dose-related concept. To determine this value, an ionization chamber is exposed to the primary beam. This chamber produces ion pairs and free electrons within it, which form a current to be measured. The standard unit of measure is the *roentgen (R),* and it is defined as *the quantity of x-ray exposure required to produce 2.08×10^9 ion pairs per cubic centimeter of air*. This quantity of ion pairs is equivalent to 2.58 x 10^{-4} C/kg. The unit *coulomb (C)* is the unit of measure of electrical charge and represents a quantity of 6.25 x 10^{18} electrons flowing per second. The unit *kilogram (kg)* represents the unit mass of air exposed. The SI equivalent of the roentgen is expressed as coulombs per kilogram (C/kg). The equivalency between these units is as follows:

$$1 \text{ R is equal to } 2.58 \times 10^{-4} \text{ C/kg } or \text{ 1 mR is equal to } 2.58 \times 10^{-7} \text{ C/kg}$$

To convert a value expressed in roentgens to coulombs per kilogram, multiply the original value by 2.58 x10^{-4}. For example, 20 R (20 × 10^1) equals 5.16 × 10^{-3} C/kg. This was solved as follows:

$$(2.0 \times 10^1)\,(2.58 \times 10^{-4}) = (2.0 \times 2.58)\,(10^{1-4}) = 5.16 \times 10^{-3} \text{ C/kg}$$

To convert a value expressed in coulombs per kilogram to roentgens, divide the original value by 0.000258 (2.58 × 10^{-4}). For example, 5 C/kg = 19,380 R. This may also be solved by keeping the values in their exponential format:

$$\frac{5 \times 10^0}{2.58 \times 10^{-4}} = (5/2.58)(10^{0-[-4]}) = (1.94)(10^{0+4}) = 1.94 \times 10^4 \text{ R or 19,400 R}$$

Practice these conversions by solving the following problems.

1. 12 R = _____ C/kg
2. 220 mR = _____ C/kg
3. 1 C/kg = _____ R
4. 0.2 C/kg = _____ R
5. 2 C/kg = _____ mR

Absorbed Dose Conversions: 1 rad = 10^{-2} Gy. The measurement of the dose received by a person exposed to radiation is based on the amount of energy deposited in the irradiated object. The unit of measure to express absorbed dose is the *rad*, which is specifically defined as *the amount of energy* (measured in ergs) *deposited per unit mass of tissue* (measured in kilograms); 1 rad equals 100 ergs per kilogram of tissue. The SI equivalent of the rad is the gray (Gy). The equivalency between these units is as follows:

$$1 \text{ rad} = 0.01 \text{ Gy } (10^{-2}) or \text{ 100 rad} = 1 \text{ Gy}$$

To convert a value expressed in rads to grays, multiply the original value by 0.01. For example, 20 rad = 0.2 Gy. This was solved as follows: 20 × 0.01 = 0.02 Gy. To convert grays to rads, divide grays by 0.01 (or multiply by 100); for example, 50 Gy = 5000 rad. Practice this conversion by solving the following problems.

1. 65 rad = _____ Gy
2. _____ rad = 4.25 Gy
3. 480 mrad = _____ Gy
4. _____ rad = 22 cGy
5. 780 mrad = _____ mGy

Dose Equivalent Calculations: Rad × QF = rem. Each type of ionizing radiation has its own characteristic properties of energy, wavelength, and particulate or nonparticulate nature. These characteristic variations lead to differences in biologic effects for equal doses of radiation exposure. To account for these differences, the term *dose equivalent* is applied and is expressed in *rem* (*r*adiation *e*quivalent in *m*an). The value for *dose equivalent* is the product of absorbed dose and a radiation quality factor (QF). The accepted quality factors for various types of radiation, according to NCRP No. 91, are as follows:

Radiation type	QF
x-rays, gamma rays, beta particles and electrons	1
thermal neutrons	5
alpha particles	20

Therefore, the dose equivalent value for 20 rad of x-rays is equal to 20 rem (20 × 1), while an equal dose of thermal neutrons is equal to 100 rem (20 × 5). Find the dose equivalent for the following.

1. 10 rad of beta exposure = _____ rem
2. 300 mrad of x-ray exposure = _____ rem
3. 5 rad of alpha exposure = _____ rem
4. 36 rad of neutron exposure = _____ rem
5. 18 rad of neutron exposure = _____ mrem

Dose Equivalent Conversion: 1 rem = 0.01 Sv. The SI unit for dose equivalent is the sievert (Sv):

1 rem = 0.01 Sv *or* 100 rem = 1 Sv

To convert a value expressed in rem to sieverts, multiply the original value by 0.01. For example, 20 rem is converted as follows: 20 × 0.01 = 0.02 Sv. To convert sieverts to rem, divide sieverts by 0.01 (or multiply by 100); for example, 50 Sv = 5000 rem. Practice this conversion by solving the following problems.

1. 22 rem = _____ Sv
2. _____ rem = 0.70 Sv
3. 542 mrem = _____ Sv
4. _____ rem = 86 cSv
5. 320 mrem = _____ mSv

Answers to Practice Problems

Numerical Prefixes

1. 0.00000005 mm; 0.00000000005 m
2. 75,000 V; 0.075 MV
3. 5400 Å; and 0.540 μm
4. 0.580 rem; 580,000 μrem
5. 15 cGy; 150 mGy

Milliampere-second Calculations

1. 6 mAs
2. 20 mAs
3. 16 mAs
4. 12 mAs
5. 9 mAs

Solving for Milliamperage or Time

1. 400 mA
2. 0.024 s or 24 ms
3. 300 mA
4. 0.08 s or 80 ms
5. 600 mA

Relationship between Milliamperage and Time

1. 0.025 s or 25 ms
2. 0.015 s or 15 ms
3. 0.03 s or 30 ms
4. 200 mA
5. 400 mA

Relationship between Milliamperage-seconds and Kilovoltage Peak

1. 69 ≈ 70kVp
2. 92 kVp
3. 36 mAs
4. 20 mAs
5. 92 kVp

Relationship between Grid Ratio and Milliamperage-seconds

1. 40 mAs
2. 25 mAs
3. 8 mAs
4. 14 mAs
5. 6.4 mAs

Relationship between Screen and Milliamperage-seconds

1. 96 mAs
2. 12 mAs
3. 12 mAs
4. 40 mAs
5. 18 mAs

Inverse Square Law

1. 92.85 ≈ 93 mR
2. 98.66 ≈ 99 mR
3. 26.23 ≈ 26 mR
4. 39 mR
5. 190.77 ≈ 191 mR

Relationship between SID and Milliamperage-seconds

1. $43.12 \approx 43$ mAs
2. $12.34 \approx 12$ mAs
3. 27 mAs
4. $15.68 \approx 16$ mAs
5. $5.14 \approx 5$ mAs

Relationship between Kilovoltage Peak and Beam Intensity

1. $148.61 \approx 149$ mR
2. $608.99 \approx 609$ mR
3. $416.38 \approx 416$ mR
4. $275.47 \approx 275$ mR
5. $309.42 \approx 309$ mR

Magnification Factor

1. $1.0769 \approx 1.08$
2. $1.125 \approx 1.13$
3. 2
4. $1.0588 \approx 1.06$
5. $1.0526 \approx 1.05$

Magnification Percentage

1. 8%
2. 13%
3. 100%
4. 6%
5. 5%

Geometric Blur

1. 0.077 mm
2. 0.035 mm
3. 0.070 mm
4. 0.052 mm
5. 0.033 mm

Film Speed

1. Film A = 10
2. Film B = $66.66 \approx 67$
3. Film C = 20

Average Gradient

1. 2.5
2. $1.166 \approx 1.17$
3. $1.296 \approx 1.3$
4. $2.916 \approx 2.92$
5. 1.94

Ohm's Law

1. 60 V
2. 3 A
3. 24 ohms
4. 3 V
5. 30 ohms

Transformer Law

1. 220 V
2. 22 V
3. 22,000 V
4. 5.5 V
5. 4:1

Relationship between Voltage and Amperage

1. 2.5 A
2. 5.5 A
3. 0.393 A = 393 mA
4. 5 A = 5000 mA
5. 0.670 A = 670 mA

Power Rating

1. 90 kW
2. 35 kW
3. 37.8 kW
4. 120 kW
5. 35 kW

Heat Units

1. 700 HU
2. $492.48 \approx 492$ HU
3. 16,243 HU
4. 20,736 HU
5. 1,056 HU

ESE—Diagnostic Exposure

1. 28.5 mR ≈ 29 mR
2. $17.75 \approx 18$ mR
3. $13.84 \approx 14$ mR
4. $37.5 \approx 38$ mR
5. $19.387 \approx 19$ mR

ESE—Fluoroscopic Exposure

1. 30 mR
2. $16.875 \approx 17$ mR
3. $12.6 \approx 13$ mR
4. 16 mR
5. $15.312 \approx 15$ mR

Exposure Conversions

1. $30.96 \times 10^{-4} = 3.096 \times 10^{-3}$ C/kg
2. 5.676×10^{-5} C/kg
3. $0.387 \times 10^4 = 3870$ R
4. $0.775 \times 10^3 = 775$ R
5. $0.775 \times 10^4 = 0.775 \times 10^4 =$ 7750 R or 7,750,000 mR

Absorbed Dose Conversions

1. 0.65 Gy
2. 425 rad
3. 0.0048 Gy
4. 22 rad
5. 7.80 mGy

Dose Equivalent Calculations

1. 10 rem
2. 300 mrem ≈ 0.300 rem
3. 100 rem
4. 180 rem
5. 90 rem ≈ 90,000 mrem

Dose Equivalent Conversions

1. 0.22 Sv
2. 70 rem
3. 0.00542 Sv
4. 86 rem
5. 3.2 mSv

THE EXAMINATION
Radiation Protection

DIRECTIONS: Each numbered question or incomplete statement below contains lettered responses. Select the **one best** response.

1. According to the wave equation, the relationship between the frequency and wavelength of electromagnetic radiation is

   (A) directly proportional
   (B) inversely proportional
   (C) direct, but not proportional
   (D) inverse, but not proportional

2. Which of the following descriptions of electromagnetic radiation photons will be the most penetrating?

   (A) Frequency of 10^3 Hz, wavelength of 10^0 meters (m), energy of 10^{-8} eV
   (B) Frequency of 10^{20} Hz, wavelength of 10^{-9} m, energy of 10^5 keV
   (C) Frequency of 10^{10} Hz, wavelength of 10^{-5} m, energy of 10^{-5} eV
   (D) Frequency of 10^{14} Hz, wavelength of 10^{-7} m, energy of 10^1 eV

3. Which of the following is a factor that differs between x-rays and gamma rays?

   (A) Electrical nature
   (B) Particulate nature
   (C) Speed in a vacuum
   (D) Source of origin

4. At what speed will electromagnetic waves travel in a vacuum?

   (A) 3×10^8 meters per second (m/s)
   (B) 3×10^{10} m/s
   (C) 186,000 m/s
   (D) 186,000 cm/s

5. The wavelength of an x-ray photon is commonly expressed in units of angstroms. An angstrom is equivalent to

   (A) 10^{-6} m
   (B) 10^{-9} m
   (C) 10^{-10} m
   (D) 10^{-12} m

6. The type of x-ray/matter interaction that will result in the total absorption of the incident photon is termed

   (A) photoelectric
   (B) photodisintegration
   (C) Compton scattering
   (D) coherent scattering

7. A photoelectric interaction between an x-ray photon and matter will result in

   (A) production of a secondary characteristic ray
   (B) scattering of the primary photon with loss of energy
   (C) scattering of the primary photon, but with retention of all its energy
   (D) absorption of the primary photon by the nucleus of an atom within the irradiated matter

8. In general, what effect will an increase in photon energy have on the probability of a photoelectric interaction?

   (A) Increased probability
   (B) Decreased probability
   (C) No effect on probability

9. Which x-ray/matter interaction produces a relatively high-energy scattered photon?

   (A) Photoelectric
   (B) Photodisintegration
   (C) Compton scattering
   (D) Coherent scattering

10. What is the energy of a scattered photon if the incident photon had an energy value of 78 keV, the ejected electron acquired 12 keV of energy, and the binding energy of the ejected electron was 1 keV?

    (A) 91 keV
    (B) 77 keV
    (C) 65 keV
    (D) 13 keV

11. Compton interactions will predominate over photoelectric interactions in the energy range of

    (A) ultra-low energy (<10 keV)
    (B) low energy (10 to 30 keV)
    (C) moderate energy (40 to 70 keV)
    (D) high energy (>70 keV)

12. A scattered photon with the greatest energy would be the one deflected from its original path at an angle of

    (A) 20°
    (B) 45°
    (C) 60°
    (D) 90°

13. Which incident photon energy will produce a scattered photon with the LEAST amount of energy?

    (A) 130 keV
    (B) 100 keV
    (C) 70 keV
    (D) 50 keV

14. The x-ray/matter interaction that results in scattering of the incident photon with no loss of energy is termed

    (A) photoelectric
    (B) photodisintegration
    (C) Compton scattering
    (D) coherent scattering

15. The x-ray/matter interactions that cause ionization of the irradiated matter include:
    1. Coherent
    2. Photoelectric
    3. Compton

    (A) 1 & 2
    (B) 2 & 3
    (C) 1 & 3
    (D) 1, 2, & 3

16. The use of positive contrast media will have what effect on the probability of photoelectric interactions?

    (A) Increased probability
    (B) Decreased probability
    (C) No effect on probability

17. The effect of photoelectric interactions on radiographic image quality will be to increase

    (A) radiographic density
    (B) radiographic contrast
    (C) recorded detail
    (D) magnification

18. What effect will an increase in photoelectric interactions have on patient dose?

    (A) Increase
    (B) Decrease
    (C) No influence

19. Which unit of measurement would be most appropriate for stating the quantity of radiation exposure as measured by an ionization chamber?

    (A) Roentgen
    (B) Sievert
    (C) Rad
    (D) Curie

20. The unit of radiation exposure known as the *rad* expresses the

    (A) quantity of electric charge produced in air
    (B) amount of energy transferred to irradiated tissue
    (C) product of absorbed dose and radiation quality factor
    (D) number of emissions from a radioactive nucleus per second

21. What is the SI (International System of Units) equivalency for radiation absorbed dose?

    (A) 2.58×10^{-4} coulombs per kilogram of air (C/kg)
    (B) 10^{-2} Gy
    (C) 10^{-2} Sv
    (D) 3.7×10^{10} becquerels (Bq)

22. The unit of radiation measurement used to indicate *dose equivalent* is the

    (A) rad
    (B) rem
    (C) gray
    (D) roentgen

23. What is the dose equivalent of an absorbed dose of 20 rads of alpha radiation?

    (A) 20 rads (0.2 Gy)
    (B) 20 rem (0.2 Sv)
    (C) 400 rads (4.0 Gy)
    (D) 400 rem (4.0 Sv)

24. What is the SI equivalency for dose equivalence?

    (A) 2.58×10^{-4} C/kg of air
    (B) 10^{-2} Gy
    (C) 10^{-2} Sv
    (D) 13.7×10^{10} Bq

25. The monitoring and measuring of a person's exposure to radiation is termed

    (A) densitometry
    (B) dosimetry
    (C) sensitometry
    (D) ALARA

26. Which of the following may be used as personnel radiation monitoring devices?

    (A) Film badges, ion chambers, scintillation crystals
    (B) Ion chambers, thermoluminescent dosimeter (TLD), Geiger-Müller (G-M) counter
    (C) TLD, film badges, ion chambers
    (D) Scintillation crystals, TLD, film badges

27. What is the active component of the TLD?

    (A) Lithium fluoride
    (B) Cesium iodide
    (C) Xenon gas
    (D) Sodium iodide

28. Which type of personnel radiation monitor may be used for the longest period of time before being read?

    (A) Film badge
    (B) Pocket ion chamber
    (C) Scintillation crystal
    (D) TLD

29. The advantages of the film badge type of radiation monitor include:

    1. It provides a permanent record of exposure
    2. It is not affected by light, heat, or humidity
    3. It provides information regarding the energy of the exposure

    (A) 1 & 2
    (B) 2 & 3
    (C) 1 & 3
    (D) 1, 2, & 3

30. The amount of radiation exposure received by a film badge is indicated by the measurement of

    (A) light produced during evaluation of film
    (B) density on the processed film
    (C) electrical discharge on the film
    (D) heat produced during processing of the film

31. A radiation monitor device should be worn by a

    (A) radiographer undergoing a radiographic procedure
    (B) nurse working in an area where mobile radiography is performed
    (C) family member assisting a patient during a radiographic procedure
    (D) radiographer performing fluoroscopic procedures

32. What is the whole-body dose equivalent limit for the occupationally exposed person according to the National Council on Radiation Protection (NCRP) Report No. 91?

    (A) 5000 mSv (500 rem)
    (B) 500 mSv (50 rem)
    (C) 50 mSv (5 rem)
    (D) 5 mSv (0.5 rem)

33. According to NCRP Report No. 91, what is the maximum dose equivalent for the occasionally (nonoccupationally) exposed worker?

    (A) 0.5 mSv (0.05 rem)
    (B) 5 mSv (0.5 rem)
    (C) 50 mSv (5 rem)
    (D) 500 mSv (50 rem)

34. What is the gestational dose-equivalent limit for exposure to the embryo/fetus of an occupationally exposed person?

    (A) 500 mSv (50 rem)
    (B) 50 mSv (5 rem)
    (C) 5 mSv (0.5 rem)
    (D) 0.5 mSv (0.05 rem)

35. How is the cumulative exposure limit calculated according to NCRP No. 91?

    (A) 50 mSv × (age − 18)
    (B) 50 mSv × age
    (C) 10 mSv × (age − 18)
    (D) 10 mSv × age

36. According to NCRP No. 91, the cumulative exposure limit for a 40-year-old radiographer who has been employed as a radiographer for only 5 years would be

    (A) 50 mSv (5 rem)
    (B) 250 mSv (25 rem)
    (C) 400 mSv (40 rem)
    (D) 2000 mSv (200 rem)

37. If a radiographer receives 100 mrads of exposure from a medical procedure, 100 mrem of background radiation, and 200 mrem from working as a radiographer, what is the total occupational dose equivalent?

    (A) 100 mrem (1 mSv)
    (B) 200 mrem (2 mSv)
    (C) 300 mrem (3 mSv)
    (D) 400 mrem (4 mSv)

38. The *cardinal rules* of radiation protection recommend the use of

    (A) maximum exposure time, distance, and shielding
    (B) automatic exposure control, fast imaging systems, and maximum shielding
    (C) minimum exposure time, maximum distance, and appropriate shielding
    (D) maximum beam restriction, minimum exposure time, and maximum distance

39. What is the material used to express shielding equivalents?

    (A) Copper
    (B) Lead
    (C) Aluminum
    (D) Tungsten

40. What is the correct method for the storage of lead aprons when they are not in use?

    (A) Hung on racks designed for this purpose
    (B) Carefully folded and stored on a shelf
    (C) Stretched out on a flat surface
    (D) Draped across the top of the processor

41. *Primary radiation* is that which is

(A) produced during photoelectric interactions
(B) emitted by the patient
(C) emitted through the window of the x-ray tube
(D) emitted through the housing of the x-ray tube

42. Which of the following indicates *primary radiation*?

(A) Photons that have been scattered during x-ray/matter interactions
(B) The major source of operator radiation exposure
(C) Photons that do not undergo x-ray/matter interactions
(D) The major component of the exit beam

43. Any surface toward which the x-ray tube may be directed during operation is referred to as

(A) a primary barrier
(B) a secondary barrier
(C) a controlled area
(D) an uncontrolled area

44. The major contributor to natural background radiation is

(A) medical x-rays
(B) radon
(C) cosmic (extraterrestrial) rays
(D) consumer products

45. Background radiation exposure includes:
1. Cosmic radiation
2. Medical x-rays
3. Fallout radiation
4. Ultrasonic waves

(A) 1, 2, & 3
(B) 2, 3, & 4
(C) 3 & 4
(D) 1 & 2

46. For a given examination, dose to which anatomic structure will be the greatest?

(A) Gonads
(B) Skin
(C) Bone marrow
(D) All the above structures receive equal doses

47. In the U.S., the average level of yearly background radiation exposure is

(A) 1 to 2 mSv (100 to 200 mrem)
(B) 2 to 3 mSv (200 to 300 mrem)
(C) 3 to 4 mSv (300 to 400 mrem)
(D) 4 to 5 mSv (400 to 500 mrem)

48. Man-made sources of radiation include:
1. Nuclear fallout
2. Medical and dental procedures
3. Building materials that emit radiation

(A) 1 & 2
(B) 2 & 3
(C) 1 & 3
(D) 1, 2, & 3

49. The *effective dose-equivalent limits* defined in NCRP No. 91 refer to what aspect of radiation exposure?

(A) Lowest level of radiation exposure achievable
(B) Average dose for radiologic examinations in the U.S.
(C) Average background radiation exposure in the U.S.
(D) Upper level radiation dose considered to have a negligible risk

50. According to NCRP No. 91, what is the annual effective dose-equivalent limit for whole body exposure for a radiation worker?

(A) 0.5 Sv (50 rem)
(B) 5 Sv (500 rem)
(C) 50 mSv (5000 mrem)
(D) 5000 mSv (500 rem)

51. According to current standards, a radiation worker's cumulative dose-equivalent limit is determined by

(A) (age − 18) × 5 mSv
(B) (age − 18) × 50 mSv
(C) age × 100 mSv
(D) age × 10 mSv

52. What would be the cumulative effective dose-equivalent limit for a 35-year-old radiation worker who has acquired 100 mSv (10 rem) of exposure over 15 years of employment?

    (A) 850 mSv (85 rem)
    (B) 350 mSv (35 rem)
    (C) 250 mSv (25 rem)
    (D) 170 mSv (17 rem)

53. If a radiation worker undergoes a medical radiographic procedure and receives a dose of 2 mSv, then receives 4 mSv from background exposure and 10 mSv from occupational exposure, how much will be deducted from this worker's cumulative effective dose equivalent?

    (A) 10 mSv
    (B) 12 mSv
    (C) 14 mSv
    (D) 16 mSv

54. The radiation protection philosophy that promotes the use of the least amount of radiation possible for medical imaging is termed

    (A) NCRP
    (B) NRC
    (C) ICRP
    (D) ALARA

55. Ionization of matter occurs at the structural level of the

    (A) atomic nucleus
    (B) atomic shells
    (C) molecule
    (D) cell

56. Linear energy transfer (LET) indicates which characteristic of ionizing radiation?

    (A) Amount of biological effect produced by irradiation
    (B) Type of biologic effect produced by irradiation
    (C) Amount of energy deposited during irradiation
    (D) Radiosensitivity of a specific tissue

57. What is the relationship between linear energy transfer (LET) and relative biologic effectiveness (RBE)?

    (A) Direct
    (B) Indirect
    (C) None

58. Which radiation type will have the highest LET?

    (A) 80-keV x-rays
    (B) 5-MeV x-rays
    (C) Gamma rays
    (D) Fast neutrons

59. Factors that contribute to radiation having a low LET include:
    1. High charge
    2. No mass
    3. High penetration

    (A) 1 & 2
    (B) 2 & 3
    (C) 1 & 3
    (D) 1, 2, & 3

60. Which type of ionizing radiation will have the LEAST biologic effect?

    (A) Alpha particles
    (B) Fast neutrons
    (C) 25 MeV x-rays
    (D) Diagnostic x-rays

61. *Direct effects* of irradiation are those that

    (A) cause immediate cell death
    (B) affect structures distant from the irradiated structures
    (C) affect the site of irradiation
    (D) cause the least biologic effect

62. Which of the following are considered types of *ionizing* radiation?

    (A) X-rays, gamma rays, alpha particles
    (B) Beta particles, gamma rays, light photons
    (C) X-rays, light photons, beta particles
    (D) Radio waves, alpha particles, beta particles

63. Indirect effects of irradiation are

    (A) those which are least damaging
    (B) the predominant type of radiation effect in biologic tissue
    (C) the result of irradiation of the DNA molecules
    (D) those which occur as a result of irradiation of macromolecules

64. Radiolysis of water molecules creates

    (A) increased radiosensitivity of the tissue involved
    (B) decreased radiosensitivity of the tissue involved
    (C) free radicals
    (D) larger water molecules

65. What is the basic concept of the *target theory* in cell survival?

    (A) The nucleus is the most radioresistant structure in the cell
    (B) A key molecule determines cell survival
    (C) Direct effects are more damaging than indirect effects
    (D) Free radicals within a cell are most susceptible to irradiation

66. Which type of cell is most sensitive to irradiation?

    (A) Red blood cells
    (B) White blood cells
    (C) Epithelial cells
    (D) Muscle cells

67. Highly radiosensitive cells would have which of the following characteristics?
    1. Immaturity
    2. High specialization
    3. High rate of proliferation

    (A) 1 & 2
    (B) 2 & 3
    (C) 1 & 3
    (D) 1, 2, & 3

68. Approximately how large a radiation dose to the gonads would cause temporary sterility in males or females?

    (A) 1 Gy (100 rads)
    (B) 2 Gy (200 rads)
    (C) 5 Gy (500 rads)
    (D) 7 Gy (700 rads)

69. Radiation effects that manifest themselves in the person exposed years after the exposure are considered to be:
    1. Early effects
    2. Late effects
    3. Somatic effects
    4. Genetic effects

    (A) 1 & 3
    (B) 1 & 4
    (C) 2 & 3
    (D) 2 & 4

70. An example of an early somatic effect of irradiation would be

    (A) leukemia
    (B) lung cancer
    (C) cataract formation
    (D) skin erythema

71. The term $LD_{50/30}$ refers to the dose level that will cause

    (A) Skin erythema in 30 percent of the population within 50 days
    (B) Skin erythema in 50 percent of the population within 30 days
    (C) Death to 30 percent of the population within 50 days
    (D) Death to 50 percent of the population within 30 days

72. Which of the following are examples of possible late somatic effects?

    (A) Cancer, skin erythema, congenital defects
    (B) Destruction of the GI tract, shortening of the life span, cataract formation
    (C) Hemorrhage, cataract formation, convulsive seizures
    (D) Cancer, congenital defects, shortening of the life span

73. The risk of congenital abnormalities is greatest if the embryo or fetus is irradiated during the

    (A) first 2 weeks following fertilization
    (B) first trimester after the first 2 weeks
    (C) second trimester
    (D) third trimester

74. The term $SED_{50/30}$ refers to the dose that will cause skin

    (A) reddening in 30 percent of the population within 50 days
    (B) reddening in 50 percent of the population with 30 days
    (C) ulceration in 30 percent of the population within 50 days
    (D) ulceration in 50 percent of the population with 30 days

75. Which of the following devices are used to protect the patient from unnecessary radiation exposure?

    (A) Collimators, filters, grids
    (B) Immobilization devices, filters, high-kVp techniques
    (C) Shields, direct exposure systems, increased SID
    (D) Short source-to-skin distance, fast screens, cones

76. Methods that will reduce the need for repeat imaging due to motion problems include:
    1. Restraining devices
    2. Short exposure times
    3. Suspended respiration

    (A) 1 & 2
    (B) 2 & 3
    (C) 1 & 3
    (D) 1, 2, & 3

77. How does filtration of the primary beam affect patient dose?

    (A) It softens the beam
    (B) It increases average beam energy
    (C) It absorbs the high-energy photons
    (D) It allows low-energy photons to pass

78. The collimator should be adjusted to a field of exposure

    (A) as large as the radiographer desires
    (B) 50 percent larger than the image receptor
    (C) 50 percent smaller than the image receptor
    (D) no larger than the image receptor

79. The minimum distance from source-to-table top for a fixed fluoroscopic unit should be

    (A) 10 inches
    (B) 12 inches
    (C) 15 inches
    (D) 18 inches

80. The maximum time that may elapse before the cumulative timer is activated on a fluoroscopic unit is

    (A) 2 min.
    (B) 5 min.
    (C) 8 min.
    (D) 10 min.

81. Methods for minimizing exposure dose during fluoroscopy include:
    1. Intermittent exposure
    2. High-kV techniques
    3. Nonintensified imaging

    (A) 1 & 2
    (B) 2 & 3
    (C) 1 & 3
    (D) 1, 2, & 3

82. For what purpose is a dose-response relationship important?

    (A) It determines the LET of various radiation types
    (B) It indicates the mean survival time following radiation exposure
    (C) It assigns quality factors to different types of radiation
    (D) It is used in the development of radiation protection policies

83. An increase in which exposure factors will cause a decrease in patient dose?

(A) Milliamperage-seconds (mAs) and kilovoltage (kV)
(B) Kilovoltage and source-to-image distance (SID)
(C) SID and milliamperage-seconds
(D) Milliamperage-seconds, kilovoltage, and SID

84. Which of the following combinations of exposure factors will cause the LEAST amount of patient exposure for approximately the same radiographic density as achieved by use of 30 mAs, 60 kV, and SID of 40 inches?

(A) 15 mAs, 60 kV, 40 inches SID
(B) 20 mAs, 70 kV, 40 inches SID
(C) 20 mAs, 70 kV, 48 inches SID
(D) 45 mAs, 60 kV, 48 inches SID

85. Which of the following situations will result in the LEAST amount of patient dose?

	Total filtration	SID	Field size	mR/mAs
(A)	2.0 mm Al	40″	10 × 12	8
(B)	2.5 mm Al	40″	14 × 17	12
(C)	3.0 mm Al	48″	4 × 4	12
(D)	2.5 mm Al	48″	14 × 17	15

86. Which of the following practices will reduce exposure to breast tissue during scoliosis imaging?
    1. Use of breast shields
    2. Use of AP rather than PA projection
    3. Use of a compensating filter

(A) 1 & 2
(B) 2 & 3
(C) 1 & 3
(D) 1, 2, & 3

87. Each of the following is a true statement regarding the use of gonadal shielding EXCEPT

(A) shields should be used when gonads are in or near the field of exposure
(B) shields should be used in place of beam collimation
(C) shields should be used on all persons in their reproductive years
(D) shields should not be used when they are likely to obscure the structure of interest

88. Which of the following will function effectively as a gonadal shield?
    1. Contact shield
    2. Lead and plastic filter system
    3. Shadow shield

(A) 1 & 2
(B) 2 & 3
(C) 1 & 3
(D) 1, 2 & 3

89. All the following are guidelines to be observed with regard to holding a patient in position during radiographic exposure EXCEPT

(A) mechanical holding devices should be used whenever possible
(B) protective apparel must be worn by any person holding a patient
(C) persons under the age of 18 should not be used to hold a patient
(D) the same person should be routinely used to hold patients

90. If a radiology department issues its radiographers only one personnel monitoring device, where should it be worn when performing routine radiography procedures?

(A) At collar level
(B) On the wrist
(C) At waist level
(D) Wherever it is convenient

91. The primary purpose for using personnel monitors is to

(A) protect the radiographer
(B) calculate the total amount of radiation a radiographer delivers
(C) monitor a radiographer's repeat rate
(D) indicate a radiographer's occupational exposure

92. The majority of the radiation survey devices, such as the G-M counter, detect radiation based on the ability of x-rays to cause

(A) certain materials to fluoresce
(B) photographic emulsion to darken
(C) water molecules to dissociate
(D) ionization of air molecules

93. Which of the following statements is true regarding the differences between primary and secondary radiation?

    (A) Primary radiation is the main source of dose to the radiographer
    (B) Primary radiation is produced within the patient
    (C) Secondary radiation has a higher energy than primary radiation
    (D) Secondary radiation requires less shielding material

Questions 94-96

For items 94-96, use the inverse square law to solve the problems.

94. By how much would a radiographer's occupational exposure be changed if the radiographer's distance from the patient increased from 1 foot to 3 feet during a fluoroscopic examination?

    (A) Decreased to 1/4 the original exposure
    (B) Decreased to 1/9 the original exposure
    (C) Increased to 2 times the original exposure
    (D) Increased to 4 times the original exposure

95. If a radiographer received an exposure of 160 mR while standing 2 feet from the patient, what would the approximate exposure be at 5 feet from the patient?

    (A) 26 mR
    (B) 64 mR
    (C) 400 mR
    (D) 1000 mR

96. The following set of technical factors produced an exposure intensity of 85 mR: 20 mAs, 70 kV, 40 inches SID, 200 speed image receptor, and 8:1 grid. What would the exposure intensity be if the SID were changed to 30 inches?

    (A) 48 mR
    (B) 64 mR
    (C) 113 mR
    (D) 151 mR

97. If a fluoroscopic unit produces an exposure intensity of 2.4 R/mA-min, what will the patient's approximate skin dose be if the examination requires 3 min of exposure at 2.2 mA?

    (A) 2 R
    (B) 5 R
    (C) 8 R
    (D) 16 R

98. Which of the following field sizes will expose the greatest area of tissue?

    (A) A 4 inch × 6 inch rectangle
    (B) Circle with 5 inch diameter
    (C) A 5 inch × 5 inch square
    (D) A 3 inch × 7 inch rectangle

99. The minimum amount of lead equivalent required for a lead apron is

    (A) 0.25 mm
    (B) 0.5 mm
    (C) 0.75 mm
    (D) 1.0 mm

100. A radiographer maintains a position during a fluoroscopy procedure that provides an exposure intensity of 325 mR/h. If the exposure time was 5 min, the total exposure would be

    (A) 5 mR
    (B) 27 mR
    (C) 65 mR
    (D) 1625 mR

101. The following statements regarding beam restrictors are true EXCEPT

    (A) the primary role is to reduce patient exposure
    (B) extension cones may be used in conjunction with collimators
    (C) the exposure factors must be decreased when using a small field size
    (D) good collimation will reduce occupational exposure as well as patient exposure

102. Which of the following sets of technical factors will produce the LEAST amount of patient dose?

	mAs	kV	SID	Receptor speed	Grid ratio
(A)	25	70	40″	200	8:1
(B)	32	70	40″	400	5:1
(C)	15	70	48″	400	10:1
(D)	10	70	36″	200	12:1

103. If a set of exposure factors for a specific radiographic unit produces an intensity of 8.4 mR/mAs at 80 kV, what would be the patient's dose if 30 mAs were used?

    (A) 19 mR
    (B) 85 mR
    (C) 190 mR
    (D) 252 mR

104. Which area of radiation dose measurement is most frequently used when referring to a patient's dose?

    (A) Skin dose
    (B) Mean marrow dose
    (C) Gonadal dose
    (D) Mean glandular dose

105. What is the maximum monthly radiation exposure dose allowed for the pregnant technologist?

    (A) 0.05 rem (0.5 mSv)
    (B) 0.1 rem (1 mSv)
    (C) 0.5 rem (5 mSv)
    (D) 5 rem (50 mSv)

106. Which radiation effect has a threshold between radiation dose and response?

    (A) Cataracts
    (B) Leukemia
    (C) Skin cancer
    (D) Shortening of life span

107. All the following are recommended practices for radiation protection to reduce the chance of exposing a pregnant patient EXCEPT

    (A) scheduling abdominal and pelvic radiographic examinations during the 10-day period following the onset of menstruation
    (B) asking all female patients of child-bearing age if they could possibly be pregnant
    (C) posting signs in waiting and radiographic rooms, in various languages, requesting patients to inform the technologist of the possibility of pregnancy
    (D) requiring all women of child-bearing age to have a pregnancy test performed

DIRECTIONS: Each group of questions below consists of lettered headings followed by a set of numbered items. For each numbered item select the **one** lettered heading with which it is **most** closely associated. Each lettered heading may be used **once, more than once, or not at all.**

Questions 108–111

Use the chart below to answer the questions.

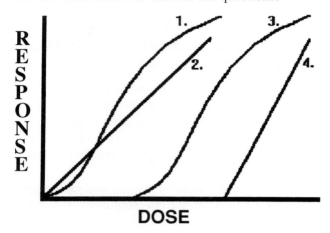

108. Which curves represent a *directly proportional* relationship between dose and response?

(A)   1 & 2
(B)   2 & 3
(C)   1 & 3
(D)   2 & 4

109. Which curve would be termed a *nonlinear, threshold* relationship between dose and response?

(A)   1
(B)   2
(C)   3
(D)   4

110. Which curve is the basis for current radiation protection policies?

(A)   1
(B)   2
(C)   3
(D)   4

111. Which curves offer a safe exposure range (no response)?

(A)   1 & 2
(B)   2 & 3
(C)   3 & 4
(D)   1 & 4

Questions 112–117

Classify each condition as a general type of radiation effect.

(A)   Genetic effect
(B)   Early somatic effect
(C)   Late somatic effect
(D)   Not associated with radiation exposure

112. Radiation induced malignancies

113. Death within 3 weeks of exposure

114. Point mutations of chromosomes

115. Effect caused only by gonadal exposure

116. Congenital abnormalities following in utero exposure

117. Blood changes resulting in increased infections, anemia, or hemorrhage

Questions 118–124

Indicate whether each of the following statements is true or false with regard to guidelines for diagnostic x-ray equipment as stated by NCRP No. 102.

(A)   True
(B)   False

118. The total filtration of the primary beam should be a minimum of 1.5 mm of aluminum for tubes capable of operating at greater than 70 kVp

119. The x-ray tube housing and collimator assembly must maintain the level of leakage radiation to less than 1 R/h at a distance of 1 m from the source

120. Stationary radiographic units must locate the exposure switch so as to require the operator to be behind a protective barrier during its operation

121. Protective devices employed to reduce operator exposure to scattered radiation during fluoroscopy should be equivalent to a minimum of 0.25 mm of lead

122. The absolute minimum for the source-to-skin distance for fluoroscopy units should be 12 inches (30 cm)

123. Mobile radiography equipment may be used even if the patient is capable of being transported to the radiology department

124. The operator of a mobile x-ray unit need not wear a protective lead apron as long as the cord attached to the exposure switch allows the operator to stand back 6 feet

Questions 125–129

Indicate how the following changes in technical factors will influence patient dose, if at all.

(A) Increase patient dose
(B) Decrease patient dose
(C) No influence on patient dose

125. Change in image receptor speed from 400 to 100

126. Change in grid ratio from 6:1 to 10:1

127. Change in field size from 10×12 to 8×10

128. Use of compensating filter compared to no filter

129. Change from small to large focal spot

Questions 130–134

Indicate whether the statements are properties of x-rays or not.

(A) True
(B) False

130. X-rays can be focused by a lens

131. X-rays carry a negative electrical charge

132. X-rays are polyenergetic

133. X-rays travel at 3×10^8 m/s in a vacuum

134. X-rays can ionize air molecules

Questions 135–142

Indicate which type of personnel monitor device is being described

(A) Thermoluminescent dosimeter (TLD)
(B) Film badge
(C) Pocket ion chambers
(D) Two of the three types above

135. Employs a luminescent crystal

136. Provides a permanent record of radiation exposure

137. Is *not* affected by heat or high humidity

138. Must be charged prior to daily use

139. Can provide an immediate exposure reading

140. Is reusable

141. Responds to radiation in a manner equivalent to that of human tissue

142. Detects x-radiation, gamma radiation, and high-energy beta particles

Questions 143–145

Estimate the average skin dose for a radiographic examination of each structure.

    (A)   10 mR
    (B)   50 mR
    (C)   200 mR
    (D)   400 mR

143.   Skull

144.   Chest

145.   Abdomen

Questions 146–150

Who will primarily benefit from the following protection practices?

    (A)   Patient
    (B)   Radiographer
    (C)   General public

146.   Increased filtration of the primary beam

147.   Gonadal shielding

148.   Protective barriers between radiography rooms and an uncontrolled area.

149.   Protective curtain on the fluoroscopy carriage

150.   Protective barrier between the radiographic unit and the control panel

Radiation Protection

Answers

1. **The answer is B.** *(Bushong, 5/e, pp 60–61. Carlton, p 37. Curry, 4/e, p 5. Selman, 8/e, pp 150–152.)* The wave equation is expressed as: wave speed = wavelength × frequency ($c = v\lambda$). Since wave speed for electromagnetic radiation in a vacuum is constant (the speed of light), the relationship between wavelength and wave frequency is inversely proportional. This means that as wavelength (the distance between adjacent wave peaks) decreases, frequency (number of waves per second) will increase. Understanding this relationship is important in further understanding photon energy and the regulation of photon energy. The diagram in the figure below demonstrates two waves: wave A represents long wavelength and low frequency, which results in low energy; wave B represents short wavelength and high frequency, which produces high energy.

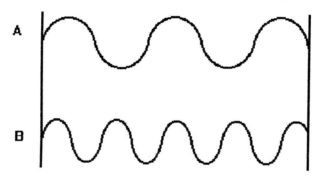

2. **The answer is B.** *(Bushong, 5/e, pp 61–63, 70–71. Curry, 4/e, pp 5–6. Selman, 8/e, pp 150–152. Thompson, pp 62–63.) Frequency, wavelength,* and *energy* are the factors that differentiate one form of electromagnetic radiation from another. In terms of penetrability, the photon with the highest frequency, shortest wavelength, and highest energy will be the most penetrating. This is the reason x-rays penetrate matter while other forms of electromagnetic radiation, such as visible light, radio waves, or microwaves do not.

3. **The answer is D.** *(Bushong, 5/e, p 64. Thompson, p 63.)* X-rays and gamma rays are virtually identical with the exception of their source of origin. X-rays are produced via the sudden deceleration of high-speed electrons in a device such as an x-ray tube. Gamma rays are a naturally occurring form of nuclear radiation arising from the nucleus of radioactive elements. Both types of radiation are nonparticulate (no mass), have a neutral electrical nature, are highly energetic, will travel at the speed of light in a vacuum, and will cause biologic and chemical effects on matter.

4. **The answer is A.** *(Bushong, 5/e, pp 56–57. Curry, 4/e, p 4. Selman, 8/e, p 150.)* Electromagnetic waves travel at the speed of light in a vacuum. The speed of light is defined in metric terms as 3×10^8 m/s or

3×10^{10} cm/s and in British terms as 186,000 miles/s. This characteristic is the same for all forms of electromagnetic radiation (visible light, radiowaves, microwaves, and so on).

5. **The answer is C.** *(Carlton, p 37. Curry, 4/e, p 5. Selman, 8/e, p 152.)* The angstrom unit of measurement is equivalent to 10^{-10} m or one ten-billionth of a meter (0.0000000001). The typical x-ray has a wavelength measurement of from 0.1 to 0.5 angstrom. This property contributes to its penetrability of matter.

6. **The answer is A.** *(Bushong, 5/e, p 175. Carlton, pp 196–198. Selman, 8/e, pp 179–181. Thompson, pp 200–201.)* The photoelectric interaction between x-rays and matter occurs when the photon energy is equal to or slightly greater than the binding energy of an inner shell electron. Therefore, this interaction results in the incident photon using all its energy and ionization of the atom. Since the x-ray photon is pure energy (no mass), the loss of all its energy ends the existence of the photon. The probability of photoelectric interactions is directly influenced by the atomic number of the matter irradiated and indirectly by the energy of the incident photon (relative to the binding energies of the electrons within the irradiated matter).

7. **The answer is A.** *(Bushong, 5/e, pp 175–176. Carlton, pp 196–198. Selman, 8/e, pp 179–181. Thompson, pp 200–201.)* During the photoelectric interaction between x-rays and matter, the incident photon gives up all its energy in the ejection of an inner shell electron. The incident photon is thus totally absorbed. The instability in the atom, created by the electron vacancy, is balanced by the movement of an outer shell electron into the inner vacancy. As this electron shift occurs, the energy difference between the orbits involved is released in the form of a secondary characteristic photon. These photons generally have very little energy and are absorbed a short distance from their origin. Therefore, these secondary rays are not significant to the formation of an x-ray image.

8. **The answer is B.** *(Bushong, 5/e, p 177. Carlton, pp 196–198. Selman, 8/e, p 181. Thompson, pp 200–201.)* The probability of photoelectric interactions is influenced by the atomic number of the matter irradiated and the energy of the photon relative to the binding energies of the electrons of the matter irradiated. More specifically, the energy of the incident photon must be equivalent to or slightly greater than the binding energy of the electron to be ejected. As the energy of the incident photon increases, exceeding the binding energy of the electron, the photon is more likely to penetrate the object or undergo a Compton interaction. Most matter, especially that of the human body, is composed of elements of low atomic number, which reduces the probability of photoelectric interactions between matter and high-energy photons.

9. **The answer is C.** *(Bushong, 5/e, pp 173–174. Carlton, pp. 200–201. Selman, 8/e, pp 181–183. Thompson, pp 202–206.)* The Compton interaction is the cause of high-energy scattered radiation. During this type of interaction, the incident photon interacts with an outer electron of the irradiated object, ejecting it from its orbit. These outer electrons are loosely bound, having minimal binding energy. Therefore, the incident photon gives up only a portion of its energy in the ionization process. The incident photon is redirected from its original path as a result of this collision. The remaining energy in the scattered photon is sufficient to undergo additional interactions or penetrate the irradiated object and contribute to the formation of the x-ray image. This scattered radiation is also the primary source of radiation exposure to operators of x-ray equipment. Photoelectric interactions result in the total absorption of the incident photon and no scatter. Coherent scatter is extremely *low*-energy scatter. Photodisintegration is the radioactive decay process.

10. **The answer is C.** *(Bushong, 5/e, p 173. Carlton, pp 200–201. Selman, 8/e, pp 181–183. Thompson, pp 202–206.)* The energy of the scattered photon is calculated as the difference between the energy of the incident photon and the binding energy of the ejected electron plus the energy acquired by the ejected electron: $E_s = E_i - (E_e + E_b)$. E_s is the energy of the scattered photon; E_i is the energy of the incident photon; E_e is the energy acquired by the ejected (recoil) electron; and E_b is the binding energy of the ejected electron. For this problem the solution would be found as follows: $E_s = 78 - (12 + 1) = 65$ keV.

11. The answer is D. *(Bushong, 5/e, p 173. Carlton, pp 200–201. Carroll, 5/e, pp 59–61. Curry, 4/e, pp 65–68. Thompson, pp 202–206.)* As photon energy increases, the photon becomes more penetrating and less likely to undergo an x-ray/matter interaction of any kind. Therefore, the probability of both photoelectric and Compton interactions decreases as photon energy increases. However, the rate of decrease is not the same for both types of interactions. As photon energy increases, the photoelectric interaction will decrease at a faster rate than will Compton interactions. The end result is that Compton interactions will predominate over photoelectric interactions in the higher energy range.

12. The answer is A. *(Bushong, 5/e, p 174. Carlton, pp 200–201. Curry, 4/e, pp 65–68. Statkiewicz-Sherer, 2/e, pp 25–26. Thompson, pp 202–206.)* The amount of energy retained by the scattered photon is determined by the incident energy of the photon undergoing the Compton interaction and the angle of deflection of the incident photon with the electron to be ejected. The scattered photon will have less energy as the angle of deflection (from the original path of the incident photon) increases. Incident photons of lower energy tend to be deflected more during the scattering event than high-energy photons. Therefore, x-rays produced in the diagnostic range of energies will most likely be deflected in a forward direction and be recorded by the image receptor.

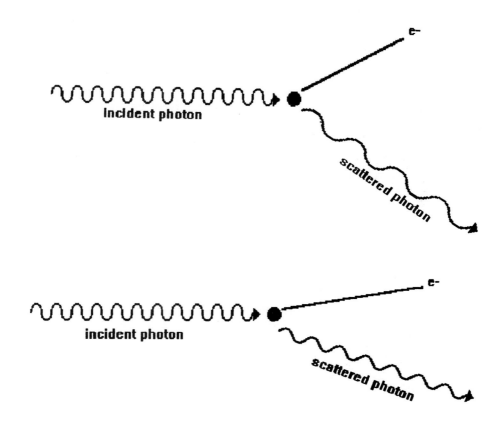

13. The answer is D. *(Bushong, 5/e, pp 173–174. Carlton, pp 200–201. Curry, 4/e, pp 65–68. Thompson, pp 202–206.)* The energies of the incident and subsequent scattered photons are directly related. As incident photon energy decreases, the energy of the scattered photon will also be less. This is due to the fact that scattered photon energy is the difference between the incident energy and the energy given up in ejecting the recoil electron; thus, if there is less to begin with, the end result must be less. Low-energy photons tend to produce a larger angle of deflection during the Compton interaction, which also decreases the retained energy for the scattered photon.

14. **The answer is D.** *(Bushong, 5/e, p 172. Carlton, p 199. Curry, 4/e, pp 61–62. Statkiewicz-Sherer, 2/e, p 28. Thompson, p 200.)* Coherent scattering (also known as Thompson, classical, or unmodified scattering) results in a scattered photon *equal* to the incident photon in energy, wavelength, and frequency and redirected from its original path. This interaction occurs at a very low (10 keV or less) energy range. The interaction does not ionize the atom, but rather excites it. The incident photon interacts with the atom as a whole (Rayleigh scattering) or with a single electron (Thompson scattering). The energy of the photon is given up to the atom and the incident photon ceases to exist. This excess energy causes vibration (excitation) of the electrons of the irradiated atom and the ultimate release of a scattered photon, identical to the incident photon, in the process of atomic restabilization.

15. **The answer is B (2, 3).** *(Bushong, 5/e, pp 172–176. Carlton, pp 196–201. Curry, 4/e, pp 61–67. Thompson, pp 200–206.)* Ionization is defined as the removal or addition of electrons from an atom. Both Compton and photoelectric interactions result in the ejection of electrons from the atoms irradiated. Compton interactions remove loosely bound electrons, which are then replaced by free electrons. Photoelectric interactions eject tightly bound inner-shell electrons, causing the atomic structure to become unstable. The vacancy is filled by the transition of outer-shell electrons. Coherent scattering interactions do not remove electrons. The energy of the incident photon is transferred to the atom, causing a state of excitation. The release of a scattered photon of energy equal to that of the incident photon restabilizes the atom.

16. **The answer is A.** *(Bushong, 5/e, pp 177, 181–182, 185. Carroll, 5/e, pp 60–62. Curry, 4/e, p 64. Thompson, pp 201–202.)* The probability of photoelectric interactions increases greatly with materials of higher atomic number. The electron density of elements of high atomic number is greater, causing the electrons to be more tightly bound to their shells and raising the probability of photoelectric interaction. The addition of iodine or barium contrast media to the anatomic structures raises their atomic number and increases the number of photoelectric interactions to roughly the equivalent of the atomic number raised to the third power. For example, soft tissue has an atomic number (Z) of 7.4, while the Z of barium is 56. The increased probability of photoelectric interactions is $(56 / 7.4)^3 = (7.56)^3 = 432$; that is, barium is 432 times more likely to undergo a photoelectric interaction than is soft tissue.

17. **The answer is B.** *(Bushong, 5/e, pp 180–181. Carroll, 5/e, pp 60–62. Curry, 4/e, p 64. Statkiewicz-Sherer, 2/e, p 33. Thompson, pp 201–202.)* Photoelectric interactions result in the total absorption of the x-ray photon, leaving no exit photon to expose the image recording medium. This results in an area of unexposure on the image and is the source of true radiographic contrast. The increase in the number of photoelectric interactions will yield an image that demonstrates a high level of differential absorption, or high contrast. The overall contrast obtained is influenced by many factors; however, if the ratio of photoelectric interactions to Compton interactions can be increased, the overall image contrast will increase.

18. **The answer is A.** *(Carroll, 5/e, pp 60–62. Curry, 4/e, p 64. Statkiewicz-Sherer, 2/e, p 31. Thompson, pp 201–202.)* The process of photoelectric interactions results in the complete absorption of photon energy by the material irradiated. This absorption of energy may cause atomic, molecular, or cellular change that could be detrimental to the organism. Increases in such energy deposits contributes to an increase in patient dose. While it is important to have a sufficient number of photoelectric interactions to demonstrate contrast between structures, this must be balanced with a sufficiently high energy (kVp) to minimize unnecessary patient dose.

19. **The answer is A.** *(Bushong, 5/e, p 15. Statkiewicz-Sherer, 2/e, pp 46, 50. Thompson, p 456.)* The roentgen is a unit of measurement of radiation "in air." It is more specifically defined as the quantity of radiation exposure to produce an electrical charge of 2.58×10^{-4} coulombs per kilogram of air (C/kg). The ionization chamber is a device that converts ionizing radiation to a corresponding electric charge (number of ion pairs created) and ultimately expresses the quantity of radiation exposure in terms of roentgens. While the other terms listed as answer options are units of radiation measurement, their use is more appropriate to other types of radiation effects, according to their various definitions.

20. The answer is B. *(Bushong, 5/e, p 15. Statkiewicz-Sherer, 2/e, p 51. Thompson, p 456.)* The *rad* originated as an acronym for *radiation absorbed dose*. It is the unit of measurement defined to express absorbed dose as a result of the amount of energy transferred from a photon to the tissue irradiated. More specifically, absorbed dose is stated as the amount of radiation required to deposit 100 ergs of energy per gram of tissue irradiated. Its SI equivalent is the gray (Gy).

21. The answer is B. *(Bushong, 5/e, p 16. Selman, 8/e, pp 187–188. Statkiewicz-Sherer, 2/e, p 51.)* The standard unit of measure for expressing radiation absorbed dose is the *rad*. Its SI counterpart is the *gray (Gy)*. One rad equals 0.01 Gy (10^{-2}). The rad represents the amount of radiant energy transferred from the x-ray beam to the tissue transversed. It is correctly used to express the amount of radiation dose delivered during the course of a diagnostic or therapeutic radiologic procedure.

22. The answer is B. *(Bushong, 5/e, p 16. Selman, 8/e, pp 504–505. Statkiewicz-Sherer, 2/e, p 52. Thompson, pp 457–458.)* Each form of ionizing radiation (nuclear or electromagnetic) has the ability to cause a biologic response. However, the response will vary with the type of radiation. *Dose equivalent* is used to account for the differences in biologic response. The standard unit of measure to express dose equivalent is the *rem*, and its SI counterpart is the *sievert*. Calculation of the dose equivalent is the product of absorbed dose and the quality factor (QF) for the type of radiation involved. According to NCRP Report No. 91, the QF for gamma, beta, and x-rays is the same: one (1). Particulate types of radiation have higher quality factors to correspond with their more reactive effect on biologic tissue; thermal neutrons have a QF of 5, and other neutrons, protons, and alpha particles have a QF of 20. These higher QF values demonstrate the increased biologic effect an equal dose of these forms of radiation will deliver compared with gamma or x-rays.

23. The answer is D. *(Selman, 8/e, pp 504–506. Statkiewicz-Sherer, 2/e, p 53. Thompson, pp 457–458.)* Dose equivalent is the product of absorbed dose and the quality factor (QF) applied to alpha particles. The correct unit of measure to indicate dose equivalent is the rem (sievert). To solve this problem, multiply 20 rads (absorbed dose) by 20 (QF of alpha) to equal 400 rem, which is equivalent to 4.0 Sv. This demonstrates the increased biologic effect of alpha exposure compared with an equal dose of x-rays, which would have a dose equivalence of 20 rem (20 × 1).

24. The answer is C. *(Bushong, 5/e, p 16. Selman, 8/e, p 505. Statkiewicz-Sherer, 2/e, p 52. Thompson, pp 457–458.)* The standard unit of measurement to express dose equivalence is the *rem* (radiation equivalent in man). Its SI counterpart is the sievert *(Sv)* and it is equivalent to 100 rem (1 rem = 10^{-2} Sv). Dose equivalence is used to indicate the biologic response of various types of radiation for an equal dose of radiation delivered. It is correctly used to report occupational exposures such as from film badges or thermoluminescent dosimeters.

25. The answer is B. *(Bushong, 5/e, p 635. Thompson, p 459.)* The monitoring and measurement of radiation exposure is termed *dosimetry* (dose measurement). Occupational exposure is measured through the use of personnel dosimeters such as the film badge, thermoluminescent dosimeter (TLD), or personal ionization chambers. Patient dose may also be measured, most commonly with the placement of a TLD type of radiation monitor in the field of exposure. The active component (lithium fluoride) of the TLD acts as a tissue equivalent for radiation exposure. *Densitometry* is the measurement of radiographic density on an exposed and processed film. *Sensitometry* is an indication of a film's response to exposure and processing. *ALARA* is an acronym for the basic radiation philosophy introduced by the ICRP, which states that all radiation exposure should be kept *as low as reasonably achievable*.

26. The answer is C. *(Bushong, 5/e, p 659. Selman, 8/e, pp 513–514. Statkiewicz-Sherer, 2/e, p 245.)* The devices employed as personnel radiation monitors are the film badge, ion chamber (pocket style), and thermoluminescent dosimeter (TLD). Each of these meets the basic requirements for consideration as personnel monitors: small, easy to wear, and sensitive to x- and gamma radiation. Each also has its own advantages and disadvantages, which radiation safety officers must evaluate in order to determine which will best fulfill the needs of monitoring those who are occupationally exposed to radiation. The use of scintillation crystals to detect radiation is employed in such devices as automatic exposure controls, CT detectors, and nuclear medicine cameras. These crystals are coupled with a photomultiplier tube, which converts the light photons produced by the crystals to electrical current, which can then be measured. G-M counters are limited to radiation monitoring of areas such as in the case of radiation leaks or spills of radiopharmaceuticals.

27. **The answer is A.**   *(Bushong, 5/e, p 660. Curry, 4/e, pp 298–299. Selman, 8/e, p 513. Statkiewicz-Sherer, 2/e, p 255.)*   The TLD is one type of personnel monitoring device available to indicate the amount of radiation exposure one receives. The active component of this device is the lithium fluoride crystal, which has luminescent properties and responds to radiation exposure by a rearrangement of its valence electrons into the trapped band of the outer shell. In this manner, the x-ray energy is stored in the crystal until it is time to be read. During analysis of the TLD, the crystal is heated and the trapped electrons are allowed back to their normal state (valance band) with an associated emission of energy in the form of light. This light is collected and measured. The amount of light produced is proportionate to the amount of radiation exposure received by the crystals. Cesium iodide and sodium iodide are luminescent crystals used in image intensifiers, gamma cameras, or CT detectors. However, these crystals emit light photons with no or minimal delay. They do not need the stimulation of high temperature to produce the light emissions. Xenon gas is used in the design of CT detectors of the ion chamber type.

28. **The answer is D.**   *(Bushong, 5/e, p 660. Statkiewicz-Sherer, 2/e, p 257. Thompson, p 461.)*   The TLD can be worn for up to 3 months without loss of information. These devices are not affected by heat and humidity as film badges are, nor by mechanical shock as pocket ion chambers are. The film badge should be replaced after 1 month of use to ensure the most accurate reading. Pocket ion chambers are the most sensitive to loss of information and should be read daily and their readings recorded before the unit is recharged. Once this is done, there is no way to retrieve the original information. Scintillation crystals are not employed in personnel monitoring devices.

29. **The answer is C (1, 3).**   *(Bushong, 5/e, pp 659–660. Statkiewicz-Sherer, 2/e, p 252. Thompson, p 461.)*   The film badge type of radiation monitor is small, lightweight, and easy to use (just clip it on!). It is also the only type that provides a permanent record of exposure. Once it is processed, the film is filed away and may be retrieved for future reevaluation. The film badge is also coupled with filters to provide an indication of the energy of the radiation to which it was exposed. Neither the TLD nor the pocket ion chamber provides a permanent record or the ability to indicate energy level. However, the film badge is sensitive to light exposure (if the film packet is damaged), heat, and humidity. Therefore, it is recommended that the film badge be used for no more than a month before being processed and analyzed.

30. **The answer is B.**   *(Bushong, 5/e, p 659. Statkiewicz-Sherer, 2/e, p 247. Thompson, p 461.)*   The design of the film badge type of radiation monitor includes a piece of dosimetry film enclosed in a light-tight packet, which is placed into a holder containing filters. As it is worn, any radiation that reaches the device exposes the film. At the end of the monitoring period, the film is processed and the level of exposure is determined by the amount of density on the film as determined by a standardized chart. As with all film exposed to radiation, the density level on the film is directly proportionate to the amount of incident radiation exposure. Light is produced and measured during analysis of the TLD device. The ion chamber indicates exposure as a result of the amount of discharge that occurs between the central electrode and the quartz fiber indicator.

31. **The answer is D.**   *(Bushong, 5/e, p 659. Carlton, p 49. Thompson, p 462.)*   The use of radiation monitor devices is limited to those persons who are routinely exposed to radiation and are likely to receive more than one-tenth the recommended exposure level during the performance of their occupational duties. Those persons who are occasionally exposed to radiation as a result of their occupation need not be monitored, but they must be removed from the exposure area or protected with lead garments if they are required to

remain with the patient (including family members). Those health care professionals who assist with radiographic procedures should be rotated so that the same person is not repeatedly exposed.

32. The answer is C. *(Bushong, 5/e, p 606. NCRP No. 91, pp 24, 48.)* NCRP No. 91, issued in 1987, states that the maximum dose equivalent for whole-body exposure of the occupationally exposed person is 50 mSv (5 rem) per year. This dose limit is in reference to *stochastic effects,* which assume a linear, non-threshold response; that is, an early response is produced at any level of radiation exposure. This value is an *upper* limit under normal conditions. Studies have shown that the average radiographer has an annual exposure of well below this dose limit. The concept of ALARA should still be the goal for all radiation exposure.

33. The answer is B. *(Bushong, 5/e, p 606. NCRP No. 91, p 48.)* The occasionally, or nonoccupationally, exposed person has a dose-equivalent limit for whole-body radiation exposure of 5 mSv (0.5 rem) per year. This value represents one-tenth the dose-equivalent limit of the occupationally exposed person. The difference in limits addresses the fact that occupationally exposed persons represent a small percentage of the population, which thereby keeps the number of radiation mutations within the entire population to an insignificant level. Also, occupationally exposed persons are trained in and employ protection methods to minimize their dose. As previously stated, all radiation exposure should be kept to levels *as low as reasonably achievable (ALARA).*

34. The answer is C. *(Bushong, 5/e, p 606. NCRP No. 91, p 48.)* The dose-equivalent limit for the gestation period for an embryo/fetus is 5 mSv (0.5 rem). Once a radiographer becomes pregnant, the dose-equivalent limit of the nonoccupationally exposed person must be followed to accommodate the embryo/fetus. The dose equivalent of the embryo/fetus is further restricted by a monthly exposure limit of 0.5 mSv (0.05 rem). The department may, but is not required to, provide a second radiation monitoring device to be worn under the lead apron at the level of the waist in order to monitor fetal exposure.

35. The answer is D. *(Bushong, 5/e, p 606. NCRP No. 91, pp 25, 48.)* The cumulative exposure limit is determined by the product of 10 mSv (1 rem) and the age of the radiation worker. This cumulative information is pertinent to the occupationally exposed person only. The current limit is a reduction in the level of cumulative exposure from previous NCRP reports and reflects the concept of keeping exposure levels low and the recognition of safety features included on modern radiographic equipment.

36. The answer is C. *(Bushong, 5/e, p 606. NCRP No. 91, pp 25, 48.)* The cumulative exposure limit is calculated as 10 mSv × age (1 rem × age) of the subject. Therefore, the solution to this problem is 10 × 40 = 400 mSv (1 × 40 = 40 rem). The measure is not based on the length of a radiographer's employment.

37. The answer is B. *(Bushong, 5/e, pp 602, 647.)* Occupational exposure is defined as the radiation a person is exposed to as a result of work activities with ionizing radiation. Dose-equivalent limits are applied only to occupationally and occasionally exposed situations, not to dose received during a medical procedure. There are no dose limits for absorbed dose as received by a patient. It is expected that the benefit of medical diagnosis outweighs the risk of the radiation exposure. Radiographic procedures should only be performed under the order of a physician. Background radiation is naturally occurring radiation in the environment to which all persons are exposed. Therefore, the solution to this question is found by considering only that exposure received as a result of occupational duties: 200 mrem (2 mSv).

38. The answer is C. *(Bushong, 5/e, p 599. Thompson, p 464.)* The cardinal rules of radiation protection are the basics and apply to the protection of both the patient and personnel. They include the use of the shortest exposure time, maximum distance between the source and the subject, and shielding of body parts not within the area of interest. Reducing exposure time refers to decreasing the amount of time the beam is on as well as minimizing the time personnel remain in a radiation area (i.e., fluoroscopy). Maximizing distance from the radiation source reduces exposure as defined in the inverse square law. Minimum source-to-skin distances are established for patient protection. Room design should allow personnel to stand back when not needed. Shielding of sensitive body parts is necessary for anyone in the radiographic room during a procedure, including patient, family, and personnel. Use of protective apparel as well as good collimation will satisfy this protection rule.

39. The answer is B. *(Bushong, 5/e, p 601. Statkiewicz-Sherer, 2/e, p 174.)* Lead is the material of choice for shielding purposes due to its high atomic number and dense molecular nature. By comparison with other materials, lead would be required in the least quantity to shield against radiation. When other materials are employed, sufficient quantities of these materials must be used to provide a level of shielding equivalent to that of lead. Aluminum is the material of choice for filters. Copper is occasionally used for filtration and tungsten is used in the construction of the tube filament and target disk.

40. The answer is A. *(Bushong, 5/e, p 665. Thompson, p 466.)* The soft lead used in the construction of lead aprons is susceptible to rough handling and can be torn or develop cracks. To avoid damaging the protective quality of lead aprons, they should be hung on racks designed for this purpose. This avoids folds and pressure, which could be damaging. Aprons should never be left crumpled on the floor or piled on top of a hot processor. They should also be inspected on an annual basis or when damage is suspected. This inspection should include an evaluation with the fluoroscope to check for radiation leaks.

41. The answer is C. *(Bushong, 5/e, p 632. Carroll, 5/e, p 13. Statkiewicz-Sherer, 2/e, p 25.)* Primary radiation is that which is emitted through the window of the x-ray tube and which is not altered as it passes through matter. It is composed of characteristic radiation and bremsstrahlung (braking radiation) resulting from electron-target interactions. Some primary radiation will exit the patient and be included in the exit beam, contributing to the radiographic image. The high energy associated with primary radiation requires higher levels of shielding to protect areas that may receive this type of exposure.

42. The answer is C. *(Bushong, 5/e, p 632. Carroll, 5/e, pp 13–14. Statkiewicz-Sherer, 2/e, p 25.)* Primary radiation refers to those photons that do not participate in x-ray/matter interactions and therefore remain the same as when they originated. The three incorrect answer options all refer to scattered radiation, which is formed by Compton interactions. Scatter is the major source of exposure for the operator of radiographic equipment and is also the most prevalent component of the exit beam.

43. The answer is A. *(Bushong, 5/e, p 632. Statkiewicz-Sherer, 2/e, p 217.)* The *primary barrier* is any surface that receives primary radiation. Therefore, any wall or floor toward which the x-ray tube may be directed and energized is considered a primary barrier. This designation is important in order to properly construct the surface with sufficient thickness of building material to meet shielding requirements. The energy of the primary beam is greater than scattered or secondary radiation. *Secondary barriers* receive scattered exposure only and do not require as much shielding as the primary barriers. The terms *controlled* and *uncontrolled areas* are used to designate the occupancy status of various areas surrounding and containing radiation-producing equipment. The occupancy status must also be considered in determining shielding requirements for construction.

44. The answer is B. *(Bushong, 5/e, p 6. NCRP No. 93, pp 55–56. NCRP No. 105, p 6. Statkiewicz-Sherer, 2/e, pp 5–9.)* Background radiation is that radiation to which all persons are exposed during their lives. This radiation arises from natural and man-made sources. Natural radiation includes cosmic radiation, which originates in outer space and interacts with the earth's atmosphere, and terrestrial (earth) elements, which are unstable and emit radioactive particles and waves during their decay process. Radon is the major terrestrial radiation that contributes to our background exposure. Over half the background exposure received (natural and man-made) is due to radon exposure. Not only are we exposed to these types of radiation from outside our bodies, but radionuclides are found in the food chain, resulting in radiation exposure from within our bodies. Man-made radiation includes medical and dental x-rays, fallout from weapons testing and nuclear accidents, and radiation-emitting consumer products.

45. The answer is A. *(Bushong, 5/e, p 6. NCRP No. 105, p 6. Statkiewicz-Sherer, 2/e, pp 5–9.)* All the factors listed in the answer contribute to background exposure except ultrasonic waves. Only forms of ionizing radiation are included in the definition of background radiation. Ultrasonic waves are mechanical in nature. Although they may vibrate enough to cause some biologic reaction, such as tissue heating, ultrasonic waves are nonionizing.

46. The answer is B. *(Bushong, 5/e, p 651. Statkiewicz-Sherer, 2/e, pp 15–17.)* For a given amount of radiation exposure to biologic tissue, the skin dose will be the greatest because it receives the entrance dose. As the radiation passes through the exposed medium, it is attenuated. The deeper structures will receive a reduced amount of exposure. Specifically, the dose to the gonads will further vary in regard to their position relative to the site of exposure. Also, for some examinations the gonadal dose for males will be much higher than for females and vice versa on other examinations. Again, this is due to the distance of the gonads from the area of exposure and the external versus internal location of the gonads, which offer a variation in the level of attenuation.

47. The answer is C. *(Bushong, 5/e, p 6. NCRP No. 93, pp 52–56. Statkiewicz-Sherer, 2/e, pp 9–11.)* The average level of background radiation exposure in the U.S. is about 3 to 4 mSv (300 to 400 mrem) per year. The majority of this irradiation is from natural sources, primarily radon at about 2 mSv (200 mrem) per year and from cosmic and other terrestrial sources at 1 mSv (100 mrem). Man-made radiation contributes to the remaining 25 percent of the background radiation, of which the majority arises from medical and dental sources. A small percentage (3 percent) arises from radiation-emitting consumer products and negligible amounts from nuclear fallout.

48. The answer is A. *(Bushong, 5/e, p 6. Statkiewicz-Sherer, 2/e, pp 10–15.)* Man-made sources of radiation include medical and dental procedures, nuclear medicine examinations, radiation-emitting consumer products, and fallout from above-ground nuclear weapons testing and nuclear accidents. These sources of radiation account for about 25 percent of the average background exposure level in the U.S. Natural sources of radiation include cosmic and terrestrial types of radiation. Terrestrial radiation results from unstable elements in the earth that emit radioactive particles and rays as they undergo nuclear decay. Building materials include some of these unstable elements to which we are routinely exposed. Other radionuclides expose us from inside our bodies as a result of their presence in our food chain. Radon emissions contribute to over 50 percent of our background exposure.

49. The answer is D. *(NCRP No. 91, pp 24–25. Statkiewicz-Sherer, 2/e, p 64.)* *Effective dose-equivalent limits* refers to the uppermost level of radiation exposure received from occupational sources or by members of the general public who receive occasional exposures. These exposures do not include background radiation or radiation for medical purposes. These limits represent the amount of exposure that, if sustained, would still have a negligible risk of causing somatic or genetic damage. However, these limits are accompanied by the recommendation for establishing a radiation protection philosophy known as ALARA.

50. The answer is C. *(Bushong, 5/e, pp 605–606. NCRP No. 91, pp 25, 48. Statkiewicz-Sherer, 2/e, pp 73–75.)* Recommendations on effective dose-equivalent limits were issued in NCRP No. 91 (1987) and superseded by NCRP No. 116 (1993). As with earlier reports, the annual dose limit for whole-body exposure for the radiation worker is 50 mSv (5000 mrem or 5 rem). The exception to this dose limit is for the pregnant radiation worker. Protection of the fetus requires the dose limit to be reduced to 5 mSv (500 mrem) and a maximum of 0.5 mSv (50 mrem) per month for the gestation period.

51. The answer is D. *(Bushong, 5/e, pp 605–606. NCRP No. 103, pp 13–14. Statkiewicz-Sherer, 2/e, pp 73–75.)* The cumulative dose-equivalent limit only pertains to the radiation worker. As part of NCRP No. 91, the cumulative dose limit was significantly reduced from one's age minus 18 times 5 rem per year to only 1 rem (10 mSv) times one's age. For example, a 42-year-old radiation worker is allowed a cumulative dose limit of 420 mSv (42 rem) under current recommendations as opposed to 1200 mSv (120 rem) as previously calculated. This limit more closely follows ALARA. Also, workers are less likely to become careless in their personal protection as a result of a false sense of security from having such a high limit.

52. **The answer is C.** *(Bushong, 5/e, pp 605–606. Statkiewicz-Sherer, 2/e, pp 71–72.)* The cumulative effective dose-equivalent limit is calculated by multiplying the worker's age by 10 mSv (1 rem). For this radiographer, the cumulative dose limit would be calculated as 35 × 10 mSv = 350 mSv. However, since this radiographer has received occupational exposure adding up to 100 mSv, this value must be deducted for a new cumulative limit of 250 mSv (25 rem).

53. **The answer is A.** *(Bushong, 5/e, p 606. Statkiewicz-Sherer, 2/e, p 71.)* Only the occupational exposure is subjected to the effective dose-equivalent limits. Only a small percentage of the total population make up the pool of radiation workers; therefore, a higher level of exposure is tolerable without appreciable risk to the genetic pool of the whole population. The potential risk from exposures received during medical procedures is outweighed by the advantages of diagnosis, assuming the radiologic examination is sufficiently warranted. The entire human population is exposed to background radiation for which such limits do not apply. Therefore, at the conclusion of the incidents stated in the question, only the 10 mSv received as part of occupational exposure would apply to the worker's cumulative effective dose-equivalent limit.

54. **The answer is D.** *(Bushong, 5/e, p 607. Statkiewicz-Sherer, 2/e, p 65.)* ALARA is the radiation protection philosophy that has been recommended since 1954. The recommendation comes from the National Council on Radiation Protection and Measurements (NCRP). The acronym stands for "as low as reasonably achievable." In contrast to the effective dose-equivalent limits, ALARA maintains that every effort should be made to obtain the best possible radiologic results with the least amount of exposure to the patient and medical personnel. The NCRP meets to review data from various scientific groups relating to radiation exposure and to make recommendations regarding radiation protection. The NRC (Nuclear Regulatory Commission) is the enforcement agency within the federal government whose function is to ensure compliance with standards set for the operation of radiation devices and protection measurements. The ICRP (International Commission on Radiological Protection) reviews data and makes recommendations pertaining to radiation protection and measurement on an international level.

55. **The answer is B.** *(Bushong, 5/e, p 523. Statkiewicz-Sherer, 2/e, pp 105–106.)* *Ionization* results from the removal or addition of orbital electrons from or to the atom. Radiation ionizes by ejecting electrons from their orbits, resulting in the formation of an ion pair consisting of a freed electron (negative ion) and a positively charged atom (missing an electron). Photons or particles with the characteristics of high energy, short wavelength, and high penetration, are able to cause ionization events. When this does occur, at the atomic level, it can have effects on the structure of molecules that may be sufficient to disrupt cellular function.

56. **The answer is C.** *(Bushong, 5/e, p 534. Statkiewicz-Sherer, 2/e, pp 49–50, 106.)* LET is the term used to indicate differences between the various types of radiation in terms of their ability to deposit energy within the irradiated medium. Specifically, LET is the amount of energy transferred from the photon/particle per linear unit of medium traversed (keV/micron). Types of radiation with a high rate of LET, such as alpha particles, will deposit large quantities of energy over a relatively short distance. This is due to their highly charged nature (+2) and their massive size (2P+2N) compared with electrons or photons, which contributes to the fact that alpha particles have low penetrability. On the other hand, x-rays and gamma rays have no mass and no charge and thus are highly penetrating, depositing only small quantities of energy as they travel. These are types of radiation with low LET.

57. **The answer is A.** *(Bushong, 5/e, pp 534–535. Statkiewicz-Sherer, 2/e, p 107.)* LET and RBE have a direct relationship; that is, those radiation types with a high LET will have a high RBE. LET is the amount of energy deposited per unit of photon travel. The deposited energy is the source of ionization, which may cause molecular and cellular disruption and possibly result in biologic effects. LET provides a means of determining quality factors for various types of radiation based on their energy deposition. RBE provides a

comparison of the biologic effects from equal doses of different types of radiation. RBE also contributes to formulating quality factors for radiation types. For example, high-LET radiation like alpha particles deposits a large amount of radiation over a small area, resulting in a significant biologic effect (e.g., skin erythema). An equal dose of high-energy x-rays with a low LET spreads its energy over a longer distance, reducing the biologic effect. The quality factor assigned to alpha particles is 20; the quality factor for x-rays is 1.

58. The answer is D. *(Bushong, 5/e, p 534. Statkiewicz-Sherer, 2/e, pp 49–50.)* High-LET types of radiation are highly charged and have mass. Because of these factors, this type of radiation is not very penetrating and more energy will be deposited over a smaller area of the material irradiated. Of the types of radiation listed, the x-rays and gamma rays have no mass and no electrical charge, making them more penetrating. The 80-keV x-rays are the least penetrating of the three photons.

59. The answer is B. *(Bushong, 5/e, pp 52–53, 534. Statkiewicz-Sherer, 2/e, p 106.)* Radiation types with low LET values have high penetration, no mass, and no charge. These characteristics describe high-energy electromagnetic photons such as x-rays and gamma rays (also considered nonparticulate radiation). Radioactive particles like alpha particles, beta particles, and neutrons also have very high levels of energy, but their mass or electrical charge or both limit their range of penetration, thus allowing more energy to be transferred over a shorter distance and awarding them higher LET values.

60. The answer is C. *(Bushong, 5/e, p 534. Statkiewicz-Sherer, 2/e, p 107.)* The amount of biologic effect is dependent on the quantity of energy deposited in the irradiated matter and the radiosensitivity of the irradiated matter. Those types of radiation with high LET will also have a greater RBE. The LET values (stated in keV/micron of tissue traversed) for the types of radiation listed are alpha 100, fast neutrons 50, diagnostic x-rays 3, and 25-MeV x-rays 0.2. Therefore, the 25-MeV x-rays should produce the least biologic effect.

61. The answer is C. *(Bushing, 5/e, p 548. Statkiewicz-Sherer, 2/e, p 108.)* The effects of an irradiation assault may manifest themselves at the site of irradiation (direct effects) or at a point distant from the irradiation site (indirect effects). Indirect effects generally occur as a result of the free radical by-products that arise from radiolysis of water molecules. Since the human body is 60 percent water, indirect effects from irradiation predominate over direct effects.

62. The answer is A. *(Bushong, 5/e, pp 52–53. Statkiewicz-Sherer, 2/e, p 105.)* Ionizing radiation includes those types of radiant energies that have sufficient energy and short wavelengths to cause ionization of atoms (removal or addition of electrons) with which they interact. These include *particulate* radiation and *electromagnetic* radiation. As the term implies, particulate types of radiation have mass and may be electrically charged. They include alpha, beta, and neutron particles. These types of radiant energy are emitted from unstable nuclei of radioactive elements during the disintegration process. They are highly energetic, but their mass limits their penetrability; thus they tend to give up their energy over a small area in the ionization process. Electromagnetic radiation has no mass and no electrical charge. However, not all electromagnetic photons are ionizing. Low-energy, long-wavelength types of electromagnetic energy are referred to as *nonionizing* radiation and include radio and television waves and the visible light spectrum. Only x-rays and gamma rays have sufficient energy to cause ionization.

63. The answer is B. *(Bushong, 5/e, p 548. Statkiewicz-Sherer, 2/e, pp 108–115.)* Indirect effects are the most common result of irradiation of biological tissue. These effects are so named because they appear distant from the actual site of interaction. Sixty percent of the human body is made up of water, which increases the likelihood of interaction of the x-rays with water molecules. The result is radiolysis of water molecules and the formation of free radicals. These free radicals are unnatural and highly reactive. They are able to move within the tissues and enter cells, causing disruptive effects to cells distant from the actual exposure site.

64. The answer is C. *(Bushong, 5/e, p 547. Statkiewicz-Sherer, 2/e, pp 111–114.)* Radiolysis (breakdown of a structure due to irradiation) of water molecules causes the formation of positive and negative water molecules. These ions can further dissociate into a hydroxyl (–) ion and hydrogen radical or a hydrogen (+) ion and hydroxyl radical. The free radicals are highly reactive and are able to move within the tissues and enter cells, disrupting their structure and function. They may also combine to form toxic agents within the cell, causing further damage.

65. The answer is B. *(Bushong, 5/e, pp 548–550. Statkiewicz-Sherer, 2/e, pp 116–117.)* The *target theory* of cell survival assumes that there is a key, or master, molecule whose irradiation would cause cell death. This theory is used to explain why some cells do not manifest injury following irradiation and others do. It is believed that if there is only one such master molecule to a cell, inactivation of this molecule would result in cell death. Since radiation interactions are random events, the master molecule would not always be directly affected. Based on these assumptions, it is believed that the DNA molecule is the master molecule for each cell. The DNA molecule is considered the control center for growth, reproduction, and function of each cell. Loss of the DNA molecule through direct or indirect irradiation would result in cell death.

66. The answer is B. *(Bushong, 5/e, pp 532–533. Statkiewicz-Sherer, 2/e, pp 120–123.)* According to the law of Bergonié and Tribondeau, cellular radiosensitivity is directly related to the cell's proliferation and metabolic rates and indirectly related to its age and degree of specialization. This means that immature, nonspecialized cells that reproduce themselves frequently are more radiosensitive than mature, highly specialized cells with a low reproduction rate or none at all. Another factor in determining radiosensitivity is the abundance of a particular cell type (or macromolecule). Large quantities of a single type of cell (or macromolecule) mean that if some are lost, many others remain to continue their function and to repopulate the area. Therefore, radiosensitive cells include blood cells and gonadal cells. Of the blood cells, the erythrocytes are the most resistant because of their relatively large number (in the millions) and longer life cycle with a less frequent reproduction cycle as compared with white blood cells. The lymphocyte is the most radiosensitive cell in the body. This type numbers only in the thousands and has a life cycle of only about 24 h, requiring it to reproduce itself frequently. Epithelial cells are moderately sensitive to irradiation while mature muscle and nerve cells are the most resistant.

67. The answer is C. *(Bushong, 5/e, pp 532–533. Statkiewicz-Sherer, 2/e, pp 120–123.)* Highly radiosensitive cells would be immature (not fully developed) and not highly specialized (undifferentiated in their function) and would frequently reproduce. This describes such cells as blood and germ cells, especially when they are in their immature states. Muscle and nerve cells are highly specialized in their function and in their mature state do not reproduce, making them highly resistant to irradiation.

68. The answer is B. *(Bushong, 5/e, pp 566–568. Statkiewicz-Sherer, 2/e, pp 124–126. Travis, 2/e, pp 123–127.)* A gonadal dose of about 2 Gy (200 rads) would be sufficient to cause temporary sterility in males or females. This is due to the radiation-induced depletion of immature spermatogonia or ova in an intermediate stage of maturity. Given time, these germ cells can repopulate and end the "sterility" status. Permanent sterility may result from exposure levels of 5 Gy (500 rads) or more to the gonads. This level of exposure is sufficient to destroy the stem cells, preventing further spermatogonia or ova from developing or maturing. Exposure of this type may be delivered during radiation therapy but is not likely as a result of diagnostic x-ray or nuclear medicine examinations. A dose of 0.1 Gy (10 rads) to the gonads may cause genetic mutations, which could manifest in an offspring as congenital defects. For this reason, gonadal shielding should be a routine part of every radiologic procedure.

69. The answer is C (2, 3). *(Bushong, 5/e, p 577. Statkiewicz-Sherer, 2/e, pp 135–136.)* Irradiation may affect somatic or germ cells of the human body. *Germ* cells are found in the gonads and contain the genetic material of the being for purposes of reproduction. *Somatic* cells refer to all other cells of the body. Irradiation of germ cells can cause genetic effects, which may be passed on and manifest themselves in future generations. *Somatic* effects are evident in the person exposed and may be either early or late. *Early effects* are the result of relatively high levels of radiation exposure and may occur within minutes, hours, days, or weeks following the exposure. The severity and time of onset is determined by the dose received and age of the person. *Late effects* are the result of low level radiation exposure and may show up months or years after exposure.

70. The answer is D. *(Bushong, 5/e, pp 562–566. Statkiewicz-Sherer, 2/e, pp 130, 135–136.)* Early somatic effects of irradiation may be evident following whole- or partial-body exposure to a relatively high dose. Whole-body exposures of 1 Gy (100 rads) or more may cause acute radiation syndrome, also known as radiation sickness. The severity of this condition and the likelihood of recovery are dose-dependent. Some signs and symptoms of acute radiation syndrome are nausea, vomiting, diarrhea, blood changes, and destruction of the gastrointestinal or central nervous systems. Limited exposure to localized areas of the body will result in the manifestation of radiation effects in the exposed area. The possible effects include skin erythema, anemia, hair loss, nausea, vomiting, and diarrhea. Cataract formation and cancers are examples of long-term somatic effects of irradiation.

71. The answer is D. *(Bushong, 5/e, pp 562–563. Statkiewicz-Sherer, 2/e, pp 134–135.)* The term $LD_{50/30}$ refers to the amount of radiation that would be lethal to 50 percent of the exposed population within 30 days of exposure to the whole body. For the adult human, the dose level to cause this effect is about 3 Gy (300 rads) whole-body exposure. The most susceptible members of the population are the young, the elderly, and the infirm at any age. A whole-body exposure of 6 Gy (600 rads) would be sufficient to cause death in the entire exposed population within 30 days. This exposure level represents the *lethal dose* to humanity with few exceptions and is stated as $LD_{100/30}$.

72. The answer is D. *(Bushong, 5/e, pp 561–562, 577–582, 588-594. Statkiewicz-Sherer, 2/e, pp 133–146.)* *Late effects* are those that appear months or years after exposure to relatively low levels of radiation. *Somatic effects* are those which manifest in the exposed person's lifetime. The various types of late, somatic effects can be grouped into four categories: carcinogenic, cataractogenic, life span-shortening, and embryologic (of which congenital defects are one type). Many studies and observation of accidentally exposed persons have provided the data to support the understanding of the effects of low level radiation exposure. The tragic nuclear accident in Chernobyl in 1986 has provided another group of people to follow and learn from regarding the long-term effects of radiation exposure.

73. The answer is B. *(Bushong, 5/e, pp 595–596. Statkiewicz-Sherer, 2/e, p 145.)* Various embryologic effects are possible following in utero exposure. During the first trimester of gestation, the fetus is the most susceptible because of the vast amount of change and organ development. The possible results include congenital abnormalities such as growth and mental retardation, structural deformity, and induction of childhood malignancy, specifically leukemia. If exposure occurs within the first 2 weeks following fertilization, the effect is considered to be "all or none." That is, either a spontaneous abortion will occur or no damage will be caused. During the second and third trimesters, the fetus is less radiosensitive than it was in the first; however, it is still susceptible to damage and in utero exposure should always be kept as minimal as possible.

74. The answer is B. *(Bushong, 5/e, p 566. Statkiewicz-Sherer, 2/e, p 45.)* The term $SED_{50/30}$ refers to the amount of exposure that will cause skin erythema (reddening) in 50 percent of the exposed population within 30 days of exposure. A dose of 6 Gy (600 rads) to the skin will cause this reaction. Skin erythema may be visible following radiation therapy exposures, but should not occur from diagnostic x-ray procedures. Originally, the SED was used as a unit of radiation measure as the only direct means of indicating a quantity of exposure. It was replaced with the roentgen (R) unit in 1928.

75. The answer is B. *(Bushong, 5/e, pp 665–668. Statkiewicz-Sherer, 2/e, pp 163–182, 184, 189.)* Patient exposure can be reduced through the implementation of various radiation protection practices. These practices include the following:

1. Reduction of the size of field of exposure through the use of a beam restrictor (collimator or cone). This action will limit the amount of tissue irradiated and the quantity of x-ray/matter interactions.

2. Increased beam quality through filtration to lower skin entrance dose.

3. The use of immobilization devices to reduce motion and need for repeat exposures.

4. The implementation of high-kV, low-mAs techniques to provide optimum penetration with the least possible quantity of exposure.

5. Contact or shadow shields to protect radiosensitive structures in or near the field of view.

6. Increased SID or source-to-skin distance according to the inverse square law, thereby reducing patient dose.

7. The use of fast intensifying screens where appropriate, to allow the least amount of exposure while obtaining satisfactory image density.

Direct exposure (nonscreen) imaging systems require excessive exposure and should not be used. Grids significantly improve image quality to warrant the increased dose necessary, but are not considered a radiation protection practice.

76. The answer is D. *(Bushong, 5/e, pp 665–669. Statkiewicz-Sherer, 2/e, pp 163–164.)* Patient motion is the primary cause of motion artifacts and often requires the image to be repeated, thus increasing patient dose. The three practices stated in the question are acceptable means of controlling patient motion. Restraining devices should be used on any patient unable to cooperate with the positioning instructions required for an examination. Short exposure times are necessary to avoid organ motion, such as peristalsis. Minimum exposure times are dependent on the maximum mA selections available and kV requirements for optimum penetration. Having patients hold their breath is necessary for any examination of the chest or abdomen.

77. The answer is B. *(Bushong, 5/e, p 630. Statkiewicz-Sherer, 2/e, pp 171–173.)* Filtration of the x-ray beam is mandatory because it minimizes the amount of low-energy (soft) photons that reaches the patient, thus reducing dose. Filtration removes low-energy photons from the beam, increasing the average beam energy and creating a more penetrating beam. Federal standards require the primary x-ray beam to pass through a minimum total filtration level of 2.5 mm of aluminum or its equivalent for tubes capable of operating at 70 kVp or higher. An insufficient level of filtration subjects the patient to unnecessary radiation exposure.

78. The answer is D. *(Bushong, 5/e, pp 629–630. Statkiewicz-Sherer, 2/e, p 169.)* The field of exposure is controlled by the adjustment of the beam restrictor device. The collimator and cone are the most commonly used devices for this purpose. The *collimator* allows the radiographer to manipulate the shutters to form any size field in a square or rectangular shape. The *cone* provides a circular opening of fixed size, thus requiring a variety of cones to accommodate a wide range of fields of exposure. With either type, the opening should not be larger than the size of the image receptor. In order to demonstrate collimation, the opening should be adjusted to be slightly smaller than the image receptor, thus providing a border of unexposed film.

79. The answer is C. *(Bushong, 5/e, p 630. Statkiewicz-Sherer, 2/e, p 191.)* The fixed, or stationary, type of fluoroscopic unit should have a minimum distance from source to table top of 15 inches (38 cm). The mobile fluoroscopic unit should have a minimum distance of 12 inches (30 cm). This standard is set to keep patient dose to a minimum according to the inverse square law.

80. The answer is B. *(Bushong, 5/e, p 631. Statkiewicz-Sherer, 2/e, p 192.)* All fluoroscopic units are required to have a cumulative timer device to track the amount of time the fluoroscope is operated. This timer should go off after 5 min and must be reset in order to continue. The purpose for this is to keep the fluoroscopist aware of the amount of exposure time being generated. This minimizes both patient and personnel exposure levels.

81. The answer is A. *(Bushong, 5/e, pp 630–631. Statkiewicz-Sherer, 2/e, pp 190–192.)* In order to minimize exposure dose during fluoroscopy, the fluoroscopist should use intermittent exposures; i.e., the exposure should be repeatedly turned on and off. The dose delivered to patient and personnel can be significantly reduced by using intermittent rather than continuous exposure. Also, high-kVp , low-mAs techniques are generally employed during fluoroscopy. At high kVp, the beam is more penetrating and less quantity (mAs) of radiation is needed. All fluoroscopy should be performed with the assistance of an image intensifier. The improved viewing conditions allow for better visual acuity and shorter examination times as compared with nonintensified fluoroscopy.

82. The answer is D. *(Bushong, 5/e, p 538. Statkiewicz-Sherer, 2/e, pp 106–107. Travis, 2/e, pp 31–32.)* Dose-response curves are constructed to graphically demonstrate the relationship between radiation exposure and biologic effects. These curves are based on scientific studies and observation of radiation effects conducted to further the understanding of such effects. Their importance in radiologic technology is twofold. First, it provides the basis for current radiation protection policies according to the assumption that low-LET radiation exposure results in a linear, nonthreshold response. Specifically, this relationship suggests that all radiation is harmful and should be kept to a minimum level. Second, dose-response relationships are employed in the planning for radiation therapy. The LET determination of a radiation type is based on its ability to deposit energy as the radiation traverses the tissue. Mean survival time is the time between radiation exposure and death of the exposed organism. The assignment of radiation quality factors is derived from the RBE function. The data for LET, mean survival time, and quality factors are not available from the dose-response chart.

83. The answer is B. *(Bushong, 5/e, pp 600, 666–667. Statkiewicz-Sherer, 2/e, pp 181–183, 228–230).* The three exposure factors stated in the question will all have an effect on patient dose, direct or indirect. Milliampere-seconds (mAs) is the controlling factor for radiation quantity. As such, it has a *directly proportionate* effect on patient dose. This means that as mAs increases, patient dose will increase by an equal amount. However, kilovoltage (kV) and SID have an *indirect* effect on patient dose. An increase in either of these factors will decrease patient dose. Higher kilovoltage selection will produce a more penetrating beam and require fewer milliampere-seconds to produce similarly exposed radiographic results as compared with a combination of low kilovoltage and high milliampere-seconds. However, since kilovoltage also controls image contrast, there is a limit as to the use of high kilovoltage. An increase in SID will decrease exposure, according to the inverse square law. This law states that as distance between the source and the object irradiated increases, exposure will decrease to the square of the distance. This is especially important in fluoroscopy, where distance from source to table top is less than in radiography because of equipment design.

84. The answer is C. *(Bushong, 5/e, pp 600, 666–667. NCRP No. 102, pp 7, 10. Statkiewicz-Sherer, 2/e, pp 181–183, 228–230.)* The three parameters stated in the question (mAs, kV and SID) will all influence x-ray intensity, thereby influencing patient dose. The best means for reducing exposure to the patient can be achieved by increasing beam energy (kV), thus allowing a decrease in the required beam intensity (mAs). The combinations of exposure factors offered as answers would have the following effects:

(A) The decrease in milliampere-seconds only will reduce patient dose and radiographic density, resulting in an underexposed image. (B) The 15 percent increase in kilovoltage will lower patient dose, but requires a 50 percent decrease in milliampere-seconds to maintain density; the change from 30 to 20 mAs is only a 30 percent difference. (C) Both the kilovoltage and SID were increased and the milliampere-seconds varied to compensate for both these changes. The result will be a decrease in patient dose while radiographic density is maintained. (D) The increase in milliampere-seconds is appropriate to compensate for the increase in SID; however, the dose to the patient will be the same as that produced by the original set of exposure factors.

85. The answer is C. *(Bushong, 5/e, pp 630, 651. Carlton, pp 518, 524. Statkiewicz-Sherer, 2/e, pp 169–172.)* Each of the factors included in the answer options for this question will influence the patient's dose. The factors that will minimize patient dose are more filtration, longer SID, smaller field of exposure, and lower tube output (mR/mAs). The conditions stated in choice C offer the highest filtration level, longest SID, and smallest field of exposure. This choice also had the second lowest tube output. When compared with the other options, this combination would produce the least amount of patient dose.

86. **The answer is C.** *(Bushong, 5/e, p 667. NCRP No. 102, p 8. Statkiewicz-Sherer, 2/e, pp 178–180.)* Imaging of the spine for a scoliosis survey is most commonly performed on young female patients whose breast tissue is in an active stage of development and thus radiosensitive. For this reason, precautions should be taken to reduce breast exposure during these procedures, which may require many radiographic examinations over the treatment period. The examination commonly requires the AP and lateral projection of the entire spine. Collimation should be employed as well as contact or shadow shielding of the breasts. It has been recommended that the PA projection be employed to drastically reduce exposure (exit dose rather than entrance dose) with a minimal amount of magnification of the spine, which may be accomplished by increasing the SID. Finally, a trough type of compensating filter may be employed to reduce the exposure intensity to the lateral aspects of the beam while maintaining sufficient exposure to the spine. Use of this device may be limited by the extent of the lateral curve of the spine.

87. **The answer is B.** *(Bushong, 5/e, p 669. NCRP No. 102, p 8. Statkiewicz-Sherer, 2/e, pp 173–174.)* The proper use of gonadal shields is important in reducing gonadal dose and the possibility of genetic effects due to irradiation. However, their use will vary with the type of examination being performed. The gonadal shielding is always employed in addition to proper collimation of the beam. Gonadal shielding should be utilized whenever the gonads are in or near the field of exposure, as long as the shield will not obscure the structures of interest. It is important to carefully place the shield so that it does not overlap the structures of interest and require a repeat image. They should also be used on all patients who are within child-bearing age, young and old.

88. **The answer is D.** *(Bushong, 5/e, p 667. Statkiewicz-Sherer, 2/e, pp 173–174.)* Any of the shield types listed in this question may be used as gonadal shields as long as they are properly positioned so as not to obscure the structures of interest. Contact shields are placed directly on the patient over the gonads. Various sizes and shapes are available to accommodate males and females, children and adults. Shadow shields are mounted on the collimator and are positioned within the primary beam so as to cast a shadow over the area to be shielded. These can be just as effective as contact shields and may be better tolerated by some patients. The newest type of shield is incorporated with a filter system and is made of clear plastic impregnated with lead; it attaches to the bottom of the collimator. The clear plastic allows the localizing light of the collimator to project onto the patient while reducing exposure. Shielding is achieved through the use of accessory pieces that contain lead shapes and magnetically attach to the filter. This configuration resembles the shadow shield.

89. **The answer is D.** *(Bushong, 5/e, p 665. NCRP No. 102, p 9. Statkiewicz-Sherer, 2/e, pp 232–234.)* Occasionally, patients are unable to cooperate with maintaining a required position for radiography. Such cases require some external means of restraining the patient. Ideally, a mechanical device should be used whenever possible. These devices would not require a person to remain in the examination room for unnecessary exposure. When such devices are not available or effective, someone must hold the patient in position. The best choice would be a relative of the patient who is older than 18 and not pregnant. When hospital personnel must be used, it should be someone other than radiology personnel. However, the same person should not be routinely called upon to hold patients. Protective apparel (aprons and gloves) must be provided to the holders and their position must be out of the primary beam as much as possible.

90. **The answer is C.** *(Bushong, 5/e, pp 662–663. NCRP No. 102, p 83. Statkiewicz-Sherer, 2/e, pp 243–244.)* The appropriate position of the personnel monitoring device should be at waist level when a protective apron is not worn, as during routine radiography. This position allows the trunk of the body to be monitored, providing data regarding the dose to the gonads. The proper location of the monitor is less well defined when a protective apron is worn. If it is left at the waist, thus under the apron, the dose recorded should be low, indicating the effectiveness of the apron. However, the unprotected radiosensitive structures

of the head and neck will be unmonitored. If the monitor is then positioned at the collar level, outside the apron during fluoroscopic or mobile procedures, the head and neck will be monitored and it is assumed the protected abdomen will have received a significantly smaller dose, if any. Ideally, two badges could be worn, one at the waist under the apron and the other at the collar outside the apron. This would require careful labeling of the respective monitors to ensure they are worn in the correct position each day. This is not a routine practice because of the increased effort in tracking these monitors as well as the increased cost. However, double badges are more commonly issued for the pregnant technologist in order to monitor fetal exposure.

91. The answer is D. *(Bushong, 5/e, p 659. NCRP No. 102, p 83. Statkiewicz-Sherer, 2/e, p 243.)* Personnel monitors are primarily issued to radiologists and radiologic technologists. The purpose of these devices is to indicate the amount of radiation exposure personnel receive as a result of the work they do. It further provides data on the effectiveness of a department's radiation protection policies and the work habits of the individual. Each type of personnel monitor has weak points of which the wearer must be aware. These devices do not directly act to protect the radiographer. Neither do they keep track of the level of exposure a radiographer delivers nor the repeat rate of the radiographer.

92. The answer is D. *(Bushong, 5/e, pp 635–636. Statkiewicz-Sherer, 2/e, p 257. Selman, 8/e, p 163.)* Since x-rays have no mass or electrical charge, they cannot be measured or detected directly. However, they do have the ability to affect matter in ways that can then be detected or measured. The majority of radiation survey devices are a type of ionization chamber and operate on the principle that x-rays are able to ionize air molecules. The basic design of such devices includes a chamber of air or gas under pressure and electrodes. Upon irradiation and ionization, the liberated electrons are conducted along a positive electrode, producing a flow of current that is measurable. Other methods of detecting radiation are based on the ability of x-rays to darken film emulsion, as in film badges, or to cause certain materials to emit light, as in photomultiplier and scintillation devices. These methods are the basis of automatic exposure control devices, CT detectors, and nuclear medicine gamma cameras.

93. The answer is D. *(Bushong, 5/e, pp 632–633, 647–648. Statkiewicz-Sherer, 2/e, pp 24–25, 215, 217.)* Primary and secondary radiation are designated according to their source of origin. Those photons that are produced as a result of an electron-target interaction within the x-ray tube and then exit the tube via the window are considered *primary* photons. Radiation that exits the tube from a point other than the window and radiates in all directions is termed *leakage* radiation. *Secondary* radiation arises from an interaction between a primary photon and matter, such as characteristic photons arising from photoelectric interactions. The interactions that produce secondary photons use most of the incident photon energy. Thus secondary photons are much less energetic than primary photons. *Scattered* radiation results from an x-ray/matter interaction that only had a slight effect on the primary photon. The effect, however, is enough to alter the original path of the photon. At no time should any part of the radiographer be in the path of the primary beam. The shielding requirements for areas receiving only secondary exposure are less than for those surfaces subjected to primary radiation. This is due to the decreased energy of secondary radiation compared with primary.

94–96. The answers are 94-B, 95-A and 96-D. *(Bushong, 5/e, pp 67–68. Statkiewicz-Sherer, 2/e, pp 228–229.)* The inverse square law is used to mathematically express the effect of distance on exposure intensity. It states that intensity is inversely proportional to the distance squared and assumes all other exposure factors are unchanged. Each of these problems may be solved using this proportion: $I_{old}/I_{new} = D^2_{new}/D^2_{old}$.

In item 94, the distance is changed from 1 foot to 3 feet. This problem asks how much the exposure will change. To solve it, find the difference in distance, invert it, and square it:

Distance increased 3 times (3/1)
Inversion and squaring = $(1/3)^2$
Solution = 1/9 the original exposure

In item 95, the distance changed from 2 to 5 feet and the original intensity was 160 mR. Using the formula, the solution is

$$\frac{160}{x} = \frac{5^2}{2^2}$$
$$\frac{160}{x} = \frac{25}{4}$$
$$25x = 160 \times 4$$
$$x = 25.6$$

In item 96, the distance changed from 40 inches to 30 inches and the original intensity was 85 mR. Using the formula, the solution is

$$\frac{85}{x} = \frac{30^2}{40^2}$$
$$\frac{85}{x} = \frac{3^2}{4^2}$$
$$\frac{85}{x} = \frac{9}{16}$$
$$9x = 85 \times 16$$
$$x = 151 \text{ mR}$$

97. The answer is D. *(Bushong, 5/e, pp 600, 653. NCRP No. 102, pp 15–16.)* Entrance skin dose from fluoroscopy procedures may be estimated by calculating the product of exposure rate per milliampere (R per min) and the actual exposure time. In this problem the exposure rate is 2.4 R/min; the mA is 2.2; and the total exposure time is 3 min. Therefore, total exposure is 2.4 R × 2.2 × 3 = 15.84 R.

98. The answer is C. *(Dennis, pp 25, 35.)* The amount of exposed tissue is determined by finding the total area within the defined field size. The area of a square or rectangle is the product of length and width (l × w); for a circle it is the product of pi and the radius squared ($\pi \times r^2$). The field sizes stated in this question would produce the following areas:

(A) 4 × 6 = 24 square inches; (B) π = 3.14, r = 2.5 inches (1/2 diameter), therefore 3.14 × 2.5^2 = 3.14 × 6.25 = 19.6 square inches; (C) 5 × 5 = 25 square inches; and (D) 3 × 7 = 21 square inches. Thus the 5 by 5 inch square field exposes the largest area of tissue.

99. The answer is B. *(Bushong, 5/e, pp 664–665. NCRP No. 102, p 18. Statkiewicz-Sherer, 2/e, pp 230–232.)* The minimum amount of lead equivalent for a protective lead apron is 0.5 mm. Lead aprons are available with 0.25, 0.5, or 1.0 mm of lead equivalency. The difference in lead equivalency directly influences the radiation attenuation factor and weight of the apron. The 0.5-mm apron provides significantly more protection than the 0.25-mm and is lighter than the 1.0 mm apron, making it the most common type in use. A minimum of 0.25 mm lead equivalent is required for lead gloves.

100. The answer is B. *(Bushong, 5/e, pp 599–600.)* Total exposure can be determined by finding the product of the exposure intensity for a particular set of exposure factors and the total exposure time. If the radiographer remained at the same distance from the radiation source during the examination, the calculation would be done as follows:

$$\frac{325 \text{ mR}}{h} = \frac{5 \text{ min}}{60 \text{ min/h}} = \frac{1625}{60} = 27 \text{mR total exposure}$$

101. The answer is C. *(Bushong, 5/e, p 234. Carroll, 5/e, p 132–133, 343. Statkiewicz-Sherer, 2/e, pp 164–166.)* Beam restrictors are employed for the primary purpose of reducing patient exposure by limiting the amount of tissue irradiated and thus reducing the number of interactions (photoelectric and Compton) that may occur. The reduction in scatter production reduces both patient and occupational exposure. Of the types of beam restrictors available, the collimator (or variable aperture) is the most widely used. This device allows any size of square or rectangular field to be produced. A wide variety of sizes of cones and diaphragms would be required to provide the same range of field sizes. Cones may still be used with collimators. They are designed to slide onto an accessory tray usually found at the bottom of the collimator. This allows the use of extension cones for even more precise beam restriction. Good collimation will also improve image quality by increasing contrast due to the decrease in Compton scattered radiation. However, an increase in milliampere-seconds may be required to compensate for the loss of density, which is also due to less scatter in the exit beam. This increase in milliampere-seconds is less significant than the exposure received from too large a field.

102. The answer is D. *(Bushong, 5/e, p 666. Carroll, 5/e, pp 342–345. Statkiewicz-Sherer, 2/e, pp 181–182.)* Patient dose is dependent on the exposure intensity produced for a particular exam. For this problem, each of the factors will influence the beam intensity. If all the factors are converted to be the same (kV, SID, receptor speed, and grid ratio) and the mAs adjusted to compensate for those conversions, then the lowest mAs will be the indicator of the lowest dose. The problem should be solved as follows:

kV: Since these figures are the same, they are not an influencing factor and are eliminated as a factor to consider.

SID: Convert 48 inches and 36 inches to 40 inches and adjust the mAs accordingly:

$$\text{Answer C}: \text{New mAs} = 15\,\text{mAs} \times \frac{40^2}{48^2} = \frac{15 \times 1600}{2304} = \frac{24000}{2304} = 10$$

$$\text{Answer D}: \text{New mAs} = 10\,\text{mAs} \times \frac{40^2}{36^2} = \frac{10 \times 1600}{1296} = \frac{16000}{1296} = 12$$

The mAs values are now (A) 25; (B) 32; (C) 10; (D) 12.

Receptor speed: Convert 200 to 400 and adjust the mAs accordingly.

$$\text{Answer A}: \text{New mAs} = \frac{25 \times 200}{400} = \frac{5000}{400} = 12.5$$

$$\text{Answer D}: \text{New mAs} = \frac{12 \times 200}{400} = \frac{2400}{400} = 6$$

The mAs values are now (A) 12.5; (B) 32; (C) 10; (D) 6

Grid ratio: Convert all to 10:1 using the grid ratio conversion factors of 2, 3, 4, 5, and 6 for 5:1, 6:1, 8:1, 10:1 (12:1), and 16:1, respectively, and adjust mAs accordingly.

$$\text{Answer A}: \text{New mAs} = \frac{12 \times 5}{4} = \frac{60}{4} = 15$$

$$\text{Answer B}: \text{New mAs} = \frac{32 \times 5}{2} = \frac{160}{2} = 80$$

Answer D : Unchanged. The grid conversion factor for 10:1 and 12:1 is the same: 5.

The final mAs values are (A) 15; (B) 80; (C) 10; (D) 6.

103. The answer is D. *(Bushong, 5/e, pp 650–653.)* Patient dose, specifically skin dose, can be estimated by knowing the tube output for a specific radiographic unit at various kVp levels. This output information is expressed as the amount of exposure (in mR or R) per mAs used (mR/mAs). This value is then multiplied by the actual mAs used to provide the patient's skin dose. For this problem, the solution is found by the following equation: $8.4 \times 30 = 252$ mR.

104. The answer is A. *(Bushong, 5/e, pp 650–651. Carlton, p 518. Statkiewicz-Sherer, 2/e, pp 194–195.)* When expressing a patient's dose from radiation exposure, the skin dose is most commonly used. This area receives the highest dose since no other tissue is present to attenuate the primary beam. As the beam traverses the patient to the specific area of interest, the body tissues attenuate the beam, reducing its intensity. Skin dose is also the only area in which radiation dose can be directly measured. This can be done by placing a TLD in the center of the field of exposure and then analyzing the dose recorded. The TLD responds to radiation in a similar manner as soft tissue would, thus making it a reliable means for measurement of patient dose. Since direct measurement of organ dose is not usually possible, it must be derived from the entrance skin dose according to the attenuation of the beam and the radiosensitivity of the specific organ.

105. The answer is A.   *(Bushong, 5/e, pp 606–607. NCRP No. 91, pp 30–31, 48. Statkiewicz-Sherer, 2/e, p 72.)* The current recommendation for exposure of the fetus limits the dose to 0.5 rem (5 mSv) for the duration of the pregnancy with a maximum monthly exposure limit of 0.05 rem (0.5 mSv). Pregnant technologists need not stop working or restrict their participation in radiologic procedures as long as all usual radiation safety practices are utilized. Many departments will issue a second personnel monitor specifically for monitoring fetal exposure, even when a protective apron is used.

106. The answer is A.   *(Bushong, 5/e, pp 579–580, 585, 590. Statkiewicz-Sherer, 2/e, pp 136, 142, 144.)* Of the possible late somatic effects, most follow the linear, nonthreshold dose/response relationship. Only cataracts have been identified as having a threshold for safe exposure. Radiation-induced cataracts may occur following an exposure level of 2 Gy (200 rad) directly to the lens of the eye. Cataract formation also follows a nonlinear pattern of development. Eye shields may be recommended for high-dose radiologic examinations of the head and neck, such as multidirectional tomography examinations.

107. The answer is D.   *(Bushong, 5/e, pp 612–615. Statkiewicz-Sherer, 2/e, pp 200–201.)* It is within the responsibility of the radiologic technologist to minimize the likelihood of inadvertent exposure of a pregnant patient. Before beginning the radiologic procedure, the radiographer should inquire as to the possibility of the patient's being pregnant. The answer to this query should be documented on the patient's requisition. There should also be signs regarding pregnancy posted around the department to encourage patients to inform the technologist of their possible pregnancy status. When possible, it is recommended that female patients have their abdominal and pelvic radiography examinations scheduled during the 10 days following the onset of their menstrual cycle. This practice is intended to limit their exposure to the time period during which women are least likely to be pregnant. If the patient indicates that pregnancy may be possible, the radiologist or referring physician or both should be consulted before proceeding with the examination. They may decide to have the patient tested prior to continuing. However, requiring all female patients to have a pregnancy test is not recommended.

108–111. The answers are 108-D, 109-C, 110-B, 111-C.   *(Bushong, 5/e, pp 538–539. Statkiewicz-Sherer, 2/e, pp 126–127.)* The graphic representation shown in these questions pertains to the various relationships that may exist between radiation exposure (dose) and the probability of an effect (response). The curves have two primary characteristics: they are either linear or nonlinear and are either threshold or nonthreshold. The linear representation is straight and therefore indicates a directly proportional relationship; this means, for example, that as the dose doubles, the likelihood of a response doubles also. The nonlinear form is less predictable in that there may be greater or lesser responses as dose is increased. This relationship may be evident when evaluating a specific response in a specific population. The presence of a threshold offers a range of safety as it indicates an area where dose produces no response. However, the nonthreshold form indicates that there is always a response. The curves demonstrated on this chart are labeled as follows: (1) nonlinear, nonthreshold; (2) linear, nonthreshold; (3) nonlinear, threshold; and (4) linear threshold. The basis for current radiation protection policies is the assumption that all exposures produce an effect and that the effect is directly proportional to the exposure; i.e., a linear, nonthreshold relationship is assumed.

112–117. The answers are 112-C, 113-B, 114-A, 115-A, 116-C, 117-B.   *(Bushong, 5/e, pp 559, 577, 596–597. Statkiewicz-Sherer, 2/e, pp 130, 136, 147.)* The categories of radiation effects are defined according to the type of cells exposed and the time frame in which the effects are manifested. Two basic cell types exist in the human body: *somatic* and *germ* (or *genetic*). Germ cells contain the DNA for reproduction. These cells are contained within the male and female gonads. Exposure of the gonads can cause point mutations in the structure of the chromosomes, which are the genetic blueprints for the organism. These effects may be evident in future generations of the exposed person. All other cells in the body are of the somatic type. Exposure of these cells may produce effects that will manifest themselves within the lifetime of the exposed person. If these effects appear shortly after the exposure, they are termed *early effects.* Such effects are the result of large doses of radiation, delivered to a large volume of tissue over a short period of time. These conditions are met in the delivery of radiation for therapeutic purposes and frequently result in such effects as nausea and vomiting, diarrhea, and blood changes such as anemia, low white blood cell count, and hemorrhage. Such exposures are planned to be confined to the least amount of tissue in order to produce minimal effects. Exposure of the whole body, as may occur following a nuclear accident, would produce more damage and a reduced chance for recovery. Radiation effects that take months or years to manifest are termed *late effects*. This type may occur as the result of small exposures delivered over a long period of time as in diagnostic radiology. The potential effects include radiation-induced malignancies (cancer), formation of cataracts, nonspecific shortening of life span, and embryologic effects. Of these, radiation's carcinogenic and embryologic effects require most consideration. Numerous population groups have been studied to support the identification of radiation as a carcinogen. The effects include cancer of the skin, bone, lung, and breast, as well as leukemia. Embryologic effects are the result of in utero exposure and include such manifestations as spontaneous abortion, congenital abnormalities, and childhood leukemia.

118–124. The answers are 118-B, 119-B, 120-A, 121-A, 122-A, 123-B, 124-B. *(Bushong, 5/e, pp. 629–631. NCRP No. 102, pp 11, 14–15, 20. NCRP No. 105, p 50. Statkiewicz-Sherer, 2/e, pp. 191, 223–227.)* Modern diagnostic x-ray equipment is designed to meet minimum standards for safety from unnecessary radiation exposure. Some of these standards follow.

Control of leakage radiation. The x-ray tube housing and collimator assembly must provide protection against exposure from leakage radiation. These devices must be designed so as to maintain leakage radiation to less than 0.1 R (100 mR)/h at a distance of 1 m from the source.

Total filtration of primary beam. This includes inherent and added sources of filtration for patient protection from low-energy, nonpenetrating photons. The amount of filtration required is based on the tube potential the unit is capable of producing. The majority of diagnostic equipment is designed to operate at greater than 70 kVp. This level of tube potential requires a minimum level of total filtration equivalent to 2.5 mm of aluminum.

Location of exposure switch. This must require the operator to be behind a protective barrier for stationary units or at a distance of 6 feet for mobile equipment. This requirement is for the protection of the operator.

Protection shields on fluoroscopy units. This includes barriers to absorb scattered radiation from the patient or table such as the bucky slot cover and leaded curtain on the fluoroscopy tower. These devices must provide a level of shielding equivalent to 0.25 mm of lead.

Source-skin dose. As stated by the inverse square law, the level of exposure is inversely proportional to the square of the distance. The minimum allowed source-to-skin distance is 12 inches (30 cm). A minimum distance of 15 inches (38 cm) is preferred.

Use of mobile equipment. This should be limited to those situations in which the patient cannot be transported to the radiology department. The conditions under which most mobile radiography is performed are less than optimum, which may affect image quality. A better quality examination is much more probable if a stationary unit is used.

Lead aprons for mobile examinations. These should be used at all times. The protection of the operator of mobile units requires the wearing of lead aprons and standing back 6 feet from the source when the exposure is made. Other shielding devices should also be part of the equipment carried for mobile examinations in order to offer the patient increased radiation protection. Any persons in the immediate area of the mobile examination should be moved away if their condition allows. If not, these persons should also be shielded.

125–129. The answers are 125-A, 126-A, 127-B, 128-B, 129-C. *(Bushong, 5/e, pp 168–170, 263, 629–630, 667. Statkiewicz-Sherer, 2/e, pp 164, 179–180, 184–187.)* The technical factors that will influence the amount of radiation required to produce an acceptable radiograph will also influence the patient's dose. These factors include beam restriction, filters, image receptors, grids, exposure factors, and repeat imaging. Focal spot size has no influence on x-ray quantity, and therefore does not influence patient dose. The speed of the image receptor has an indirect effect on patient dose; that is, an increase in system speed will require less exposure and reduced dose. Grid ratio and field size have a direct effect on patient dose. As these factors increase, the exposure to the tissue increases as does dose. Compensating filters are employed to modify the intensities of the x-ray beam and thus provide a more even exposure of objects that vary in thickness. This prevents overexposure of small structures in the effort to adequately expose the larger structures. The overall effect is reduced exposure to parts of the object irradiated.

130–134. The answers are 130-B, 131-B, 132-A, 133-A, 134-A.   *(Bushong, 5/e, pp 52, 63–64. Carlton, pp 39–40. Carroll, 5/e, p 13. Thompson, p 63.)*   X-rays are a form of electromagnetic (EM) energy, as are radio, television, and light rays. Some of the properties that differentiate x-rays from other forms of EM energy are as follows.

1. X-rays cannot be focused by a lens (as visible light can be). However, x-rays may be collimated.

2. X-rays have no electrical charge. They are not influenced by electrical or magnetic fields.

3. The x-ray beam is made up of photons, each with its own energy determined by the electron-matter interaction that produced it. Polyenergetic means "many energy values." The maximum energy an x-ray can have is determined by the peak kilovoltage set on the control panel. Therefore, an x-ray photon can have an energy value anywhere between 0 and the peak kiloelectron volt produced by electron acceleration in the x-ray tube.

4. As is true for all forms of EM radiation, the speed at which x-rays travel in a vacuum is a constant value. That speed is equivalent to the speed of light, which can be expressed as 186,000 miles/s, 3×10^8 m/s, or 3×10^{10} cm/s.

5. X-rays are able to ionize matter. The ability of x-rays to ionize air molecules is utilized in the design of instruments for the measurement of x-rays. The typical ionization chamber has a quantity of air (or gas) within it and contains two charged plates (one positive, one negative); alternatively, it may contain a single electrode that is positively charged while the walls of the chamber are negatively charged. Upon irradiation, the air is ionized, creating ion pairs. The freed electron is attracted to the positive terminal and the remaining atom (positive ion) is attracted to the negative terminal. The result is a flow of current (electrons) along the positive electrode, which can be measured or used to discharge a capacitor. This device is commonly used in the construction of automatic exposure control devices, radiation detectors for CT equipment, and ion chambers for radiation detection and measurement.

135–142. The answers are 135-A, 136-B, 137-A, 138-C, 139-C, 140-D, 141-A, 142-D.   *(Bushong, 5/e, pp 659–663. Statkiewicz-Sherer, 2/e, pp 258–259. Thompson, p 461.)*   The luminescent material lithium fluoride is the active element of the thermoluminescent dosimeter (TLD). In response to radiation exposure, the valence electrons of the lithium fluoride are raised to the trapped band, where they will remain until heated and returned to their normal state. This movement back to the valence band produces the emission of light photons proportionate to the energy stored by the crystal. The TLD type of radiation monitor is the most durable as it is not affected by mechanical shock such as from dropping, as the pocket ion chamber is. Neither is it affected by heat or high humidity, as both the film badge and pocket ion chambers are. The heat required to stimulate the light emission of the lithium fluoride crystals is at least 190° C. The TLD is the only type of radiation monitor device that has a tissue-equivalent response to radiation exposure. For this reason, the TLD may be used to provide patient dose information for specific radiologic examinations. This may be done by placing the TLD on the patient's skin or in conjunction with a radiographic phantom.

The film badge is the only type of radiation monitor that provides a permanent record of the radiation exposure. This is achieved by storage of the processed piece of film once it has been analyzed. Should the need arise, the film can be retrieved and reread. Readings from the TLD and pocket ion chambers must be recorded immediately, as the reading process destroys the data. The dosimetry film used in the film badge must be replaced once it has been read. At the end of the monitoring period, the exposed film is processed and the density level indicates the exposure level. The film cannot be reused, but is filed for future reference. Both the ion chamber and TLD devices may be reused once they have been read and cleared of data (the ion chamber must also be recharged).

The film badge and TLDs are capable of detecting high-energy beta particles, as well as gamma rays and x-rays. Pocket ion chambers detect only gamma rays and x-rays.

The pocket ion chamber type of radiation monitor responds to radiation exposure as any ion chamber would; that is, as the air in the chamber is irradiated, ionization of the air molecules occurs, releasing electrons for movement. Prior to use, the pocket dosimeter is charged to cause a repulsion between the central electrode and the quartz fiber indicator. As ionization occurs, the charge within the chamber is neutralized, allowing the indicator to move towards the central electrode and providing a reading. The pocket ion chamber is also the only type of radiation monitor that can be read immediately following an exposure to radiation. Each exposure will proportionately discharge the charged chamber, and the exposure level will be indicated by viewing the calibrated scale through the eyepiece. Pocket ion chambers may be calibrated in units of roentgens or milliroentgens.

143–145. The answers are 143-C, 144-A, 145-D. *(Ballinger, 7/e, vol 1, p 26. Bushong, 5/e, p 651. Thompson, p 486.)* The actual skin dose for various examinations will be determined by the specific radiographic unit, imaging system, and accessory devices used to produce an image. However, the doses stated in this question are representative of the actual dose range. Chest imaging requires the least amount of exposure of the structures listed. This is due to the low-density components that make up the majority of the thorax—specifically, the lungs. Also, most chest imaging is performed using high-kilovoltage techniques, which further contributes to a low skin dose of about 10 mR. Denser structures, such as the skull and abdomen, will require increased exposures. Both use about the same kilovoltage level (mid 70's), but the increased thickness of the abdomen would translate into a higher skin dose of about 400 mR compared with about 200 mR for skull radiography. A skin dose of about 50 mR would be delivered for imaging of extremities.

146–150. The answers are 146-A, 147-A, 148-C, 149-B, 150-B. *(Bushong, 5/e, pp 664–667, Statkiewicz-Scherer, 2/e, pp 171, 174, 215–217, 224–225, 232.)* Many radiation protection practices are beneficial to both the radiographer and the patient. Any practice that reduces the production of scattered radiation will decrease dose to both patient and radiographer. Such practices include minimizing field size, use of high-kilovoltage techniques, use of high-speed imaging systems, and decreasing repeat exposures. Filtration in the beam and gonadal shields are for the protection of the patient. The protective curtain on the fluoroscopy carriage and the barrier that separates the control panel from the radiographic unit are in position to protect the radiographer. The general public should be protected from occasional or frequent exposure by the proper design and use of protective barriers between any source of radiation and any area classified as *uncontrolled occupancy*. Also, when a patient needs to be held during an exposure, it should not be done by a radiographer, but a member of the general public. This person should be over 18 years of age, not pregnant, and wear proper protective apparel such as lead aprons and gloves.

Operation and Maintenance of Equipment

DIRECTIONS: Each numbered question or incomplete statement below contains lettered responses. Select the **one best** response.

151. Which of the following components would be considered part of the cathode assembly of an x-ray tube?
    1. Filament
    2. Target
    3. Focusing cup

    (A) 1 & 2
    (B) 2 & 3
    (C) 1 & 3
    (D) 1, 2, & 3

152. The size of the focal spot is determined by the

    (A) milliampere station selected
    (B) kilovoltage level selected
    (C) size of the target disk
    (D) size of the filament coil

153. The material of choice for the construction of a long-lasting filament is

    (A) molybdenum
    (B) copper
    (C) tungsten
    (D) lead

154. The primary purpose of the target disk in the x-ray tube is to

    (A) provide a source of electrons
    (B) provide the site of energy conversion
    (C) increase the heat loading capability of the tube
    (D) maintain a finely focused stream of electrons

155. Which of the following describes the construction of the modern rotating target disk for a routine diagnostic x-ray tube?

    (A) Tungsten-rhenium surface on a molybdenum base
    (B) Tungsten disk imbedded in a copper block
    (C) Molybdenum surface on a tungsten base
    (D) Lead coating on a copper base

156. The diameter of the rotating target disk will influence the operation of the x-ray tube by having

    (A) a direct effect on head-loading capability
    (B) an inverse effect on heat-loading capability
    (C) a direct effect on focal spot size
    (D) an inverse effect on focal spot size

157. What is the advantage of the rotating target disk over the stationary target?

(A) Construction of smaller x-ray units
(B) Less expense in manufacture
(C) Smaller effective focal spot
(D) Greater heat-loading capability

158. The standard speed of a rotating target is approximately

(A) 1500 rpm
(B) 3000 rpm
(C) 5000 rpm
(D) 10,000 rpm

159. Which combination of target characteristics would produce the maximum heat-loading capability?

(A) 3-inch disk, standard-speed rotation, 1.2-mm focal spot
(B) 4-inch disk, high-speed rotation, 0.6-mm focal spot
(C) 5-inch disk, standard-speed rotation, 0.6-mm focal spot
(D) 3-inch disk, high-speed rotation, 1.2-mm focal spot

160. For what purpose is there a negative electrical charge on the focusing cup?

(A) To attract the electrons to the filament
(B) To repel the electrons from the target
(C) To attract the electrons to the focusing cup
(D) To draw the electrons together into a stream

161. According to the *line focus principle*, what effect, if any, will an increase in the bevel on the target disk have on the size of the actual and effective focal spots?

(A) A direct effect on the actual and an inverse effect on the effective spot
(B) No effect on the actual and an inverse effect on the effective spot
(C) An inverse effect on the actual and no effect on the effective spot
(D) A direct effect on both actual and effective focal spots

162. Which of the following is the correct equation for calculating heat units?

(A) FSS (focal spot size) × mAs × kV
(B) SID × FSS × mAs
(C) mAs × kV × C (generator type)
(D) SID × kV × C (generator type)

163. The function of an x-ray tube rating chart is to determine the

(A) status of heat loading on the target
(B) safety of a specific combination of milliamperes, time, and kilovoltage
(C) amount of heat loading on the tube housing
(D) correct exposure factors for a radiographic examination

164. The reasons for using tungsten as the prime component of the target disk in the general purpose x-ray tube are its

(A) high melting point and high atomic number
(B) high atomic number and low atomic weight
(C) high molecular density and low atomic number
(D) good heat dissipation and low atomic number

165. The specific component in the x-ray circuit that allows for the regulation of kilovoltage is the

(A) high-tension transformer
(B) low-tension transformer
(C) autotransformer
(D) step-up transformer

166. What units of measurement does the term *volt* indicate?

1. Number of electrons flowing per second
2. Electromotive force
3. Potential difference

(A) 1 & 2
(B) 2 & 3
(C) 1 & 3
(D) 1, 2, & 3

167. What is the direction of the flow of electrons in a circuit?

    (A) Negative to positive
    (B) Positive to negative
    (C) Anode to cathode
    (D) Low point to high point

168. What is the unit of measure that indicates *electrical current*?

    (A) Volt
    (B) Ohm
    (C) Watt
    (D) Ampere

169. According to Ohm's law, what is the relationship between potential difference (voltage), current (intensity), and resistance in an electrical circuit?

    (A) Current is directly proportional to potential difference and inversely proportional to resistance
    (B) Current is inversely proportional to both potential difference and resistance
    (C) Current is inversely proportional to potential difference and directly proportional to resistance
    (D) Current is directly proportional to both potential difference and resistance

170. A circuit with a voltage of 120 V, a current of 200 mA, and a resistance of 150 ohms will produce a power output of

    (A) 24000 watts
    (B) 18000 watts
    (C) 30 watts
    (D) 24 watts

171. What is the voltage in a circuit of 10 amperes and 60 ohms?

    (A) 0.167 V
    (B) 6 V
    (C) 160 V
    (D) 600 V

172. What is the power rating of a generator capable of operating at 600 mA and 120 kV?

    (A) 720 kilowatts (kW)
    (B) 72 kW
    (C) 5 kW
    (D) 0.2 kW

173. A circuit constructed so that current runs through each electrical device consecutively is what type of circuit?

    (A) Parallel
    (B) Alternating
    (C) Series
    (D) Direct

174. True statements regarding the properties of magnets include which of the following?
    1. Magnetic materials are described as having the ability to attract iron objects
    2. Magnetic moments are randomly aligned in magnetized materials
    3. The unit of measure of magnetic force is the tesla

    (A) 1 & 2
    (B) 2 & 3
    (C) 1 & 3
    (D) 1, 2, & 3

175. True properties of magnets include which of the following?
    1. All magnets have positive and negative charges
    2. All magnets have north and south poles
    3. The force of attraction or repulsion between two magnets is inversely proportional to the square of the distance between the magnets and directly proportional to the product of the magnitude of each magnet

    (A) 1 & 2
    (B) 2 & 3
    (C) 1 & 3
    (D) 1, 2, & 3

176. Which of the following will produce a magnetic effect?

    (A) A product containing rubber or plastic elements
    (B) A moving electrical charge
    (C) A stationary electrical charge
    (D) An open electrical circuit

177. What is the process by which excess electrical charges may leave the surface of a conductor, thereby making it neutral?

    (A) Friction
    (B) Electrification
    (C) Grounding
    (D) Repulsion

178. True statements regarding the laws of electrostatics include

    (A) like charges attract, unlike charges repel
    (B) concentration of electrical charge is greatest where the curvature is greatest
    (C) the strength of the force between two charges is directly proportional to the square of the distance and inversely proportional to the product of their magnitudes
    (D) electrical charges reside at the internal core of the conductor

179. The electrification process achieved by placing an uncharged body within the electrostatic field of a charged body is termed

    (A) friction
    (B) contact
    (C) induction
    (D) static

180. Rectification is employed in the x-ray circuit to

    (A) increase voltage in the high-tension transformer
    (B) heat the filament of the x-ray tube
    (C) simplify circuitry of the x-ray generator
    (D) convert alternating current (AC) to pulsating direct current (DC)

181. A fully rectified, single-phase generator employs how many solid-state rectifiers?

    (A) 2
    (B) 4
    (C) 6
    (D) 12

182. The advantages of three-phase power over single-phase power include:
    1. More efficient x-ray production
    2. Higher milliamperage
    3. Shorter exposure times

    (A) 1 & 2
    (B) 2 & 3
    (C) 1 & 3
    (D) 1, 2, & 3

183. The specific device employed to alter incoming line voltage before it can be converted to kilovoltage is the

    (A) autotransformer
    (B) step-up transformer
    (C) step-down transformer
    (D) rectification system

184. Which device is used to regulate the voltage applied to the filament circuit?

    (A) Autotransformer
    (B) Step-up transformer
    (C) Step-down transformer
    (D) Rectification system

185. What is the relationship between current and voltage in a transformer?

    (A) Directly proportional
    (B) Inversely proportional
    (C) Directly proportional to the square of the difference
    (D) Inversely proportional to the square of the difference

186. A transformer with 50 turns on the primary coil and 1000 turns on the secondary coil and an input voltage of 120 V would have an output voltage of

    (A) 6 V
    (B) 6 kV
    (C) 2.4 V
    (D) 2.4 kV

187. The technique that allows for dynamic imaging of anatomic structures is

    (A) tomography
    (B) fluoroscopy
    (C) stereoscopy
    (D) subtraction

188. The purpose of employing *image-intensified* fluoroscopy is to

    (A) raise the level of image brightness
    (B) decrease the patient dose during fluoroscopy
    (C) enlarge the image for better viewing
    (D) act as a means of storing the image

189. The image intensifier converts the exit beam to other forms of electromagnetic energy in which of the following orders?

    (A) X-rays to electrons to light to x-rays
    (B) X-rays to light to x-rays to electrons
    (C) X-rays to light to electrons to light
    (D) X-rays to light to x-rays to light

190. Which component of the image intensifier is stimulated by the exit beam to produce light photons?

    (A) Output phosphor
    (B) Input phosphor
    (C) Photocathode
    (D) Electrostatic lenses

191. What does the term "brightness gain" refer to in fluoroscopy?

    (A) Automatic regulation of milliamperage and kilovoltage selection
    (B) The size of the image produced by the image intensifier
    (C) The ability to view the image using scotopic vision
    (D) The increased light level created by the image intensifier

192. How is brightness gain determined?

    (A) Product of minification and flux gain
    (B) Sum of minification and flux gain
    (C) Product of kilovoltage, milliamperage, and type of generator
    (D) Ratio of amount of information recorded to information available

193. If a fluoroscopic procedure employed an image intensifier with an input phosphor (IP) of 25 cm and an output phosphor (OP) of 2.5 cm and used exposure factors of 110 kV, 2 mA for 3 min, the minification gain would be

    (A) 100
    (B) 220
    (C) 330
    (D) 660

194. What material is used for the input phosphor of the modern image intensifier?

    (A) Calcium tungstate
    (B) Cesium iodide
    (C) Zinc cadmium sulfide
    (D) Gadolinium

195. What is the role of the electrostatic lenses in the image intensifier?

    (A) To convert incident x-rays to light photons
    (B) To convert light photons to electrons
    (C) To convert electrons to light photons
    (D) To direct electrons from the cathode to anode end

196. For an image intensifier with an output phosphor of 2.5 cm, an input phosphor of 17 cm, and flux gain of 150, what will the approximate brightness gain be?

    (A) 7000
    (B) 5000
    (C) 3000
    (D) 1000

197. The component of the image intensifier to which a television camera is coupled in order to view the image on a television monitor is the

    (A) input phosphor
    (B) output phosphor
    (C) photospot camera
    (D) electrostatic lenses

198. On which type of medium is the fluoroscopic image able to be recorded?

    1. Cine film
    2. 105-mm film
    3. Conventional radiographic film
    4. Magnetic tape

  (A) 1 & 3
  (B) 2 & 4
  (C) 1, 2, & 3
  (D) 1, 2, 3, & 4

199. What is the purpose of the television monitoring system employed in fluoroscopy?

  (A) To monitor patients when they are left alone
  (B) To view the fluoroscopic images
  (C) To record the fluoroscopic images
  (D) To entertain the patient

200. What is the advantage offered by dual or tri-focus image intensifier tubes?

  (A) Brighter image
  (B) Less patient dose
  (C) Ability to create a magnified image
  (D) Lower exposure factors

201. The role of the beam-splitting mirror in the configuration of the image intensifier and the TV monitoring system is to divide the

  (A) input image between the photocathode and output phosphor
  (B) electrons from the photocathode between the input and output phosphors
  (C) output image between TV camera and photospot camera
  (D) x-ray beam between the input and output phosphors

202. The systematic approach to ensuring an optimum level of performance with a minimum of radiation exposure to patients and personnel is the definition of

  (A) quality assurance
  (B) quality control
  (C) troubleshooting
  (D) ALARA

203. If an x-ray beam is created using exposure factors of 80 kV, 600 mA, and 0.016 s and yields an exposure output of 240 mR, what would the mR/mAs be?

  (A) 2.5
  (B) 25
  (C) 250
  (D) 2500

204. Using the table below, select the answer that is true regarding acceptable linearity levels as stated by their mR/mAs values.

mA station	mR/mAs
100	30
200	28
300	40
400	36

  (A) Linearity is acceptable between 100 and 200
  (B) Linearity is acceptable between 200 and 300
  (C) Linearity is NOT acceptable between 300 and 400
  (D) Linearity is acceptable between all consecutive mA stations

205. A spinning top device may be used to evaluate

  (A) filtration
  (B) grid alignment
  (C) exposure timer
  (D) exposure output

206. Which of the following test results is within the range of tolerance for the component evaluated?

  (A) A selected kilovoltage of 80 yields a measured kilovoltage of 86
  (B) A stated focal spot of 0.6 mm measures 0.9 mm
  (C) X-ray/light field alignment varies by 3 cm toward the head of the table at SID of 40 inches
  (D) A spinning top test yields 8 dots for selected exposure time of 0.05 s

207. The half-value layer (HVL) of an x-ray beam indicates

(A) accuracy of positive beam limitation
(B) beam quality
(C) exposure linearity
(D) collimator/x-ray field alignment

208. The components of the automatic exposure control that should be monitored by quality control testing include:
    1. Exposure compensation for various kilovoltage peak selections
    2. Back-up timer response
    3. Minimum timer response

(A) 1 & 2
(B) 2 & 3
(C) 1 & 3
(D) 1, 2, & 3

209. The primary purpose of including a repeat analysis as part of a quality assurance program in radiology is to determine

(A) how much film to purchase
(B) which quality control tests to perform
(C) the most common source of error
(D) the need for changes in staffing

210. What action should be taken if the results of a quality control procedure do not meet minimum standards?

(A) Call in a service engineer
(B) Inform the chief radiologist
(C) Record the results for future reference
(D) Repeat the quality control procedure

211. What would be a likely cause for an increase in the half-value layer (HVL) over a period of 2 years?

(A) Repeated use of very high milliamperage with a small focal spot
(B) Inappropriate use of the positive beam limitation
(C) Buildup of tungsten plating on the window of the x-ray tube
(D) Failure to adequately warm up the x-ray tube prior to use

212. How many half-value layers (HVLs) would be required to reduce a beam intensity of 342 mR to 43 mR?

(A) 1
(B) 2
(C) 3
(D) 4

213. What relationship, if any, exists between half-value layer (HVL) and beam quality?

(A) Direct
(B) Indirect
(C) No relationship

214. Which of the following statements is true regarding optimum viewing conditions for radiographic images?

(A) Background or ambient lighting should be as bright as possible
(B) The color of the light produced by view-boxes is not important
(C) Individual light bulbs should be replaced as they burn out
(D) All viewboxes in the department should produce the same light level

215. Which component can be evaluated by means of a visual check only?

(A) Grid alignment
(B) Table locks
(C) Viewbox light intensity
(D) Film-screen contact

216. A properly functioning exposure timer on a three-phase radiographic unit would demonstrate an

(A) arc of 6° for an exposure time of 0.017 s
(B) arc of 9° for an exposure time of 0.05 s
(C) image of 2 dots for an exposure time of 0.017 s
(D) image of 12 dots for an exposure time of 0.05 s

217. The test tools that may be used to evaluate the size of the focal spot include:
    1. Pinhole camera
    2. Slit camera
    3. Star resolution pattern

    (A) 1 & 2
    (B) 2 & 3
    (C) 1 & 3
    (D) 1, 2, & 3

218. The condition of a lead apron is evaluated by

    (A) visual inspection
    (B) wearing a personal ion chamber under the apron during fluoroscopy and checking it for a reading
    (C) scanning the apron with an ultraviolet light source for cracks
    (D) fluoroscoping or radiographing the apron at high kilovoltage

219. In comparison with a single-phase unit, how will a three-phase power source influence the x-ray emission spectrum?
    1. Increase quantity
    2. Increase quality
    3. Decrease quantity
    4. Decrease quality

    (A) 1 & 2
    (B) 1 & 4
    (C) 2 & 3
    (D) 3 & 4

220. The goal of the rectification system is to produce

    (A) pulsating alternating current (AC)
    (B) nonpulsating AC
    (C) pulsating direct current (DC)
    (D) nonpulsating DC

221. What type of component is used as a rectifier in modern radiographic units?

    (A) Valve tube
    (B) Vacuum tube
    (C) Semiconductor diode
    (D) Scintillation crystal with photomultiplier

222. Which of the following is an advantage of a three-phase generator over a single-phase?

    (A) Less expensive
    (B) Less complex
    (C) Higher milliamperage selections
    (D) Higher kilovoltage selections

223. What device is responsible for maintaining the flow of electrons from cathode to anode in an x-ray tube?

    (A) Induction motor
    (B) Rectifiers
    (C) Step-up transformer
    (D) Step-down transformer

224. When using the automatic exposure control, which of the following must be selected?
    1. Minimum reaction time
    2. Back-up time
    3. Optimum kilovoltage peak

    (A) 1 & 2
    (B) 2 & 3
    (C) 1 & 3
    (D) 1, 2, & 3

225. An optimally calibrated AEC should be able to automatically

    (A) adjust the kilovoltage for the part being imaged
    (B) adjust the exposure time for the part thickness
    (C) select the minimum back-up time
    (D) select the appropriate combination of sensor chambers

226. If the AEC is used to radiograph L5–S1 in the lateral position and the image is underexposed, what may be the cause?

    (A) Plus density was selected
    (B) Center chamber was positioned over the spine
    (C) Center chamber was positioned posterior to L5–S1
    (D) Minimum reaction time

227. A properly operating AEC will automatically compensate for all the following EXCEPT

   (A) screen speed
   (B) kilovoltage peak
   (C) thickness of the anatomic part
   (D) pathologic conditions that affect exposure

228. On what type of imaging equipment would automatic exposure control be commonly available?
   1. Diagnostic
   2. Fluoroscopic
   3. Mammographic

   (A) 1 & 2
   (B) 2 & 3
   (C) 1 & 3
   (D) 1, 2, & 3

229. In which areas of specialty imaging is fluoroscopy commonly employed?

   (A) Tomography and mammography
   (B) Angiography and mammography
   (C) Computed tomography and cardiac catheterization
   (D) Angiography and cardiac catheterization

230. Which imaging technique allows the part of interest to be viewed in sections?

   (A) Fluoroscopy
   (B) Tomography
   (C) Cinefluorography
   (D) Xeroradiography

231. If AP chest tomograms are to be obtained to demonstrate a structure located 10 cm posterior to the sternum in a patient who measures 25 cm, at what level should the fulcrum be set?

   (A) 10 cm
   (B) 15 cm
   (C) 20 cm
   (D) 25 cm

232. The waveform produced by a battery-operated mobile x-ray unit most closely resembles that of a

   (A) half-wave rectified generator
   (B) full-wave rectified generator
   (C) three-phase generator
   (D) capacitor-discharge generator

233. Which statement is true regarding battery-operated mobile x-ray units?

   (A) They must be plugged into an AC outlet during exposure
   (B) Kilovoltage drops over the course of the exposure
   (C) They produce a constant potential (output)
   (D) They employ a DC chopper to create an AC waveform

234. All the following statements pertain to equipment requirements of *both* fixed and mobile radiographic equipment EXCEPT

   (A) the exposure switch is attached to a 6-foot cord
   (B) the protective housing must keep leakage exposure to less than 100 mR/h at 1 m from the source
   (C) the equipment should include some form of beam restriction
   (D) the equipment should provide total filtration of 2.5 mm of aluminum or equivalent

235. In which part of the x-ray circuit will the rectification system be located?

   (A) Prior to the autotransformer
   (B) Between the autotransformer and the primary side of the high-tension transformer
   (C) In the filament circuit
   (D) Between the secondary side of the high-tension transformer and x-ray tube

236. What is meant by an "entrance type" of automatic exposure control device?

(A) The amount of exposure is determined before the x-ray tube is energized
(B) The exposure is detected just before it enters the patient
(C) The exposure is detected before it reaches the image receptor
(D) The exposure is measured as it leaves the x-ray tube

237. Which of the following are considered beam restriction devices?

(A) Grids, cones, and filters
(B) Cones, collimators, and diaphragms
(C) Collimators, diaphragms, and filters
(D) Collimators, filters, and grids

238. The components included in the basic design of a variable-aperture collimator include:
1. Four shutters that operate as one unit
2. Four shutters that operate in pairs
3. Light localizing system
4. Compensating filter

(A) 1 & 3
(B) 1 & 4
(C) 2 & 3
(D) 3 & 4

239. The modern collimator device is capable of producing what types of field shapes?
1. Rectangular
2. Square
3. Circular

(A) 1 & 2
(B) 2 & 3
(C) 1 & 3
(D) 1, 2, & 3

240. Which device is employed to remove scattered radiation from the exit beam?

(A) Added filtration
(B) Compensating filter
(C) Beam restrictor
(D) Grid

241. Which system is responsible for maintaining a proper level of illumination of the fluoroscopic image?

(A) Automatic exposure control
(B) Automatic gain control
(C) Automatic brightness control
(D) Automatic beam limitation

242. The automatic brightness control (ABC) component of a fluoroscopic system provides automatic adjustment of what factors?

(A) X-ray field size
(B) Kilovoltage and milliamperage
(C) Amplification of the video signal
(D) Termination of exposure

243. An automatic brightness control (ABC) system would be included in a

(A) dedicated chest radiographic unit
(B) dedicated mammography unit
(C) fluoroscopic unit
(D) computed tomography unit

244. The usual range of milliamperage used for fluoroscopy is

(A) 1 to 5 mA
(B) 5 to 10 mA
(C) 10 to 50 mA
(D) 200 to 400 mA

245. What level of milliamperage is used to *record* a fluoroscopic image?

(A) 1 to 5 mA
(B) 5 to 10 mA
(C) 10 to 50 mA
(D) 200 to 400 mA

246. Each of the following is a characteristic of a spot-film camera used for the recording of fluoroscopic images EXCEPT

(A) the camera has the ability to provide rapid serial imaging
(B) the camera uses a film format measuring between 70 and 105 mm
(C) the patient dose is less than for traditional cassette-type spot films
(D) the image is produced by direct x-ray exposure

247. The advantages of cassette-type spot-film systems over spot-film camera systems for recording the fluoroscopic image include:
    1. More efficient framing of image onto film
    2. Higher framing frequency
    3. Better resolution for same exposure time

    (A) 1 & 2
    (B) 2 & 3
    (C) 1 & 3
    (D) 1, 2, & 3

248. Which types of artifacts are the result of damage to screens or cassettes?
    1. High-density crescent marks
    2. Regularly repeating high-density marks
    3. Random low-density specks
    4. Localized blurring

    (A) 1 & 2
    (B) 2 & 3
    (C) 3 & 4
    (D) 1 & 4

249. Which of the following may cause artifacts on the radiographic image?
    1. Dirt on the radiographic table
    2. Bandages over the anatomic structure of interest
    3. Dried contrast media on the cassette front

    (A) 1 & 2
    (B) 2 & 3
    (C) 1 & 3
    (D) 1, 2, & 3

250. Which of the following conditions will most likely result from excessive rotor "boost" or preparation time prior to x-ray exposure?

    (A) Increased rotor speed
    (B) Cracked glass envelope
    (C) Vaporization of the target disk
    (D) Excessive heating of the filament

DIRECTIONS: Each group of questions below consists of lettered headings followed by a set of numbered items. For each numbered item select the **one** lettered heading with which it is **most** closely associated. Each lettered heading may be used **once, more than once, or not at all.**

Questions 251–254

Use the radiographic rating charts below to determine whether the following combinations of exposure factors are safe or not.

(A) Safe
(B) Unsafe

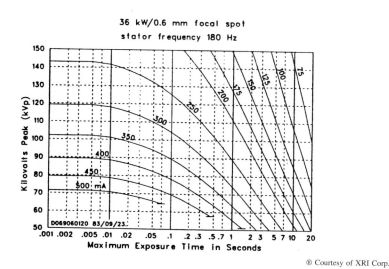

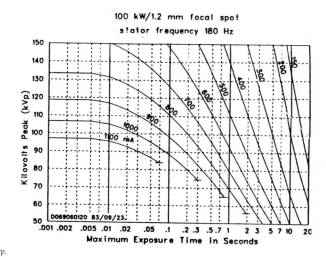

® Courtesy of XRI Corp.

251. 300 mA, 0.2 s, 90 kV, small focal spot

252. 800 mA, 0.5 s, 100 kV, large focal spot

253. 300 mA, 1 s, 85 kV, small focal spot

254. 800 mA, 20 ms, 120 kV, large focal spot

Questions 255–259

Match each description with the correct component of an x-ray tube. Use the diagram of an x-ray tube below as needed.

(A)   Filament
(B)   Focusing cup
(C)   Rotor
(D)   Target
(E)   Window

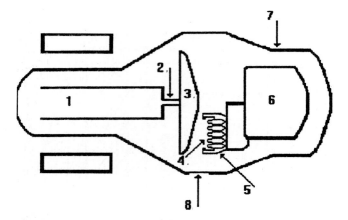

255.   What is the component labeled number 3?

256.   What component is responsible for restricting the electron stream from spreading out?

257.   What is the component labeled number 5?

258.   What component causes the target disk to rotate during tube operation?

259.   What component is labeled number 8?

Questions 260–264

Match each description with the correct term.

(A)   Direct current
(B)   Alternating current
(C)   Incoming voltage
(D)   Single-phase power
(E)   Three-phase power

260.   The form of current when it flows in a sine wave

261.   The source of current to the input voltage for the autotransformer

262.   The waveform with a frequency of 360 cycles per second

263.   The waveform with 100 percent ripple

264.   The flow of current at a constant peak potential

Questions 265–270

Indicate the minimum frequency for performing quality control testing on each of the components of radiographic imaging below.

(A) Daily
(B) Weekly
(C) Semiannually
(D) Annually

265. Accuracy of kilovoltage peak stations

266. Quality of beam

267. Film processor

268. Alignment of x-ray and light field

269. Linearity of exposure

270. Darkroom fog

Questions 271–275

Indicate the acceptable range of variation for each component.

(A) ± 2 percent
(B) ± 5 percent
(C) ± 10 percent
(D) ± 50 percent

271. Linearity of exposure

272. SID indicator

273. Size of focal spot

274. Kilovoltage peak

275. Reproducibility of exposure

Questions 276–279

Identify the appropriate test tool for evaluation of each component.

(A) Wisconsin test cassette
(B) Wire mesh
(C) Dosimeter
(D) Star resolution pattern

276. Film-screen contact

277. Linearity

278. Focal spot size

279. Kilovoltage peak

Questions 280–283

Use the following data from a repeat film survey to find each approximate repeat rate. The total number of processed films was 1542.

Reason for rejection	Number
Positioning errors	28
Overexposure	68
Underexposure	60
Artifacts	7

(A) Less than 2 percent
(B) 3 to 5 percent
(C) 6 to 8 percent
(D) 9 to 11 percent

280. Repeat rate for overexposed films

281. Repeat rate for positioning errors

282. Total repeat rate for this collection period

283. Repeat rate for all exposure errors

Questions 284–290

For each condition, select the most probable cause.

(A)   Poor film-screen contact
(B)   Loss of imaging system speed
(C)   Artifacts
(D)   Fogged film

284.   Caused by blue-sensitive film combined with green emitting screens

285.   Caused by trapped air within a cassette

286.   Detected by scanning of the surface of intensifying screens with an ultraviolet light

287.   Controlled for by routine cleaning with an antistatic product

288.   Detected by making a radiograph of a wire mesh test device

289.   Exhibited as localized areas of blurriness

290.   Caused by yellowing or staining of a screen surface over time.

Questions 291–295

Identify the tomographic term being referred to in each question.

(A)   Zonography
(B)   Focal plane
(C)   Fulcrum
(D)   Angle/amplitude

291.   Path the tube travels during exposure

292.   Point around which the tube and image receptor move

293.   Tomographic technique that results in thick slices

294.   Regulator of the thickness of the section imaged

295.   Indicator of the anatomic structures that will be in maximum focus

Questions 296–300

Match each description with the correct tomographic tube motion.

(A)   1 to 10° linear
(B)   11 to 50° linear
(C)   30° circular
(D)   48° hypocycloidal

296.   Would result in the thickest section in focus

297.   Would provide the best quality blur

298.   Is most likely to cause phantom, or false, images as a result of displacement of a blurred image

299.   Would be the most effective in demonstrating small structures such as the inner auditory canals

300.   Is most commonly used during intravenous urography (IVU) procedures

Operation and Maintenance of Equipment

Answers

151. The answer is C (1, 3). *(Bushong, 5/e, pp 117–119. Curry, 4/e, pp 11–12. Selman, 8/e, p 205.)* The cathode assembly of the x-ray tube is the negative terminal of the diode and functions to provide the electrons for acceleration and bombardment, as needed in the production of x-rays. The specific components that serve this need are the filament, which is heated to the point of thermionic emission and releases a cloud of electrons, and the focusing cup, which acts to keep the electron cloud directed as a stream onto the focal spot of the target. The target itself is the site of electron bombardment and is a component of the anode assembly of the x-ray tube.

152. The answer is D. *(Bushong, 5/e, p 119, Curry, 4/e, pp 12–13. Selman, 8/e, p 206.)* Focal spot size is chiefly determined by the size of the filament coil. Most modern x-ray tubes are dual-focused, offering a large and small filament to produce, respectively, large or small electron streams to ultimately bombard the target disk. When a small filament is selected, less area on the target disk will be involved in the bombardment. In addition to the size of the filament, the angle of the target bevel and the design of the focusing cup are contributing factors to the effective focal spot size. The milliampere selection is of importance in selecting the appropriate focal spot size in terms of heat loading, but does not actually determine focal spot size. The kilovoltage selection plays no role in focal spot size.

153. The answer is C. *(Bushong, 5/e, p 118. Curry, 4/e, p 11. Selman, 8/e, p 205.)* Tungsten is the material of choice for construction of the filament chiefly because of its high melting point (3370° C). As part of the thermionic emission process, the filament will be heated to the point of incandescence by a high amperage current flowing through it. Repeated exposure of the filament to high heat loads may cause the filament to become thin owing to vaporization and eventually break, causing an incomplete circuit. Metals of lower melting points would not withstand this type of heat loading.

154. The answer is B. *(Bushong, 5/e, p 120. Curry, 4/e, p 13.)* The role of the target disk within the anode assembly of the x-ray tube is to provide a surface for electron bombardment and the conversion of kinetic energy to electromagnetic energy (x-rays and heat). The filament and focusing cup within the cathode assembly act as the source of electrons and a means of maintaining a finely focused electron stream, respectively. Although the overall heat-loading capability is influenced by the size of the focal spot, which is the actual area of electron interaction, the target disk is the site of electron bombardment.

155. The answer is A. *(Bushong, 5/e, p 120. Cullinan, 2/e, pp 43–44. Curry, 4/e, p 17. Selman, 8/e, pp 210–211.)* Modern general purpose x-ray tubes are constructed with rotating disks made of molybdenum or graphite base to which a tungsten layer is added and then coated with rhenium. Tungsten is the desired material for the production of x-rays in the useful energy range for medical imaging. In order to reduce the overall weight of the disk, the tungsten is layered on a base of lighter weight material such as molybdenum or graphite. This reduction in weight will allow for greater speeds during rotation of the disk. The graphite is also a more effective conductor of heat and thereby improves a tube's heat-loading capability. The addition of the rhenium to the tungsten surface aids in providing a more durable surface and less pitting due to repeated electron bombardments. Early x-rays tubes, with stationary targets, were constructed of a small button of tungsten imbedded in a copper block. The copper was effective in conducting heat away from the target area. Molybdenum targets are commonly used in special purpose tubes such as for mammography in order to produce x-rays in the desired energy range.

156. The answer is A. *(Bushong, 5/e, p 121. Cullinan, 2/e, p 43. Curry, 4/e, p 15. Selman, 8/e, pp 211–212.)* The diameter of the target disk has a direct effect on the heat-loading capability of the x-ray tube. The primary purpose of constructing rotating targets is to increase the area for electron bombardment from a *focal spot* to a *focal track*, thereby providing more surface area for heat dissipation. As the diameter of the disk increases, the focal track also increases. Another factor in overall heat-loading capability is the mass of the target, which also has a direct effect. The size of the focal spot (or track) is determined by the size of the electron stream (and its influencing factors).

157. The answer is D. *(Bushong, 5/e, pp 120–121. Cullinan, 2/e, pp 42–43. Curry, 4/e, pp 14–15. Selman, 8/e, pp 210–212.)* The advantage of the rotating target disk over the stationary target is the increase in heat loading. Rotating the target disk changes the focal spot to a focal track, increasing the total area that may be bombarded during operation of the x-ray tube. This allows the heat load to be spread out and better tolerated by the x-ray tube. The mechanism needed to cause the target to rotate is not found in the stationary target tubes and thus will add to the cost of such a unit. The size of the focal spot is determined by the size of the electron stream and not the target disk itself.

158. The answer is B. *(Bushong, 5/e, p 121. Curry, 4/e, p 14. Selman, 8/e, p 211.)* For a current of 60 Hz, the standard rotation speed of a target disk is 3000 to 3600 rpm (about 60 rotations per second). At this speed, an exposure of 1/60 of a second would be spread out across the entire disk surface and allow for better heat dissipation than the stationary target, which would require the entire heat load to be delivered to a single area. High-speed x-ray tubes are available with rotation speeds of approximately 10,000 rpm.

159. The answer is D. *(Bushong, 5/e, pp 119–121. Curry, 4/e, p 15. Selman, 8/e, pp 210–212.)* Numerous factors must be considered in determining the ability of an anode to effectively dissipate heat generated during energy conversion. These factors are the diameter of the target disk, the rotation speed of the disk and the focal spot size, all of which have a direct effect on heat dissipation. The length of the focal track can be stated as the product of the focal area and the disk circumference. The circumference for the diameters stated in the answers are calculated as follows:

Diameter (inches)	Diameter (mm)	Radius	Circumference
3″	76.2 mm	38.1 mm	239.27 mm
4″	101.6 mm	50.8 mm	319.00 mm
5″	127.0 mm	63.5 mm	398.90 mm

Assuming the focal spots are square, their area would be as follows:

$$1.2 \times 1.2 = 1.44 \text{ mm}^2 \quad \text{and} \quad 0.6 \times 0.6 = 0.36 \text{ mm}^2$$

The total area of the targets stated in the answers would be:

(A) 3″ disk with 1.2 mm² focal spot: 239.27 × 1.44 = 344.55 mm.
(B) 4″ disk with 0.6 mm² focal spot: 319.00 × 0.36 = 114.84 mm.
(C) 5″ disk with 0.6 mm² focal spot: 398.9 × 0.36 = 143.60 mm.
(D) 3″ disk with 1.2 mm² focal spot: 239.27 × 1.44 = 344.55 mm.

A further gain in heat dissipation of about 2.75 times is achieved with the high-speed rotation over standard speed. Therefore, the combination listed in answer option D will provide the greatest amount of heat dissipation and thus increase the tube's heat-loading capability.

160. The answer is D. *(Bushong, 5/e, p 118. Curry, 4/e, p 12. Selman, 8/e, pp 205–206.)* As the electrons are released during thermionic emission, they form a cloud around the filament. The natural tendency of the electrons is to be repulsed by one another owing to their like electrical charge (negative). This would cause spreading of the electrons rather than the desired fine stream. The negative charge on the focusing cup supersedes the individual negative charges and keeps the electrons tightly focused. Once the potential difference is applied, the electrons are accelerated away from the cathode to the anode.

161. The answer is B. *(Bushong, 5/e, p 124. Curry, 4/e, p 13. Selman, 8/e, p 211.)* The angle of the bevel on the target disk will have an effect on the size of the *effective* focal spot only. As stated in the line focus principle, x-ray tubes designed with a variation in the bevel angle will alter the effective focal spot directly, while maintaining the area of the actual focal spot for effective heat dissipation. The size of the *actual* focal spot is determined by the size of the electron stream, which is not altered by the target bevel. General-purpose x-ray tubes are manufactured with bevel angles up to 20°. Special-purpose x-ray tubes, such as for angiography or mammography, may have a bevel as steep as 6°, providing a smaller effective focal spot. While the decrease in the size of the effective focal spot is desirable for imaging purposes, the steeper bevel will also restrict the amount of field size covered. The figures below illustrate bevels with a shallow angle *(left)* and a steep angle *(right)*.

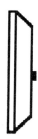

162. The answer is C. *(Bushong, 5/e, pp 142–143. Curry, 4/e, pp 20–21. Selman, 8/e, p 220.)* Heat units are the product of the current flowing from the cathode to anode (mA), the potential difference applied to the x-ray tube (kV), the duration of the exposure (s), and the correction factor for the type of generator used (C). This is expressed mathematically as mA × time (s) × kV × C. The value for C is determined as follows: single phase, fully rectified, C = 1; three phase, 6 pulse, C = 1.35; and three phase, 12 pulse, C = 1.41.

163. The answer is B. *(Bushong, 5/e, p 141. Cullinan, 2/e, pp 44–47. Curry, 4/e, pp 20–23. Selman, 8/e, pp 217–219.)* Various types of rating charts are supplied with the purchase and installation of new x-ray tube. They are designed to assist the radiographer in the safe operation of the x-ray tube. The tube rating chart is supplied to demonstrate the safe combination of exposure factors, including milliamperes, time, kilovoltage, generator type, focal spot size, and target rotation speeds. Radiographic units are also equipped with an overload protection circuit to ensure that an appropriate combination of exposure factors is not inadvertently used. Such an oversight could cause serious damage to the x-ray tube. The *anode* and *housing cooling curves* are used to keep track of the cumulative heat loading on the target and housing, respectively, over a period of time. Such tracking provides information on the amount of time the radiographer should wait between exposures, especially when numerous exposures are being made.

164. The answer is A. *(Bushong, 5/e, p 121. Curry, 4/e, pp 14, 33–34. Selman, 8/e, p 208.)* Tungsten is the most desirable material for the target disk for several reasons. Its high melting point (about 3370° C) extends the life of the target and limits the effects of the tremendous amounts of heat generated during bombardment. Its high atomic number (Z = 74) contributes to the increased production of both bremsstrahlung (braking) and characteristic types of x-ray. It is a good conductor of heat, although copper is better. The tungsten is layered on a molybdenum or graphite base and coated with rhenium for greater endurance.

165. The answer is C. *(Bushong, 5/e, pp 127–128. Cullinan, 2/e, pp 13–16. Curry, 4/e, pp 39–40. Selman, 8/e, pp 130–131.)* Kilovoltage selection is controlled by the autotransformer, which is located on the primary side of the x-ray circuit. The autotransformer allows the incoming line voltage to be varied up or down through the process of electromagnetic self-induction. In this manner, the autotransformer acts as both a step-up and step-down transformer. As kilovoltage selection is made, the appropriate portion of the windings on the autotransformer is included in the circuit and will produce an output voltage according to the autotransformer law: $V_s/V_p = A_s/A_p$, where V is the voltage ratio for the secondary to primary sides of the circuit and A is the number of total turns to the number of turns included in the circuit. The output voltage from the autotransformer becomes the input voltage to the primary side of the high-tension transformer.

166. The answer is B (2, 3). *(Bushong, 5/e, p 79. Carlton, pp 73–74. Curry, 4/e, p 37. Selman, 8/e, pp 69–70.)* The term *volt* is the unit of measure that indicates potential difference and electromotive force. Specifically, the *volt* is defined as the amount of electrical pressure that causes 1 ampere of current to flow in a circuit with a resistance of 1 ohm. This electrical pressure is the result of a difference in electrical potential: a point of excess electrons versus a point of electron deficiency within an electrical circuit. The greater this difference, the greater the force to drive the electrons (current) between the negative and positive terminals. This force has the ability to convert electric energy to mechanical energy. Therefore, the term *volt* may be applied to indicate potential difference or electromagnetic force (EMF). The number of electrons flowing per second in a circuit is termed *amperage*.

167. The answer is A. *(Carlton, pp 72–73. Selman, 8/e, pp 68–70, 75. Thompson, pp 91–92.)* The flow of electrons in a circuit is always from a point of excess electrons to a point deficient in electrons. The terminal with an excess of electrons has a large quantity of negative charges and is thus termed the *negative terminal*. The terminal deficient in electrons is termed the *positive terminal* because of its *lack* of negative charge. The electrons are the components of the atom that are "free" to move under certain conditions, and their nature is to repel like charges (each other) while being attracted to opposite charges (positive terminal). Therefore, the flow of electrons may be described as from negative to positive terminals, from a point of excess electrons to a point deficient in electrons, or from cathode to anode.

168. The answer is D. *(Bushong, 5/e, p 81. Carlton, p 73. Selman, 8/e, p 70. Thompson, pp 91–92.)* The ampere is the unit of measure that indicates the quantity of current or the number of electrons flowing per second in a circuit. Specifically, the ampere is equivalent to 1 coulomb (C) of electric charge flowing per second past a given point in a circuit having a potential difference of 1 volt (V) and a resistance of 1 ohm (Ω). The term *coulomb* is the SI unit for electric charge and is equal to 6.25×10^{18} electrons. The volt is the unit of measure of potential difference, the ohm is the unit of measure of electrical resistance, and the watt is the unit of measure of electrical power.

169. The answer is A. *(Bushong, 5/e, p 81. Carlton, p 77. Selman, 8/e, pp 71–72. Thompson, pp 94–95.)* The relationship between the three elements of an electric circuit are as follows: current (intensity) is directly proportional to the voltage and inversely proportional to the resistance of the circuit. That is, as voltage increases, the amount of current flowing will also increase, assuming the resistance stays the same; and as the resistance of the circuit increases, the amount of current flowing will decrease, assuming the voltage stays the same. This relationship is known as Ohm's law and is mathematically expressed as

$$V = I \times R \ \ or \ \ I = \frac{V}{R} \ \ or \ \ R = \frac{V}{I}$$

170. The answer is D. *(Bushong, 5/e, pp 85–86. Carlton, pp 77–78. Selman, 8/e, p 84. Thompson, pp 102–103.)* The amount of power generated by a circuit is the product of the voltage and amperage in that circuit and is expressed in watts. Specifically, the watt is defined as 1 ampere of current flowing in a circuit with a potential difference of 1 volt. In this problem, the current was stated in milliamperage and must be converted to amperes for calculation. Therefore, the solution is determined as follows:

$$120 \text{ V} \times 0.2 \text{ A} = 24 \text{ W}$$

Resistance plays no role in calculating power.

171. The answer is D. *(Bushong, 5/e, p 81. Carlton, pp 76–77. Selman, 8/e, p 73. Thompson, pp 94–96.)* According to Ohm's law the voltage may be found for the whole circuit or a branch of a circuit. Ohm's law states that voltage is equal to the product of amperage and resistance. Therefore this problem is solved as follows: $10 \times 60 = 600$ V.

172. The answer is B. *(Bushong, 5/e, pp 85–86. Carlton, p 77. Selman, 8/e, p 84. Thompson, pp 192–193.)* The power rating of a generator is calculated by finding the product of the maximum voltage and amperage capable of being produced by an electrical unit. To properly determine this value for this question, the given units in milliamperage and kilovoltage should be converted to amperage and voltage, respectively. Since each conversion requires an equal movement of the decimal point (three places to the left), the value will be the same even if conversion is not done. The solution is found as follows:

$$120,000 \text{ V} \times 0.6 \text{ A} = 72,000 \text{ W (72 kW)}$$
$$or$$
$$120 \text{ kV} \times 600 \text{ mA} = 72,000 \text{ W (72 kW)}$$

173. The answer is C. *(Bushong, 5/e, p 81. Carlton, pp 78–79. Selman, 8/e, pp 76–78. Thompson, pp 96–97.)* Circuits may be constructed as a series circuit or a parallel circuit. The difference between these is that in a series circuit current flows through each electrical component consecutively, one after the other, while in a parallel circuit the current is divided among the devices, flowing simultaneously through each component. This difference in type of circuit influences the voltage distribution across each electrical component and also the function of the circuit as a whole. For example, in a series circuit, if the flow of current is interrupted at some point in the circuit, no current will reach the remaining components. In a parallel circuit, if one component malfunctions, current will still be able to reach the other components.

174. The answer is C (1, 3). *(Bushong, 5/e, pp 86–89. Carlton, pp 87–89. Thompson, pp 108–110.)* The general definition of magnetism is the ability of certain materials to attract iron objects. Magnets exist naturally in nature and as man-made objects. The elemental component of a magnetic material is the presence of magnetic moments. The presence and distribution of these moments determines the magnetic nature of an object. Natural magnets, such as the earth and lodestones, have their magnetic moments uniformly aligned. Certain materials have magnetic potential, but are not always in a magnetic state. This is caused by a random orientation of magnetic moments within the materials. Processes such as magnetic induction and electromagnetism can be utilized to cause these random magnetic moments to uniformly align themselves and exhibit magnetic properties. The SI unit of magnetic field strength is the tesla (T), which is more commonly utilized than its associated unit, the gauss (G); 1 T = 10,000 G.

175. The answer is B (2, 3). *(Bushong, 5/e, p. 89. Carlton, pp 88–89. Selman, 8/e, pp 87–88. Thompson, pp 108–110.)* The laws of magnetism include (1) all magnets have a north and a south pole; if a magnet is broken in half, each half will acquire its own north and south poles; (2) unlike poles attract and like poles repel; and (3) the strength of magnetic force is inversely proportional to the square of the distance between the poles and directly proportional to the product of each pole's magnitude (strength). The property of "charge" applies to electrostatics, not magnetism. Although, many of the properties and laws pertaining to electrostatics and magnetism are similar, the terminology is different and specific to each.

176. The answer is B. *(Bushong, 5/e, pp 87–88. Carlton, p 86. Selman, 8/e, pp 96–97. Thompson, p 110.)* As demonstrated by Oerstead's experiment, an electrical charge in motion will create a magnetic field perpendicular to its direction of travel. This magnetic presence can be detected by the placement of a magnetic compass in the vicinity of an electrical circuit. When the circuit is open, no current is flowing and the compass aligns itself with the earth's magnetic field. When the circuit is closed, current flows through the conductor, generating magnetic flux, and the compass needle will react by aligning itself with the magnetic field. Movement of the compass with respect to the conductor will cause the compass needle to move to maintain this alignment and will be perpendicular to the electron flow. Materials composed of wood, glass, rubber, or plastic are considered to be nonmagnetic materials because their magnetic moments are not freely able to align themselves. Stationary charges possess an electrical field, but do not have a magnetic field until they are set into motion.

177. The answer is C. *(Bushong, 5/e, pp 74–75. Carlton, p 64. Selman, 8/e, p 59. Thompson, p 88.)* In order to prevent electrical shock, electrical devices need to be grounded in some manner. This generally means that a pathway exists to allow excess electrons to move away from a conductor with a negative charge or for electrons to be acquired by a conductor with a positive charge. This pathway is achieved by way of a connection with the earth, which acts as a reservoir for electrons; excess electrons may move to this reservoir or electrons may leave the earth to add electrons where there is a deficit. Electrification is the process of conferring an electrical charge on an uncharged body. Friction is one method of electrification. It is created by rubbing together two objects, which results in the removal of electrons from one (positive body) to the other (negative body). Repulsion is an electrostatic or magnetic force whereby two like charges or like magnetic poles push each other away.

178. The answer is B. *(Bushong, 5/e, pp 75–78. Carlton, pp 65–66. Selman, 8/e, pp 59–61. Thompson, pp 88–89.)* The laws of electrostatics are as follows: (1) Two types of charges exist in nature: positive and negative charges. Like charges repel each other while unlike charges are attracted to each other. (2) The force of attraction or repulsion between two electrical charges is inversely proportional to the square of their distance and directly proportional to the product of their magnitude. (3) Electrical charges exist on the external surface of a conductor and are equidistant owing to mutual repulsion. (4) The concentration of electrical charge is greatest where the curvature of the conductor is greatest. (5) Negative charges are free enough to move along a conductor while positive charges (atomic nuclei) are bound by the structure of the atom.

179. The answer is C. *(Bushong, 5/e, pp 74–75. Carlton, pp 66–69. Selman, 8/e, pp 56–58.)* Electrification is the process of causing an uncharged body to acquire an electrical charge. The three methods of electrification are *friction, contact,* and *induction.* Friction results in the transfer of electrical charge from one body to another by rubbing them together. This action removes electrons from one body (making it positive) and adds electrons to the other (making it negative). Contact electrification involves placing a charged body in physical contact with an uncharged body. The result will be the movement of charges from the charged body to the uncharged body, which will cause both objects to have the same charge. Induction electrification utilizes the electrostatic field surrounding the electric charge. Placing an uncharged body within the electrostatic field, but not touching the charged body, causes a movement of electrons toward or away from the charged body, according to the laws of electrostatics. The effect of induction will be for the uncharged body to acquire the opposite charge of the charged body.

180. The answer is D. *(Bushong, 5/e, pp 134–135. Carlton, pp 108–112. Curry, 4/e, pp 42–48. Selman, 8/e, p 139. Thompson, pp 176–180.)* Rectification is the process of converting alternating current to pulsating direct current. The x-ray tube is not a symmetric diode; the structure of the cathode and anode differ greatly. The flow of electrons must be in one direction only (cathode to anode) in order to produce high-energy x-rays. In early tubes, which were not rectified, the production of x-rays only occurred during one-half of the cycle, utilizing only 60 pulses per second rather than 120 pulses or more per second as with modern radiographic units. The incorporation of four solid-state rectifiers into the circuit maintains the flow of current in one direction only. The result is an increase in x-ray production, utilizing a minimum of 120 pulses per second. These added components increase the complexity of the x-ray circuit, as well as the size, although modern solid-state rectifiers are much smaller than the original valve tube rectifiers.

181. The answer is B. *(Bushong, 5/e, pp 136–137. Carlton, p 113. Curry, 4/e, pp 47–48. Selman, 8/e, p 143. Thompson, pp 179–180.)* Four solid-state rectifiers are used to provide a fully rectified waveform from a single-phase generator. These devices are located on the secondary side of the high-tension transformer. The rectification process allows for the production of x-rays during each cycle of alternating current, effectively doubling x-ray production over half-wave or nonrectified units. The use of only two rectifiers would produce a half-waveform. Three-phase, full-wave rectified units use 6 or 12 rectifiers to produce an even more efficient waveform and higher x-ray production than the single-phase units.

182. The answer is D (1, 2, 3). *(Bushong, 5/e, pp 137–139. Carlton, pp 125–126. Curry, 4/e, pp 48–51. Selman, 8/e, pp 256–258. Thompson, pp 118–121.)* The advantages of three-phase generators compared with single-phase generators include all the answer options. Three-phase generators supply three lines of voltage to the unit, each out of phase with the other. As voltage begins to decline in the first line, the second is reaching its peak, and so it continues with the third line. The result is less voltage drop and more high-energy x-rays produced. Maintaining the high level of voltage applied to the x-ray tube increases acceleration of the electrons and increases the tube current. Modern three-phase generators are capable of up to 2000 mA. The increased milliamperage will allow the use of extremely short exposure times.

183. The answer is A. *(Bushong, 5/e, pp 133–134. Carlton, pp 104–109. Curry, 4/e, pp 37–40. Selman, 8/e, pp 123–126, 130–132. Thompson, pp 126–130.)* Transformers are the devices used to regulate voltage. The x-ray circuit employs an autotransformer as well as step-up and step-down types of transformers. The autotransformer is capable of increasing or decreasing the voltage applied to it. This type is used to regulate the incoming line voltage to the proper level, which is then applied to the high-tension transformer to be stepped-up to the kilovoltage range. A step-up transformer is used in the high-tension circuit. As its name implies, this device increases or steps up the input voltage according to the turns ratio between the primary and secondary coils. If a transformer has a turns ratio of 500:1 (secondary:primary) and the input voltage from the autotransformer is 150 V, the output voltage will be 75,000 V, or 75 kV. The step-down transformer is employed in the filament circuit, where low voltage is required. Since this type of transformer has a turns ratio of less than 1, the output voltage will be less than the input voltage.

184. The answer is C. *(Bushong, 5/e, p 129. Carlton, pp 129–130. Curry, 4/e, p 40. Thompson, pp 187–189.)* The heating of the filament in the x-ray tube is controlled by the filament circuit. Proper filament heating requires a relatively high current and low voltage compared with the tube current and voltage between the cathode and anode. These requirements are achieved by a step-down transformer in the filament circuit. The step-down transformer has a turns ratio of about 1:10 or 20. As milliamperage selection is made at the control panel, voltage, supplied to the filament circuit by the autotransformer, is lowered to about 5 to 10 V. With the lowered voltage, current will increase to the desired level, according to the inverse relationship that exists between current and the transformer turns ratio ($I_p/I_s = N_s/N_p$).

185. The answer is B. *(Bushong, 5/e, p 102. Carlton, p 105. Curry, 4/e, pp 38–39. Selman, 8/e, p 126. Thompson, p 129.)* Ideally, the power should remain constant on both the primary and secondary sides of a transformer, that is, what goes in should come out. Power is defined as the product of current and voltage. Therefore, as voltage is varied by a transformer, current must vary inversely in order to maintain power level. This relationship is stated mathematically as $V_s/V_p = I_p/I_s$.

186. The answer is D. *(Bushong, 5/e, p 102. Carlton, p 105. Curry, 4/e, p 38. Selman, 8/e, p 129. Thompson, pp 128–129.)* The role of the transformer is to vary voltage, based on the principles of electromagnetic induction. This is achieved by increasing or decreasing the number of turns (coil windings) on the secondary side of the transformer with respect to the number of turns on the primary side. The relationship between number of turns and voltage is directly proportional and is mathematically stated as $V_s/V_p =$

N_s/N_p, where V = voltage; N = number of turns (windings); s = secondary coil; and p = primary coil. Solution of this problem is found as follows: x/120 = 1000/50; 50x = 120,000; x = 2400 V (2.4 kV).

187. The answer is B. *(Bushong, 5/e, p 352.)*   Dynamic imaging provides a means for viewing anatomic structures in motion; that is, it shows how they function. Fluoroscopy allows the radiologist to indirectly observe physiologic motion within the gastrointestinal system or the flow of blood through arteries and veins. Such imaging is obtained through the use of a fluoroscope, which includes a fluorescent screen and an optics system for viewing the image. Continuous or pulsed irradiation of the patient provides a fairly continuous image of structures as they function. Fluoroscopy has changed greatly from the early days with tremendous improvement in the quality of the images and reduction of dose delivered to patient and personnel. Tomographic techniques are used to image the body in planes or sections in order to avoid looking through structures above or below the area of interest. Motion of the tube and image receptor are employed to obtain the images; however, the images are static, not dynamic. Stereoscopy is another technique employed to better visualize structures in regard to their relationship with other structures in the area of interest; however, it also yields static images. Subtraction techniques are used to photographically or electronically remove unwanted information from the image for better viewing of the desired structures. This technique may be employed with fluoroscopy, but the fluoroscope provides the means of dynamic imaging, not the subtraction techniques, which are used to enhance static images.

188. The answer is A. *(Bushong, 5/e, pp 352, 355.)*   The incorporation of the image intensifier in the construction of the modern fluoroscope is necessary to achieve fluoroscopic images of an intensity level bright enough for optimum viewing. The original fluoroscopes produced such low levels of light that the image had to be viewed in complete darkness in order to visualize maximum information. By raising the brightness level of the image, "daytime" viewing becomes possible and with it improved visual acuity. The use of image-intensified fluoroscopy does not lower radiation dose, nor does it store the image. Some intensifiers will have the option of producing a magnified image, but this is not the primary purpose of the image intensifier.

189. The answer is C. *(Bushong, 5/e, p 357.)*   The image intensifier is employed in fluoroscopy for the primary purpose of increasing the light level of the image and thereby improving viewing conditions. Nonintensified fluoroscopy produced a faint image on a fluoroscopic screen. The low light level of this image required complete darkness in order to enhance the use of the eye's scotopic viewing mechanism—the use of the rods of the eye. The result was poor visual acuity of the structures imaged. The incorporation of the image intensifier provides a method of amplifying the fluoroscopic image. This is achieved by converting the image to an electronic signal (electrons), which can be accelerated (acquiring large amounts of kinetic energy), and directing it into a very small fluoroscopic screen (output phosphor). The result of these two actions (flux gain and minification gain) is the transfer of a large quantity of energy onto a small area, producing many more light photons than were previously available. The components of the image intensifier first convert the exit photons to light photons, then to electrons, and finally back to light photons. The use of the image intensifier provides a much brighter fluoroscopic image, which may be viewed in daylight conditions (photopic vision). This improves the level of visual acuity and decreases patient anxiety about being in the dark during fluoroscopic procedures.

190. The answer is B. *(Bushong, 5/e, pp 356–357. Curry, 4/e, pp 166–170.)*   The image intensifier is a lead-lined tube, mounted above the patient on a C-arm, for use during fluoroscopy. Like the x-ray tube, this tube has cathode and anode ends and a glass envelope that maintains a vacuum around its internal components. Moving from the cathode to the anode, the components of the image intensifier include the following: (1) *Input phosphor*—A fluorescent screen of 4 to 10 inches in diameter, which is coated with cesium iodide and responsible for converting the exit beam to a representative light image. (2) *Photocathode*—A photosensitive layer of antimony and cesium, mounted very close to the input phosphor, which emits a proportionate number and distribution of electrons upon stimulation by the light from the input phosphor. (3) *Electrostatic lenses*—These are distributed along the length of the image intensifier tube and act to focus the electron stream from the photocathode onto the output phosphor. (4) *Output phosphor*—A fluorescent screen of about 1 inch in diameter, coated with zinc cadmium sulfide, which is bombarded by the electron stream to produce a minified and much brighter version of the image originally formed on the input phosphor. The acceleration of the electrons across the image intensifier is achieved by the potential difference applied between the cathode and anode ends of the device.

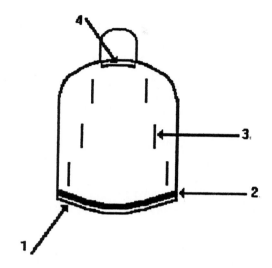

191. The answer is D.   *(Bushong, 5/e, p 357. Curry, 4/e pp 170–171.)*   The term "brightness gain" indicates the degree of amplification of the light level of the fluoroscopic image provided by the image intensifier. This is the primary reason for the use of image intensifiers. The brightness gain is the product of the flux gain (kinetic energy acquired by the accelerated electrons) and the minification gain (the square of the ratio of the input phosphor to the output phosphor). The flux gain value is constant for each image intensifier. However, the minification gain may vary in dual or trifocus tubes, which allow the size of the input phosphor to be altered.

192. The answer is A.   *(Bushong, 5/e, p 357. Curry, 4/e, pp 171–172.)*   Brightness gain is the product of minification and flux gain. Flux gain is a constant value and indicates the acquired energy of the electrons as they were accelerated from the cathode to the anode of the image intensifier, as regulated by the potential difference applied. The minification gain is the square of the ratio between the diameters of the input and output phosphors $(IP/OP)^2$. Dual or trifocus image intensifiers allow the manipulation of the amount of the input phosphor used for imaging and thus vary the minification gain. For an image intensifier with a flux gain of 50, an input phosphor of 12 inches and an output phosphor of 1 inch, the brightness gain would be 7200 times brighter than nonintensified imaging:

Brightness gain (BG) = minification gain (MG) × flux gain (FG)
MG = $(IP/OP)^2$ or $(12/1)^2 = 144$
FG = 50
BG = 144 × 50
BG = 7200

193. The answer is A.   *(Bushong, 5/e, p 357. Curry, 4/e, p 171.)*   Minification gain is the square of the ratio of the diameters of the input and output phosphors of the image intensifier. As this ratio increases, the minification gain increases. Since minification gain is a factor in the overall brightness gain achieved by an image intensifier, the larger ratio will provide a brighter image. In this problem, minification gain is calculated as follows:

$$\left(\frac{IP}{OP}\right)^2 = \left(\frac{25}{2.5}\right)^2$$
$$= 10^2$$
$$= 100$$

194. The answer is B. *(Bushong, 5/e, p 356. Curry, 4/e, pp 166–167.)* Modern image intensifiers employ cesium iodide as the material for the input phosphor. This compound is preferred over the previously used zinc cadmium sulfide because of its better k-edge match with the average energies of the exit x-ray beam. Improved k-edge matching increases the absorption efficiency of the phosphor, and, therefore, a thinner coating of the phosphor can be used for the same level of illumination, but with an increased level of image resolution. Zinc cadmium sulfide is still used for the output phosphor.

195. The answer is D. *(Bushong, 5/e, p 357. Curry, 4/e, p 168.)* The electrostatic lenses mounted within the image intensifier between the cathode and anode ends direct the electrons as they are accelerated across the tube. The electron distribution arises from the photocathode and is representative of the exit x-ray beam. These electrons are accelerated (acquiring energy) and will interact with the much smaller output phosphor to produce a brighter image. The electrostatic lenses ensure that the electrons maintain appropriate position as they are accelerated and also act to focus them onto the output phosphor screen to provide an image representative of the information originally contained in the exit x-ray beam.

196. The answer is A. *(Bushong, 5/e, p 357. Curry, 4/e, pp 171–172.)* The amount of amplification of the light level achieved by the image intensifier is termed *brightness gain* (BG). This factor is the product of the flux gain (FG) and minification gain (MG). For the conditions set in the question, brightness gain would be calculated as follows:

$$BG = FG \times MG$$
$$FG = 150$$
$$MG = \left(\frac{17}{2.5}\right)^2 = 6.8^2 = 46.24$$
$$BG = 150 \times 46.24$$
$$= 6936 \text{ (or about 7000 times brighter)}$$

197. The answer is B. *(Bushong, 5/e, pp 359, 361. Curry, 4/e, pp 175–176.)* In order to view the fluoroscopic image, a system, either mirror-optics or television, must be employed. The mirror-optics system included a series of lenses and a mirror for indirect viewing of the output phosphor screen. This system, although less complex than television monitoring, provided a small area for only one viewer to see. The closed-circuit television system is more commonly used. This system incorporates a TV camera, coupled to the output phosphor; a control unit; and a TV monitor for final viewing of the image. The TV camera converts the light image from the intensifier to a video signal, which is then transmitted via cable through the control unit and on to the TV monitor, where the video signal is reconverted back to a light image.

198. The answer is D (1, 2, 3, 4). *(Bushong, 5/e, p 358. Curry, 4/e, pp 186–191.)* The fluoroscopic image can be recorded on various types of media. Conventional radiographic film loaded in cassettes is used in the spot film device of the image intensifier. During fluoroscopy, the cassette is stored in a protective area, out of the exit x-ray beam. To record an image, the cassette is moved into position between the patient and the intensifier and the film is directly exposed to the exit beam. Modern image intensifiers can accommodate a wide range of cassette sizes (including 14 × 17) and can provide multiple exposures to one film. Another form of fluoroscopic image recording uses the photospot camera, which records the image from the output phosphor of the intensifier onto a smaller film format such as 90-, 100- or 105-mm films. The camera allows for increased framing frequencies and less patient exposure than conventional spot filming. For some radiographic procedures, extremely fast framing frequencies are required to film such structures as the coronary vessels during opacification, as in cardiac catheterization. Such imaging uses a cine camera. Like a movie camera, cine uses a smaller frame film (16 or 35 mm) and the images are recorded at frequencies up to 60 frames per second. After processing, the film is viewed using a projector, which can present the individual frames at such a rate as to demonstrate the motion of the structures imaged. Both the photospot and cine cameras are connected to the output phosphor of the image intensifier through a lens or fiberoptics mechanism. A beam-splitting mirror is incorporated into the design to allow a portion of the image (about 10 percent) to go to the TV camera in order to allow continued monitoring of the image during filming. Most recently, the fluoroscopic image is being recorded onto magnetic tapes or disks and onto optical laser disks. These systems record the image from the TV video signal.

199. The answer is B. *(Bushong, 5/e, p 359. Carlton, pp 561–564. Curry, 4/e, p 175.)* The television monitoring system allows the radiologist to indirectly view the fluoroscopic image in real time (as it is being created). This system replaced the earlier methods of viewing the image, which included direct viewing of the fluoroscopic screen and indirect viewing by means of a mirror-optics system. The TV monitoring system enables other electronic components to be interfaced with the fluoroscopic unit, such as a video tape recorder or computer. These components provide means of recording or storing the image other than conventional film formats.

200. The answer is C. *(Bushong, 5/e pp 358–359. Curry, 4/e, pp 173–174.)* The availability of dual or trifocus image intensifiers provides the option of varying the amount of the input phosphor used for imaging. By reducing the area of the input phosphor, there is less information projected onto the output phosphor, making the image larger (magnified) than it would be using the entire diameter of the input phosphor. For example, on a dual focus tube (25/17 cm), if the entire 25-cm diameter area is used, a wider field of view of the irradiated anatomy is projected and compressed onto a 2.5-cm (standard diameter) output phosphor. If the 17-cm mode is selected, only the image on the central 17 cm of the input phosphor is projected onto the output phosphor, with less compression of the image. The side effect of this technique is the change in brightness gain due to less minification gain (25 cm IP = 100 MG; 17 cm IP = 46 MG). This loss in brightness gain is compensated for via the automatic brightness control, which increases the exposure factors to maintain the desired light level, but also increases patient dose.

201. The answer is C. *(Bushong, 5/e, pp 361–362. Curry, 4/e, p 191.)* The inclusion of a beam-splitting mirror in the optics system of the image intensifier is to allow the continued viewing of the fluoroscopic image during recording of the image. This device is positioned between the TV camera and the recording camera (photospot or cine). The system may allow the retraction of the mirror from the path of the TV camera when image recording is not occurring. Usually, about 10 percent of the light from the output phosphor is allowed to reach the TV camera, with the remainder being used to expose the film.

202. The answer is A. *(Bushong, 5/e, p 429. Carlton, pp 439, 452. Gray, p 1. NCRP No. 99, p 1.)* The definition stated in this question pertains to quality assurance, the concept of evaluating and analyzing the factors of radiologic services for the purpose of improving those services. The main goal is the best possible diagnostic information with the least amount of risk (exposure) to patients and personnel. Quality control refers to specific actions to provide the evaluation of the components and the analysis process. There are many quality control procedures within a quality assurance program. Troubleshooting is the organized approach to identifying a problem in order to resolve it effectively. ALARA is the radiation protection philosophy recommended by the NCRP for keeping radiation exposure to patients and personnel "as low as reasonably achievable" while obtaining optimum radiographic results.

203. The answer is B. *(Carlton, p 445. Carroll, 5/e, pp 359–360.)* The process of determining mR/mAs requires the exposure output value (usually stated in mR) to be divided by the mAs value. This expression is useful in comparing exposure output for different milliampere stations, thus providing an indication as to the calibration status of the milliampere stations. For this problem, the mAs value must be determined by multiplying mA and time (600 × 0.016 = 9.6 mAs). Then the exposure output is divided by the mAs (240 / 9.6 = 25 mR per mAs). Changes in the accuracy of the milliampere stations or the exposure times will alter this value and influence image quality and patient dose.

204. The answer is A. *(Bushong, 5/e, p 433. Carlton, p 445. Carroll, 5/e, pp 359–360. NCRP No. 99, pp 72–73.)* The acceptable range for variation in exposure linearity should be within ±10 percent for consecutive mA stations (i.e., the station just above or below the one being evaluated). According to this standard, analysis of the data in the table would yield the following results:

The 30 mR/mAs value at the 100 station would require its adjacent stations to have values between 27 and 33; thus linearity exists between 100 and 200.

The 28 mR/mAs value at the 200 station would require its adjacent stations to have values between 25.2 and 30.8; thus linearity does not exist between 200 and 300.

The 40 mR/mAs value at the 300 station would require its adjacent stations to have values between 36 and 44; thus linearity exists between 300 and 400.

205. The answer is C. *(Bushong, 5/e, pp 432–433. Carlton, p 445. NCRP No. 99, pp 70–71, 195.)* The spinning top device is used to evaluate the accuracy of the exposure timer on single-phase equipment. This device consists of a solid disk containing a small hole and mounted on a pivot to allow free movement of the disk. As the disk turns during radiation exposure, each pulse is recorded as a dot on the film. For a 60-cycle current, 120 pulses are present per second of exposure. The number of dots expected to be recorded for an accurate timer is determined by multiplying the exposure time to be tested by 120; e.g., 0.1 s × 120 = 12 dots expected. The acceptable range for variation is ±5 percent of the selected time. The exposure timer on three-phase equipment must be evaluated using an electronic synchronous device.

206. The answer is B. *(Bushong, 5/e, pp 431–433. Carroll, 5/e, pp 357–359, 362, 365, 368. NCRP No. 99, pp 63, 69–70, 73.)* The acceptable range of variation for the factors included in this question are (A) ±5 percent for kilovoltage; (B) + 50 percent for focal spot size; (C) 2 percent of SID for x-ray/light field alignment; and (D) ±5 percent for exposure timer. The 80-kV station may range between 76 and 84 kV and still be considered acceptable; thus 86 is out of tolerance. The stated 0.6-mm focal spot can be as large as 0.9 mm and still be within limits. For the average SID of 40 inches (100 cm) the x-ray/light field alignment must be within 2 cm in any direction. A spinning top test for the 0.05 s time stop should yield 6 dots (120 pulses s × 0.05 s = 6) ±1 dot for variance; thus, 8 dots indicates a longer than desired exposure time.

207. The answer is B. *(Bushong, 5/e, pp 430–431. Carroll, 5/e, pp 363–364. NCRP No. 99, pp 61–63.)* The importance of determining the half-value layer (HVL) of the x-ray beam is that it is an indication of the beam quality. Beam quality is synonymous with the penetrability of the beam, which influences both patient dose and image quality. Kilovoltage and filtration levels are the factors that determine beam quality. Therefore, changes in HVL can indicate changes in kilovolt peak (kVp) calibration or filtration level. Since kilovolt peak can be more directly determined and filtration cannot, HVL is primarily used to evaluate filtration, assuming kilovoltage calibration is within tolerance. General purpose x-rays tubes, which are capable of operating at 70 kV or higher, are required to have a minimum HVL of 2.34 mm of aluminum or equivalent when tested at 80 kVp. A lower HVL would indicate excessive skin dose to patients. Over time, changes in the x-ray tube (tungsten plating) result in higher HVL values. To a point, this is acceptable, as skin dose will be lowered, but ultimately image quality (contrast) will begin to suffer because of hardening of the beam.

208. The answer is D (1, 2, 3). *(Bushong, 5/e, p 435. Carroll, 5/e, p 374. NCRP No. 99, pp 74–76.)* Automatic exposure control (AEC) devices perform many functions and they must be evaluated for accuracy on an annual basis. The role of the AEC is to terminate the exposure when sufficient radiation has been measured to produce a predetermined level of radiographic density (around 1.0 to 1.2_D). This function includes the AEC's ability to provide the desired level of exposure for various patient thicknesses and at various kilovoltage peak levels. Also, all the sensors (chambers) and density control levels should be monitored to ensure that they function optimally. A back-up timer is included to provide a maximum level of exposure in the case of improper equipment set-up. The FDA recommends that the back-up timer not allow exposures to exceed 600 mAs. The AEC also has limitations in terms of the shortest exposure that can be provided. Determining this factor will assist the technologist in selecting a more appropriate combination of exposure factors for small patients, in whom overexposed images may be due to the minimum response time. A range of tolerance does not apply to all the AEC functions, but in general radiographic densities should be within ±10 percent (0.1_D) of each other.

209. The answer is C. *(Carlton, pp 450–452. Carroll, 5/e, pp 350–355. NCRP No. 99, pp 26–28.)* A repeat analysis is a study of the radiographic images discarded for being unsatisfactory for any number of reasons. It is also referred to as a "retake" or "reject" analysis and as such will include film discarded for reasons other than examination errors (e.g., fogged or outdated film). As part of a repeat analysis, all discarded films are categorized by the error that caused them to be discarded, such as positioning error, overexposure, underexposure, and so on. This analysis will indicate specific imaging rooms, radiographers, and examinations that require corrective action. This information should then be used to warrant service on suboptimum imaging equipment and to provide instruction to radiographers for improving their performance. The repeat rate is calculated as the percentage of discarded films out of the total number of films processed. On average, repeat rates for imaging centers are around 7 percent nationally. Repeat rates should be kept to less than 10 percent.

210. The answer is D. *(Gray, p 21.)* Quality control test procedures are performed by individuals and are at risk for systematic or random errors. Therefore, any time negative results are produced by a quality control test, the test should be repeated to ensure the results are due to the component that is being evaluated and not the way in which the procedure was performed. Achieving the same results from a second test provides more evidence that the error is in the component rather than the test procedure. It is desirable to have quality control tests performed by the same person and in the same manner to reduce the influence of subjective or procedural error in the test process. Once the suboptimum data are confirmed, prompt action should be taken to correct the component.

211. The answer is C. *(Carroll, 5/e, pp 363, 368–369. Selman, 8/e, p 218.)* An increase in HVL would be an indication of a change in beam quality due to a change in kilovoltage or total beam filtration. Since kilovoltage can be evaluated and eliminated as a probable cause more directly, the problem is most often due to an increase in beam filtration. This can occur as a result of a build-up of vaporized tungsten from the filament that settles on the inside of the window of the x-ray tube when the tube is allowed to cool. Small increases in beam quality will further reduce a patient's skin dose without influencing image quality, but continued increases in such filtration will be evidenced by a loss of density and contrast. Repeated use of high milliamperage stations can result in a condition termed focal spot "blooming" in which there is spreading of the electron stream and subsequent increases in the actual and effective focal spot size. The physical structure of the positive beam limitation contributes to the amount of total beam filtration, but its use (proper or improper) has no influence on beam quality. Proper warm-up procedures will prevent the x-ray tube from delivering a high heat load onto a cold target, which could cause the target to crack. This type of damage to the tube may affect x-ray quantity, but not quality.

212. The answer is C. *(Bushong, 5/e, pp 165–167. Selman, 8/e, pp 172–175.)* Half-value layer (HVL) is defined as the amount of aluminum required to reduce beam intensity to one-half its original value and is stated in terms of millimeters of aluminum. The HVL is used to monitor changes in beam quality, usually as a result of changes in filtration over time. The data are acquired by recording exposure levels in mR while varying the amount of aluminum sheets in the path of the beam from 0 to 5.0 mm. The exposure readings are plotted on a chart as a function of the amount of aluminum in the beam. A line is then drawn from the vertical axis (exposure readings) of the graph over to the curve formed by the data acquired. A line is drawn from that point perpendicular to the horizontal axis (aluminum thicknesses). This point indicates the HVL. For this problem, the answer may be found by noting how many times the original value is divided in half to reach the new value. Each division step is equal to 1 HVL:

$$\frac{342}{2} = 171 \text{ mR (1 HVL)}$$

$$\frac{171}{2} = 86 \text{ mR (2 HVLs)}$$

$$\frac{86}{2} = 43 \text{ mR (3 HVLs)}$$

213. The answer is A. *(Bushong, 5/e, p 167. Selman, 8/e, pp 172–175.)* The relationship between HVL and beam quality is direct. HVL is used to evaluate beam quality by indicating the amount of aluminum required to reduce beam intensity through attenuation. Higher beam quality is more penetrating and less likely to be attenuated; therefore, it requires an increased amount of aluminum to lower beam intensity to the desired level. For example, a radiographic unit may require 2.5 mm of aluminum to reduce beam intensity when using 70 kV, but when kilovoltage is increased to 100, the HVL would increase to about 3.7 mm of aluminum.

214. The answer is D. *(Carlton, pp 449–450. Carroll, 5/e, p 374.)* Viewboxes are part of the imaging chain in that they provide the desired conditions for viewing the radiograph. For this reason, they must be maintained. Regular cleaning of the surface will improve viewing conditions and limit pseudoartifacts from marks on the viewbox. The light level for all viewboxes must be consistent throughout the department. To accomplish this, the same type and color of light source must be used. As light bulbs age, they may change color or have darkened ends, reducing the light level. Light bulbs should be changed at this point, and all the bulbs should be changed at the same time. Ambient light should be low in order to cut glare and enhance viewing conditions.

215. The answer is B. *(Bushong, 5/e, pp 437–440. NCRP No. 99, pp 65–66.)* Visual checks of certain components of imaging and ancillary radiographic equipment are a form of quality control. For example, the locks on the table, tube, and upright bucky should be adjusted to their locked and unlocked positions to see if they work. Another example would be the checking and cleaning of cassettes and screens. The other answer options require a testing tool and procedure. A grid alignment tool is available to check the table bucky grid for alignment with the centered x-ray beam. A film is exposed with the tube centered and laterally off-center. When the film is processed, the density is evaluated for uniformity. The light intensity of a viewbox is measured with a light meter. Film-screen contact is evaluated with a wire mesh contact grid.

216. The answer is A. *(Carroll, 5/e, p 357. Gray, pp 107–110. NCRP No. 99, p 70.)* The exposure timer on a three-phase radiographic unit cannot be evaluated using the spinning top. That device is for single-phase equipment only. An electronic synchronous device or digital dosimeter with a timer mode is needed to evaluate the three-phase timer. The synchronous device produces an image of an arc, which can be measured using a protractor that comes with the device. This timer test tool makes one complete revolution per second and a 360° area of exposure on the film. Fractional exposure times will yield an equivalent arc. The size of the expected arc can be determined by multiplying the exposure time by 360°. For the exposure time of 0.017, an arc of 6° (360 × 0.017 = 6) would indicate timer accuracy. If the unit was single-phase and a spinning top test performed, 2 dots (120 × 0.017 = 2) would indicate accuracy. The exposure time of 0.05 would produce an arc of 18° (360 × 0.05 = 18) or 6 dots (120 × 0.05 = 6) if a spinning top was used.

217. The answer is D (1, 2, 3). *(Bushong, 5/e, p 431. Carroll, 5/e, pp 368–369. NCRP No. 99, p 65.)* Evaluation of the focal spot size may be made with a pinhole camera, slit camera, or star resolution pattern. Each has its own level of accuracy. The slit camera is recommended by the National Electrical Manufacturers Association (NEMA); this agency sets the measurement standards for focal spot size. The star pattern is a resolution grid that is radiographed using a slight magnification factor. The resultant image is viewed and the area in focus is measured with a millimeter ruler to provide the actual length and width of the focal spot. It is more accurate than the pinhole camera. The pinhole camera is a radiopaque device with a small hole in the center, which acts to finely collimate the beam before it is recorded on a direct-exposure imaging system. The area of density on the exposed and processed radiograph is measured with calipers and represents the size of the actual focal spot.

218. The answer is D. *(Bushong, 5/e, p 665. Thompson, p 410.)* All protective apparel should be evaluated for loss of integrity that may cause unnecessary exposure to patients or personnel. This evaluation should be performed on an annual basis or whenever questions arise as to the quality of the aprons, gloves, or gonadal shields. This test method involves radiographing or fluoroscoping each piece of apparel with high kilovoltage (>100) to demonstrate areas of radiation leakage. When such areas are located, the surface should be marked to identify them; one must then consider whether the apparel should continue to be used. Visual inspection of aprons or gloves may suggest leaks, which then should be confirmed by radiation exposure. Scanning with an ultraviolet light may aid in the visual inspection. If there is concern regarding a piece of protective apparel, the apparel should not be used on patient or personnel until it has been evaluated.

219. The answer is A (1, 2). *(Bushong, 5/e, pp 160-162. Carroll, 5/e, pp 119–120. Thompson, pp 118–121.)* The radiographic unit is dependent on alternating current to utilize the transformer in the production of the high voltages required for x-rays. The nature of alternating current is such that the EMF provided varies in intensity from zero to a peak potential then drops to zero and reverses its course. Single-phase radiographic units employ rectified alternating current so that the flow of electrons is always in the same direction through the x-ray tube (cathode to anode). As a result of the building and dropping of EMF, production of useful x-rays does not occur in a continuous manner, as evidenced by the 100 percent ripple factor on single-phase alternating current. Three-phase power incorporates three lines of current, each slightly out of synchrony with the previous. As EMF begins to decline in the first line, the flow of current in the second is reaching peak, and as it drops, the third line peaks. This action repeats continuously and results in a reduced ripple factor, more continuous x-ray production, and more high-energy photons. As shown in the curves below, the emission spectrum of three-phase generators shows an increase in x-ray quantity and quality over single-phase generators.

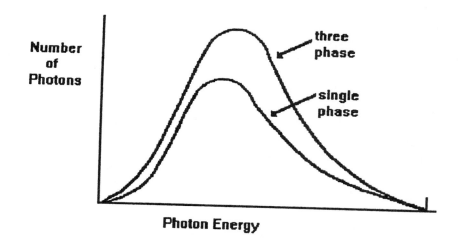

220. The answer is C. *(Bushong, 5/e, p 104. Carlton, pp 108–109.)* The rectification system in the x-ray circuit is included to maintain the direction of the flow of current through the x-ray tube from cathode to anode. This action creates two positive pulses per cycle of AC rather than the usual one positive and one negative pulse per cycle. Since current flow is now in the same direction it is said to be "direct" rather than "alternating." However, unlike true DC, EMF is not constant, but still builds to a peak and then drops back to zero. For this reason, rectified AC is referred to as "pulsating DC." In three-phase, 6- or 12-pulse power, the ripple factor is reduced, producing a waveform more closely resembling DC. The ripple factors vary as follows: single-phase = 100 percent; three-phase, 6-pulse = 13.5 percent; and three-phase, 12-pulse = 3.5 percent.

221. The answer is C. *(Bushong, 5/e, pp 104–105, 665. Carlton, pp 109–110.)* Modern x-ray equipment employs solid-state semiconductor diodes as rectifiers. These silicon-based components are a combination of n-type and p-type semiconductors. When placed in a circuit, these rectifiers will allow the flow of current under specific conditions. In this manner, they can determine the direction of current flow in the x-ray tube. Prior to the introduction of solid-state components, vacuum tubes (also known as valve tubes) were used as rectifiers. These miniature "x-ray" tubes were bulky and subject to frequent failure. Scintillation crystals coupled with a photomultiplier form a device capable of detecting radiation. Such devices are used in automatic exposure controls (phototimers), nuclear medicine equipment, and detector arrays in CT equipment.

222. The answer is C.   *(Curry, 4/e, p 51. Selman, 8/e, pp 263–267.)*   Three-phase generators are desirable because of their ability to provide a nearly constant potential and thus more continuous x-ray production. The result of this ability is the delivery of a higher quantity (about double) of x-rays per exposure time over single-phase generators. This allows the use of higher milliamperage stations (up to 1200) with very short exposure times (as low as 1 ms). Such capabilities have advanced the radiologic specialty areas of angiography and cardiography. Although the three-phase waveform also results in the production of more high-energy x-ray photons, thus slightly increasing average beam energy, there is no influence on the maximum kilovoltage peak. The kilovoltage range available is determined by the power supplied to the high-tension transformer from the autotransformer. The circuitry required to generate this kind of power is more complex and expensive than that for single-phase generators.

223. The answer is B.   *(Bushong, 5/e, pp 103–104. Carroll, 5/e, pp 121–122.)*   The operation of the transformer requires alternating current (AC) that constantly reverses its direction of flow, thus creating a changing magnetic field. The production of x-rays requires electrons to flow from the cathode and bombard the target at the anode. If true AC were applied to the x-ray tube and electrons allowed to flow from the anode to the cathode, the filament would be destroyed. Therefore, during the negative pulse of the AC cycle of a nonrectified waveform, there is no flow of electrons and x-ray output is low. This limitation was improved upon with the incorporation of rectifiers in the x-ray circuit to keep the flow of current through the x-ray tube from cathode to anode during both pulses of an AC cycle. The standard single-phase radiographic unit employs four solid-state semiconductor rectifiers to double the x-ray output over the nonrectified unit. Three-phase units employ 6 to 12 rectifiers in their circuits. An induction type of motor is used to rotate the target disk of the x-ray tube anode in order to increase heat loading, while maintaining the vacuum within the tube. Transformers are designed to vary voltage either up (step-up) or down (step-down).

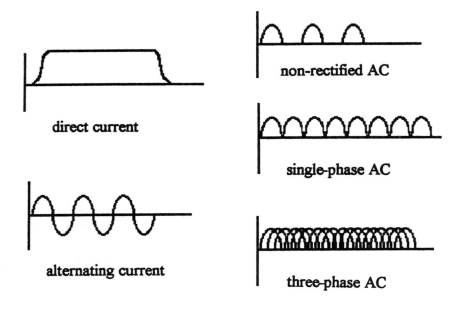

224. The answer is B (2, 3).   *(Bushong, 5/e, pp 130–132. Curry, 4/e, pp 57–59. Thompson, p 120.)*   The automatic exposure control (AEC) device has many factors to consider. These factors include the back-up time, the sensors or chambers, the optimum kilovoltage peak for the part, and the appropriate density selection. The back-up timer is the exposure time set to manually terminate the exposure should there be a problem with the set-up of the AEC. It is recommended that the back-up time be set at approximately twice the expected exposure time. The general use of 1 s as a back-up time is excessive for those examinations that would never approach such a long exposure time if manually operated, e.g., chest radiography. Most AEC devices offer three separate sensors or chambers, which may be selected individually or in various combinations to best sample the radiation required to satisfactorily expose various parts of the body. These chambers are generally arranged in a pattern that offers one chamber in the center of the x-ray beam (and image receptor) and one on each side of, and slightly above, the center. In the majority of radiographic examinations, the part of interest is placed in the center of the field over the center chamber, which is activated alone. The AEC then detects the radiation and terminates the exposure when a predetermined level has been reached. Some anatomic structures, like the chest in the PA view, require the use of one or two side chambers to sample the exposure from the lungs rather than the mediastinum, as would occur if the center chamber was selected. Although the AEC should provide adequate exposure, within a range of kilovoltage peaks, the optimum kilovoltage for the part being exposed must be selected to obtain the proper contrast and minimum exposure to the patient. Although the *normal* density selection is made for most images, the AEC does offer the ability to slightly increase or decrease the density for specific anatomic structures. Minimum reaction time is a limitation of the AEC and not a factor controlled by the radiographer.

225. The answer is B. *(Bushong, 5/e, pp 130–132. Carlton, pp 502–507. Carroll, 5/e, pp 332–336. Gray, p 102. Thompson, pp 183–186.)* The purpose of the AEC device is to automatically terminate the exposure once a predetermined level of exposure has been detected. The images obtained should have a consistent level of radiographic density, regardless of the thickness of the part. Many radiographic units select the highest milliamperage station for the kilovoltage peak selected, thus providing the shortest exposure time possible for the examination. Some units require the radiographer to select the milliamperage, which again should be the highest possible for the kilovoltage peak and focal spot size selected. In order to obtain the appropriate level of image contrast and minimum amount of patient exposure, the optimum kilovoltage peak for the part being radiographed must be selected by the operator. The successful operation of the AEC requires careful and proper centering of the part and selection of the sensor chamber compatible with the part of interest. The radiographer may select any combination of the three sensors to supply optimum sampling of radiation exposure to the part. If the anatomy is not in proper relationship with the activated sensor, the radiation detected may be inappropriate for the part, resulting in an improperly exposed image. A back-up time must also be set by the radiographer, which will act to manually terminate the exposure in case the AEC is improperly set up.

226. The answer is C. *(Bushong, 5/e, pp 130–132. Carlton, pp 502–507. Carroll, 5/e, pp 332–336. Gray, p 102. NCRP No. 99, pp 74–76. Thompson, pp 183–186.)* Achieving the desired results when using the AEC depends on the selection of the correct subcomponents of the AEC and proper positioning and centering of the part of interest. An underexposed image is the result of premature termination of the exposure. Assuming the AEC is capable of optimum operation, underexposure may occur for the following reasons: minus density selection is made, incorrect sensor chamber is selected, there is insufficient back-up time, or there is incorrect positioning of the structure of interest over the selected sensor chamber. The density selections are available to make slight increases (plus density) or decreases (minus density) in radiographic density from the predetermined "normal" level (this is generally about 1.0 to 1.2_D). The center chamber should be selected for imaging of the spine (including L5–S1) in the lateral position. If a side chamber is selected, the radiation sampling would be of either the abdomen (anterior to the spine) or free air (posterior to the spine). The area of interest would be underexposed, especially so if no anatomic structure is over the selected sensor. The back-up time should be about twice that of the expected exposure time. If it is set at less than the expected exposure time, the image will be underexposed. Finally, the part of interest must be correctly positioned and centered over the sensor selected. This is especially important in the centering of the lateral spine. If the sensor is posterior to the spine, the lack of material to attenuate the beam will result in early termination of the exposure and an underexposed image. Running into minimum reaction time occurs when the part is very small or the kilovoltage is high, requiring the shortest possible exposure time, which still may be too much and cause an overexposed image.

227. The answer is A. *(Carlton, pp 502–507. Gray, p 102. NCRP No. 99, pp 74–76.)* The AEC device is employed to provide radiographs with consistent density regardless of part thickness or various disease processes that may alter the structure of the part. This does assume that the AEC is properly calibrated and the part correctly positioned and centered over the selected sensor chamber. The AEC will also compensate for the kilovoltage set by increasing exposure time (and patient dose) when lower than optimum kilovoltage is set and decreasing exposure time when high kilovoltage is set. The effect of beam penetrability (controlled by kilovoltage) on x-ray quantity is the reason for this influence. However, since image contrast is also influenced by beam penetration (as well as patient dose), the radiographer should make every effort to set the optimum kilovoltage for the part being radiographed. The AEC will not automatically adjust for varying screen speeds. It is calibrated for a specific screen speed expected to be used with that equipment. Some units have the ability to vary the sensitivity of the AEC for use with more than one speed screen. However, this requires manual selection by the operator.

228. The answer is D (1, 2, 3). *(Bushong, 5/e, pp 130–131, 337, 435. Carlton, pp 544–545.)* The AEC device may be commonly found on just about all types of imaging equipment including diagnostic, fluoroscopic, mammography, dedicated chest radiography, and angiography. The inclusion of AEC for mobile radiography is available as an option to routine mobile imaging. For these units, the sensor chambers are part of a paddle that is positioned behind the cassette during the imaging procedure. All AEC devices must be properly used and calibrated in order to gain the benefits possible. Annual evaluation of the AEC should be performed to ensure optimum operation.

229. The answer is D. *(Adler, pp 6–8. Bushong, 5/e, pp 325, 336, 352, 364. NCRP No. 102, p 13.)* Fluoroscopy is used for dynamic imaging, that is, to visualize motion. This imaging option is commonly employed to examine the gastrointestinal tract and the circulatory system, the latter as performed in angiography and cardiac catheterization. Tomography, computed tomography, and mammography are all types of radiographic imaging that employ specific equipment. Each results in a static, or stationary, image. Static images are also possible with fluoroscopic equipment.

230. The answer is B. *(Bushong, 5/e, pp 325, 344, 352, 364. Carlton, p 574. Carroll, 5/e, pp 393, 405, 414, 421.)* The technique that demonstrates an anatomic structure in sections is termed *body section radiography*, more commonly known as *tomography*. This technique employs controlled motion of the x-ray tube and image receptor to blur structures above and below a specific plane of interest. The structures located on the plane of interest will be in maximum focus. Varying the plane of interest allows the visualization of the structures in sections or layers. Computed tomography (CT) is a sophisticated, computer-assisted advancement of tomography. Fluoroscopy is an imaging technique that allows visualization of structures in motion (dynamic imaging). Cinefluorography employs a movie camera to record motion on film and is part of a system for imaging the coronary vessels. Xeroradiography, an imaging process commonly used for mammography in the late 1970s and 1980s, is not widely available today. The technique employed an imaging plate coated with a semiconductor material that was treated with an electrical charge prior to imaging. The exit beam would create an electrostatic image on the plate, which then went through a dry processing procedure to yield a hard copy image on plastic-coated paper. The highlight of this technique was the ability to demonstrate images with extremely wide latitude.

231. The answer is B. *(Bushong, 5/e, pp 328–330. Carlton, pp 557, 581–583. Carroll, 5/e, pp 417–419. Curry, 4/e, pp 247–252).* Assuming a variable-type fulcrum tomography unit is employed, the zero fulcrum level would be even with the table top. As the fulcrum level is raised, the focal plane moves from the posterior aspect of the body to the anterior. For this patient, the anterior surface of the body would be 25 cm from the table top. To image the area of interest, the fulcrum would need to be set at the level of 15 cm above the table. If the patient were in the prone position, the fulcrum setting would be 10 cm.

232. The answer is C. *(Carlton, pp 544–545, 549. Carroll, 5/e, p 387. Thompson, pp 190–191.)* Battery-operated mobile x-ray units are compact, cordless units that use large nickel-cadmium batteries as a power source for movement of the unit and x-ray production. The direct current from the batteries is converted to a form of AC by means of a DC chopper. (AC is the required form of power for transformer operation, which supplies the high voltage required for x-ray production.) The output result of this high-frequency (about 1000 pulses per second) waveform is equal to or slightly higher than three-phase, 12-pulse generators with minimal ripple factor. Half-wave generators suppress the flow of current during the second half of the AC cycle and thus have a very low output at only 60 pulses per second. Full-wave or single-phase units make use of both pulses per cycle, thus raising the frequency to 120 pulses per second. This still produces a 100 percent ripple factor. The capacitor-discharge generators produce a constant potential initially, which drops off to zero as the unit is discharged during use.

233. The answer is D. *(Carlton, pp 544–545, 549. Curry, 4/e, pp 51–52. Thompson, pp 190–191.)* Various types of generators are available to operate the mobile radiographic units. These include the battery-powered, capacitor-discharge units and medium- or high-frequency generators. Battery-powered units employ large nickel-cadmium batteries. The DC supplied by the batteries must be converted to AC or pulsed prior to reaching the high-tension transformer in order for the transformer to operate and produce the high voltage required for x-ray production. This is achieved by means of a DC chopper, which acts to interrupt the DC and creates a high-frequency pulse that is further increased by the transformer, producing an output equal to or higher than three-phase, 12-pulse generators. These units do not need to be plugged into an AC source during exposure. Between uses, however, they should be plugged in to recharge the batteries. Capacitor-discharge generators are charged to store a preset potential prior to use. During x-ray exposure, the capacitor discharges and produces a constant potential initially, which then drops at a rate of about 1 kV/mAs.

234. The answer is A. *(Bushong, 5/e, p 630. NCRP No. 102, pp 2–25.)* The basic requirements of all radiographic equipment (fixed and mobile) are the same. This includes requirements for total filtration, beam restriction, and protection against leakage radiation. The position of the exposure switch is the main difference between radiographic and mobile equipment. Fixed radiographic units have the control panel located behind a protective shield. The exposure switch must be positioned so as to require the operator to be behind the shield in order to make an exposure. Conversely, the exposure switch on mobile units must be attached to a cord that allows the operator to stand back a minimum of 6 feet when making the exposure. This is in compliance with the basic principles of radiation protection—minimize time and maximize distance and shielding.

235. The answer is D. *(Bushong, 5/e, pp 134–137. Curry, 4/e, p 42. Selman 8/e, pp 265–266, 270.)* The rectification system is connected between the secondary side of the high-tension transformer and the x-ray tube. Its function is to receive the high voltage and maintain the flow of current through the x-ray tube from cathode to anode. The components involved are solid-state diodes. There may be as few as one or two diodes for half-wave rectification, four diodes for full-wave (single-phase) generators, and six or twelve diodes for three-phase generators.

236. The answer is C. *(Bushong, 5/e, p 131. Curry, 4/e, pp 57–58.)* Automatic exposure controls (AECs) may be described according to their location in the imaging chain relative to the image receptor; that is, they may be located in front of (entrance) or behind (exit) the image receptor. Because of their small size and radiolucency, ionization chamber AECs are most commonly entrance types. Their position in front of the image receptor triggers the termination of the exposure when sufficient ionization has discharged a preset capacitor. The photomultiplier AECs may be used as either entrance or exit types. These devices consist of a radiolucent detector coated with a phosphor material to convert the exit beam to light. The light is then picked up by a photomultiplier, which converts the light to electrons and amplifies the signal. The current is used to charge a capacitor to a predetermined level at which point the exposure is terminated.

237. The answer is B. *(Bushong, 5/e, p 239. Curry, 4/e, p 93. Selman, 8/e, pp 411–415.)* Beam restriction devices are used to limit the size of the beam to the desired area of x-ray exposure, thus minimizing patient dose. These devices are attached to the x-ray tube housing at the point where primary radiation exits the tube. The components that act in this manner are diaphragms, cones (including flared and cylinder type), and collimators (variable aperture). Diaphragms are flat pieces of lead with a specific size and shape cut out in their center. They are placed close to the tube port to restrict the primary beam to the size and shape of the opening. Cones are flared or straight tubes of lead that are also mounted to the tube housing at the port, but extend below the tube. As with diaphragms, an assortment of cone sizes must be available to permit the desired field size for various examinations and patients. The most widely used type of beam restrictor is the collimator, which is a single device, permanently attached to the tube housing and capable of forming a full range of sizes in a square or rectangular shape to correspond to the various sizes of image receptors. Additionally, these devices include a light-localizing system to aid in centering the patient with the x-ray beam and the image receptor. Regardless of which type of beam restrictor is used, care must be taken to ensure that the size of the x-ray field is never larger than the size of the image receptor.

238. The answer is C (2, 3). *(Bushong, 5/e, p 243. Curry, 4/e, p 93. NCRP No. 99, p 194. Selman, 8/e, p 415.)* The variable-aperture collimator is the most widely used type of beam restrictor device. As its name implies, the opening can be changed to form any size square or rectangular field to suit the requirements of the examination. The components of a collimator include two sets of shutters, each with four leaded leaves that operate in pairs, longitudinally and transversely. The uppermost set of shutters is very close to the tube port and provides collimation of off-focus radiation, which contributes to poor recorded detail due to geometric blur. The second set of shutters is positioned at the lowest point in the collimator and is responsible for sizing the x-ray beam. The shutters may be controlled either manually or automatically. Also included in the collimator is a light localizing system that allows a light field, representative of the x-ray field, to be projected onto the patient for centering and alignment purposes. This system includes a mirror in the path of the x-ray beam and a light bulb off to the side. The mirror is positioned to reflect the light onto the patient. Accurate placement of the mirror is mandatory to ensure proper congruence between the light field and the field of exposure. Evaluation of the alignment should be conducted on a semiannual basis. Grids and filters are accessory devices with specific purposes different from those of beam restrictors. The common feature between them is that proper use of both beam restrictors and grids will yield improved radiographic contrast on the images, and both filters and beam restrictors will lower patient dose.

239. The answer is A (1, 2). *(Bushong, 5/e, pp 243–244. Curry, 4/e, p 93. Selman, 8/e p 415.)* The collimator device is more correctly termed a *variable-aperture* type of beam restrictor. As compared with cones and diaphragms, a single collimator is capable of producing a full range of field sizes in a square or rectangular shape. This is achieved by the ability to operate the shutters in pairs, longitudinally and transversely. If these shutters operated as one unit, only square fields could be produced. This size and shape flexibility is advantageous in matching the field of exposure to the size and shape of the image receptor. Earlier versions of the variable-aperture collimator had numerous lead leaves arranged in a circular fashion resembling the iris of a camera. The result was a circular field of exposure, like those produced by flared and cylindrical cones. Since all image receptors are square or rectangular, proper alignment of the circular field on the rectangular or square image receptor produced either areas of wasted film in order to include the entire field of exposure or overexposure of the patient to include the entire film area (see diagram below).

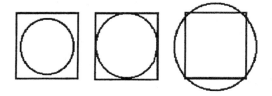

The size of the field of exposure should never be larger than the size of the image receptor.

240. The answer is D. *(Bushong, 5/e, pp 248–249. Selman, 8/e, p 389.)* Of the devices listed, only the grid will remove scattered radiation from the exit beam, which leaves the patient and exposes the image receptor. In order to do this, the grid is positioned between the patient and the image receptor. Beam restrictors lower the amount of scatter produced by limiting the volume of tissue irradiated, thus lowering the quantity of scattered radiation in the exit beam. Filters increase average beam energy by removing low-energy photons from the primary beam. Higher average beam energy results in a lower photoelectric:compton (PE:C) ratio; therefore, excessive filtration lowers radiographic contrast because of increased beam penetrability.

241. The answer is C. *(Carlton, p 559. Carroll, 5/e, p 395. Curry, 4/e, p 185. Gray, pp 126–127. NCRP No. 99, p 201.)* The quality of the fluoroscopic image is controlled by the level of x-ray exposure available to produce the light image within the image intensifier. Increased levels of exposure will impart more energy to the phosphors of the image intensifier and produce more illumination (a brighter image) and vice versa. As the patient changes position, the thickness of the tissue irradiated varies; this requires adjustment in the exposure factors (kilovoltage and milliamperage) to accommodate these changes and maintain a consistent level of image brightness. This function is performed for the operator by the automatic brightness control (ABC) system of the fluoroscopic unit. Evaluation of the ABC should be performed on a semiannual basis to ensure that proper levels of radiation exposure are not being exceeded. Automatic gain control systems are employed to adjust the video signal to maintain a proper level of image brightness on the TV monitor. This device does not alter the exposure factors. Automatic exposure control is used to terminate x-ray exposure during image recording on film or photospot cameras. Automatic beam limitation devices are generally available to properly size the x-ray beam to coincide with the size of the image receptor, but do not alter exposure factors.

242. The answer is B. *(Carlton, p 559. Carroll, 5/e, p 395. Curry, 4/e, p 185. Gray, pp 126–127.)* The *automatic brightness control (ABC)* is incorporated into the fluoroscopic unit to alter the exposure factors of kilovoltage or milliamperage as needed to accommodate variations in tissue thickness. This automatic adjustment will maintain an acceptable level of illumination of the image. The ABC will also directly influence the patient dose with the increases or decreases in exposure factors. The incorporation of the TV and video systems will also usually include an *automatic gain control (AGC)*, which adjusts the amplification of the video signal between the TV camera and monitor. Since the AGC does not alter exposure factors, increasing the gain level may produce more noise rather than image improvement. However, the AGC does respond more quickly than the ABC. The automatic termination of the exposure is controlled by the *automatic exposure control (AEC)* or phototimer, and restriction of the x-ray field may be automatically controlled by a *positive beam limitator*.

243. The answer is C. *(Carlton, p 559. Carroll, 5/e, p 395. Curry, 4/e, p 185. Gray, pp 126–127.)* Automatic brightness control (ABC) is required on equipment that employs an image intensifier, such as a fluoroscopic unit. Radiographic units such as those for dedicated chest or mammography examinations produce static images and require manual adjustment of exposure factors for subsequent images in altered positions. Computed tomography units produce a pulsed beam using high kilovoltage and milliamperage and image a section of tissue from angles all around the area of interest; thus, no change in patient position is required. The image is displayed on a cathode ray tube (CRT), and image enhancement is possible without changing the exposure to the patient.

244. The answer is A. *(Bushong, 5/e, p 352. Carroll, 5/e, p 396. Curry, 4/e, p 187.)* During fluoroscopy, the milliamperage is kept relatively low while the exposure time is long compared to routine radiographic imaging. The milliamperage used for fluoroscopy may range from 1 to 5 mA. This low level of current produces a very dim image, which is amplified by the use of image intensification. Minor adjustments in milliamperage are made by the automatic brightness controller to accommodate changes in the part thickness as the patient moves. Exposure time is directly controlled by the fluoroscopist, who must remain aware of the amount of time elapsing as this will directly influence patient dose. Five-minute timers must be set at the beginning of each fluoroscopic examination and reset if the examination exceeds the 5-min period.

245. The answer is D. *(Bushong, 5/e, pp 364. Carroll, 5/e, p 398. Curry, 4/e, p 187.)* The fluoroscopic monitoring of an examination is conducted at a low milliamperage level, ranging from 1 to 5 mA. When the fluoroscopic image is to be recorded, the milliamperage must be increased to the usual range for radiographic imaging: 200 to 400 mA. This is required to reduce the exposure time needed to produce an optimum image without motion blur. This increase in milliamperage is necessary for either traditional spot filming or photospot cameras.

246. The answer is D. *(Bushong, 5/e, p 364. Carroll, 5/e, pp 402–403. Curry, 4/e, p 187.)* Spot-film cameras (also known as photospot cameras) are commonly used in place of the traditional cassette-type spot film to record the fluoroscopic image. This camera uses either roll film in 70-, 90-, or 105-mm frame sizes or 100-mm cut film. Both roll and cut film cameras allow the rapid imaging of anatomic structures compared with cassette-type spot film, which must have sufficient time to move into proper position. Spot-film cameras employ a transport mechanism to advance each film frame for the next image. Roll film cameras offer the most rapid filming frequency of up to 12 frames per second. The smaller image format of the spot-film camera also reduces the patient's dose compared with cassette-type spot films. The spot-film camera is coupled with the image intensifier and receives its exposure from the output phosphor. A beam-splitting mirror is positioned between the TV and spot-film cameras, allowing a small portion (about 15 percent) of the light to go to the TV system and the remainder to expose the spot film. Cassette-type spot films are moved into position between the patient and the image intensifier and thus are directly exposed to x-rays.

247. The answer is C (1, 3). *(Bushong, 5/e, p 364. Carroll, 5/e, pp 402–403. Curry, 4/e, p 187.)* Both systems of recording the fluoroscopic image are widely available. Each has its advantages and disadvantages. For the characteristics listed, cassette-type spot films offer more efficient framing capability than spot-film cameras. Framing refers to utilization of the film frame with the image. Both cassette-type and spot-film cameras provide a film frame that is either square or rectangular. However, a better match of x-ray field to film frame is possible with the direct x-ray field, collimated to a square or rectangle, than with the fixed, round image provided by the output phosphor of the image intensifier for the spot-film cameras. The larger image format provided by the cassette-type spot film will also provide better resolution, based on the characteristics of screen speed and film-screen contact, than will spot-film cameras, whose resolution is determined by the image intensifier. However, the use of spot-film cameras can reduce the required exposure time, thus reducing motion blur and raising the resolution level. The most significant advantage of spot-film cameras over cassette types is their higher framing frequency, which allows for rapid imaging.

248. The answer is C (3, 4). *(Bushong, 5/e, pp 231–233, 444. Carroll, 5/e, pp 212, 482–483. Selman 8/e, pp 285–288.)* Artifacts that result from dirt or damage to screens or cassettes generally manifest as white, or low-density, areas due to the prevention of light from reaching the film. Such conditions as dirt or dust or chips on the screen surface would produce these low-density areas. Another common artifact is caused by poor film-screen contact due to damaged cassette hinges or frame, loss of integrity of the foam backing material, or the presence of a foreign object within the cassette. High-density artifacts may be the result of light leaks into the cassette, but these are random, not regularly occurring, marks. High-density crescent marks are most often caused by fingernails and rough handling of the film. Regularly occurring marks are generally the result of a problem with the transport system of the automatic processor.

249. The answer is D (1, 2, 3). *(NCRP No. 99, pp 183–185.)* Artifacts are images of objects within or around the anatomic structure of interest that are not part of that structure. This includes any occurrence within the imaging chain that obscures optimum visualization of the structures. The list of possible sources of artifacts is very long and includes all the situations listed in this question. Any component within the imaging chain that is likely to retain dirt or debris must be cleaned on a regular basis and whenever artifacts are noted. This includes cleaning of image receptors, inside (for dirt and dust) as well as outside (dirt, dried blood, or contrast media on the cassette front), as well as cleaning of the radiographic table or upright bucky. Each of these factors will obstruct either the exit x-ray beam or light from the intensifying screens, resulting in an area of no exposure and failure to demonstrate an anatomic structure. Any removable object on the patient should be removed, e.g., jewelry, dentures, and clothing with buttons or snaps. A patient who arrives with bandages or an immobilization device must be radiographed as is, unless the removal of such materials is authorized by the referring physician. When these devices cannot be removed, their presence should be noted on the requisition for the radiologist's reference.

250. The answer is D. *(Bushong, 5/e, pp 139–141. Selman, 8/e, p 216.)* The exposure control of modern x-ray units is a two-stage switch that accelerates the rotor mechanism of the rotating anode up to speed and then allows the actual exposure of x-rays. Proper operation of the x-ray tube requires the target disk to be rotating at full speed before the exposure is made. If the exposure is made too soon, the heat load will be deposited over a small area, possibly pitting or melting the disk surface. However, holding the switch at the rotor stage can be harmful to the tube also. Such excessive "boost" or preparation times are common when trying to make an exposure at a precise moment as required with infants. The problem with this practice is the increased heating of the filament, which leads to vaporization of the filament, thinning of its diameter, and eventual breakage of the thin wire. The life of the rotor bearings also decreases with increased rotor operation. Therefore, the excessive preparation time may ultimately lead to bearing damage and unstable target rotation. Increased heat loads to the target, as a result of high tube currents, long exposures, and repeated exposures without sufficient cooling, can lead to vaporization of the target and tungsten plating on the glass envelope. A loss of tube vacuum due to a crack in the glass envelope can be caused by excessive heating of the tube insert or, more commonly, an interruption in the electrical balance within the tube due to arcing caused by the buildup of tungsten on the wall of the glass envelope.

251–254. The answers are 251-A, 252-B, 253-B, 254-A. *(Bushong, 5/e, pp 141–142. Curry, 4/e, pp 20–22. NCRP No. 99, p 68. Selman, 8/e, pp 217–219.)* Radiographic tube rating charts are employed to determine the safety of a selected combination of exposure factors for a specific x-ray tube. Each x-ray tube manufactured and installed will come with its own rating chart based on the specific characteristics of that tube. Rating charts should also be consulted to determine the proper operation of the overload protection circuit. To determine the safety of the exposure factors in these questions, first locate the correct chart according to the focal spot size used: chart A for small (0.6 mm) and chart B for large (1.2 mm). Next locate the exposure time and kilovoltage peak on the vertical and horizontal axes and follow their respective lines to the point of intersection. The milliamperage stations represented by the curves *above* that point are safe for this combination of time and kilovoltage peak. The milliamperage curves *below* that point are unsafe.

255–259. The answers are 255-D, 256-B, 257-B, 258-C, 259-E. *(Bushong, 5/e, p 116. Curry, 4/e, p 16. Selman, 8/e, p 212.)* The numbered components on the diagram are as follows: (1) rotor component of the induction motor, which rotates the target disk during tube operation; (2) anode stem, which supports the target disk on rotating target tubes; (3) target disk, which is the site of electron bombardment; (4) filament, which heats up to emit electrons; (5) focusing cup, which restricts the electrons from spreading out as they travel to the anode; (6) cathode assembly; (7) glass envelope, which forms a vacuum around the tube components; and (8) window of glass envelope, which allows primary photons out of the tube assembly.

260–264. The answers are 260-B, 261-C, 262-E, 263-D, 264-A. *(Bushong, 5/e, pp 107–109. Carlton, pp 73, 124–125, 130–131. Curry, 4/e, pp 48–50. Thompson, pp 99–100, 114–115, 168–169, 178–182.)* Electric current is either direct or alternating. Direct current (DC) is described as the flow of current in one direction at a constant peak potential. The battery is the primary source of DC. This waveform starts at zero and rises to its peak potential (determined by the source) and stays at the voltage level until power is interrupted, at which time voltage returns to zero. This waveform has no ripple, no drop in voltage, and thus no changing magnetic field (as needed to operate a transformer).

Alternating current (AC) is always reversing the direction of current flow, causing the EMF to increase and decrease in the process. Like DC, AC increases from zero potential to a peak voltage level, but instead of maintaining that level, it immediately begins to decrease back to zero. At this point, the polarity of the terminals reverses and current flows in the opposite direction, again to a peak level, then dropping back to zero. The waveform created by this changing flow of current is referred to as a *sine* wave. For each cycle of AC, one positive pulse (above the graph line) and one negative pulse (below the line) are created. The standard frequency of AC is 60 cycles per second, 2 pulses per cycle, for a total of 120 pulses per second. In terms of x-ray production, the basic AC waveform is very inefficient. X-rays may only be produced during the positive pulse of the cycle (when electrons are flowing from cathode to anode). Also, it has a ripple factor of 100 percent. As the voltage rises to a peak potential and then decreases back to zero, very low-energy x-rays or no x-rays are being produced. As the voltage nears the peak level, x-rays of sufficient energy will be produced. Full-wave, *single-phase* rectification of this waveform inverts the negative pulse to a positive pulse for more efficient x-ray production. This modification produces a waveform that represents pulsating DC. *Three-phase* power is generated to produce an even more efficient source of x-rays. It is commonly used in many radiographic units and is achieved by supplying three separate lines of voltage, each slightly out of synchrony with the others. The net result is 6 to 12 pulses of current per cycle instead of 2 pulses per cycle as with basic AC. The frequency is still 60 Hz, so the total number of pulses is 360 to 720 per second. The effect of three-phase power on the waveform will be less ripple (13.5 to 3.5 percent compared with 100 percent) and a flow of current that maintains a near constant potential difference (less voltage drop). The source of input voltage to the autotransformer is the *incoming line voltage*, which is supplied by the electrical service to the radiographic room. In the U.S., the standard electrical service used for radiographic equipment has a frequency of 60 Hz at about 220 V. This voltage supplied to the autotransformer will then increase or decrease as determined by the kilovoltage peak selector. The output voltage from the autotransformer will become the input voltage to the primary coil of the high-tension transformer. (See figure in answer 223.)

265–270. The answers are 265-D, 266-D, 267-A, 268-C, 269-D, 270-C. *(Bushong, 5/e, pp 430–431, 433, 439–443, 627. Carlton, pp 442, 444–446. NCRP No. 99, pp 46–55, 61–64, 69–73, 191–196.)* Quality control procedures should be performed on specific components of the radiographic imaging system on a schedule determined by (1) the significance each component has on image quality, (2) the complexity of the test procedure, and (3) the likelihood of a variance to occur. Monitoring and maintenance of the film processor is the best example of the advantages to be achieved by a consistent quality control routine. Every image is subjected to the ups and downs of the processor. There are numerous systems within the processor that affect the final image. By ensuring optimum operation of the processor, it ceases to be a factor in poor image quality. For this reason, the processor should be monitored on a daily basis and adjusted to optimum operating levels before any images are processed. This will significantly reduce the number of repeat images and save on patient exposure and use of equipment and supplies. Once established, the daily monitoring process requires very little time and can avoid costly downtime.

Evaluation of the collimator should be performed at least twice a year or whenever the x-ray tube or collimator has been serviced. Such items as the alignment of the x-ray to light fields or x-ray to image receptor, central ray perpendicularity, and accuracy of the PBL can be evaluated with this procedure. The light field, used for centering, is projected via a mirror mounted in the collimator, which can be misaligned by rough handling or jarring of the tube head. Problems with alignment of the x-ray and light field will be evidenced by "cone-cutting" of structures supposedly included in the light field. A simple means of evaluation is placing a cassette in the bucky, centering it to the beam, adjusting the light field to be smaller than the film size, and then placing a penny on each of the four corners of the light field and one in the center marking the central ray. The film is then exposed and processed. Evaluation of the image should demonstrate each of the pennies equidistant from the edges of the film and the exposed area of the film located in the center of the film. The acceptable limit for variation is ± 2 percent of the SID. This translates to 2 cm of variation for a 100-cm (40-inch) SID.

The control of darkroom fog is necessary to prevent increased levels of base plus fog density on the unexposed film and to ensure a safe environment for the handling of all film. The primary sources of fog in the darkroom include improper "safelights" and white light leaks. Evaluation of the darkroom, particularly the safelights, should occur twice a year and whenever the safelights have been serviced. Safelights need to be checked for proper type of filter, correct wattage of light bulbs, and correct color for the types of film being handled in a particular darkroom. A simple method to determine the presence of safelight fog uses a piece of film that has received a minimum exposure to radiation in order to sensitize the film. Turn off all lights, including safelights, and place the exposed film on the work counter with half of it covered with a sheet of cardboard. This half of the film will remain covered during the rest of the test. A second piece of cardboard covers three-fourths of the uncovered side of the film. The safelights are turned on. After 1 min of safelight exposure, the second cardboard is lowered to uncover half of the test side of the film. This process is repeated twice more, for a total of four sections of the uncovered side of the film being exposed to the safelights for 4, 3, 2, and 1 min. The safelight-exposed half of the film is then compared with the unexposed half. Density levels should not be greater than 0.05 for the section representing 1 min of safelight exposure and preferably for the section exposed 2 min.

Evaluation of the kilovoltage peak stations should be conducted on an annual basis or any time the x-ray generator has been serviced. This is to ensure that the kilovoltage being selected is what is being applied between the terminals within the x-ray tube. Changes in kilovoltage peak affect the quality of the beam produced, which in turn influences patient dose and image contrast. A technologist may perform a noninvasive evaluation of various kilovoltage stations with a kilovoltage peak test cassette, such as the Wisconsin or Ardran-Crooks test cassettes. Diagnostic equipment should be calibrated to provide actual kilovoltage peak levels with ± 4 kilovoltage peak of the selected kilovoltage station.

The evaluation of beam quality provides information regarding the filtration levels of the x-ray tube, assuming the kilovoltage is properly calibrated. Filtration is an important factor to monitor because of its influence on patient dose. Insufficient levels of filtration will increase a patient's skin dose. A minimal-to-moderate increase in filtration will decrease patient dose without influencing image quality. Filtration is evaluated by determining the HVL at one or more kilovoltage stations and this should be performed at least annually and whenever the x-ray tube or collimator has been serviced. HVL is found by recording output levels in milliroentgens while introducing increasing amounts of aluminum sheets into the x-ray beam. By charting these values, one can determine the amount of filter material (aluminum) required to reduce the beam intensity to half its original value. For diagnostic tubes able to operate at 70 kV or higher, the minimum HVL should be 2.3 mm of aluminum when using the 80 kV station. Specific HVLs for other kilovoltage stations are available for a more thorough evaluation of the tube's filtration.

Exposure linearity is the ability to produce the same level of output in milliroentgens (within ± 10 percent) for a specific milliampere-second value using various milliamperage and time stations. The noninvasive method of evaluation requires using a dosimeter and recording the output values (in milliroentgens) for exposures made at the various milliamperage stations. These data can provide information regarding the calibration of the milliamperage stations, assuming the exposure times are accurate. If the time stations are not accurate, linearity may still be determined by keeping the same time stop, varying the milliamperage (yielding different milliampere-second values), and then finding the milliroentgen per milliampere-second value for analysis of linearity. For either method, the acceptable limit for variation is ± 10 percent for consecutive milliamperage stations. Evaluation of linearity should be performed at least annually and whenever the x-ray generator or control panel has been serviced. When possible, more frequent monitoring of radiographic components will alert personnel to important changes at an earlier point than will adhering to the minimum frequency schedule.

271–275. The answers are 271-C, 272-A, 273-D, 274-B, 275-B. (*Bushong, 5/e, pp 431–433. Carroll, 5/e, pp 357–359, 362, 365, 368. NCRP No. 99, pp 63, 69–70, 73.*) An important component of any quality assurance program is the analysis of data obtained from the quality control test procedures. All acquired data should be compared against the standards for each piece of equipment and the recommended range of variation. Any component found to be out of tolerance must be corrected and retested. The range of variation differs for each component:

Component	Tolerance
SID indicator, light field/x-ray field alignment, center x-ray field/image receptor	±2% of SID
Exposure timers, exposure reproducibility, kilovoltage peak	±5% of selected value
Exposure linearity, room-to-room output consistency	±10% of selected value
Focal spot size	+50% of stated size

276–279. The answers are 276-B, 277-C, 278-D, 279-A. *(Bushong, 5/e, pp 232, 431–432. Carroll, 5/e, pp 359–363, 370, 373.)* The test tools available for the technologist's use in performing quality control procedures are of the noninvasive type. The Wisconsin test cassette and Ardran-Crooks test cassette are available for the evaluation of beam energy. Specific data pertaining to both the kilovoltage peak setting and HVL can be derived with these tools. A wire mesh device is used to evaluate the level of film-screen contact by demonstrating localized areas of blurriness in the mesh pattern. The focal spot may be evaluated using the pinhole camera or a star resolution pattern. The star resolution pattern is the more accurate of the two. The exposure linearity of an x-ray unit is evaluated through its ability to produce a consistent level of output for a specified milliampere-second value. This is determined by using a dosimeter and recording the output values for various milliamperage and time combinations that produce the same milliampere-second value.

280–283. The answers are 280-B, 281-A, 282-D, 283-C. *(Bushong, 5/e, p 437. Carlton, pp 450–452. Carroll, 5/e, pp 350–355. NCRP No. 99, pp 26–28.)* In order to obtain a realistic assessment of the repeat rate for an imaging department, the repeat analysis should be conducted for at least 1 month, preferably up to 3 months. During this monitoring period, all discarded films are kept and categorized according to the reason for their being discarded. Also the total number of films processed should be tracked using counters fitted to the processor feed tray. These devices tally the number of films entering the process. This number should be recorded on a weekly basis and then the counter reset to zero. To determine the total repeat percentage, the total number of discarded films is divided by the total number of films processed, and the result is multiplied by 100. To find the percentages for various causes of repetition, the individual repeat number is divided by the total number of films processed. For the data provided in this question, the following calculations should be performed:

Total repeat percentage:
    Total number of discarded films = 163
    $163/1542 = 0.1057 \times 100 = 10.57\%$
Repeat percentage for positioning errors:
    $28/1542 = 0.018 \times 100 = 1.8\%$
Repeat percentage for overexposure errors:
    $68/1542 = 0.044 \times 100 = 4.4\%$
Repeat percentage for underexposure errors:
    $60/1542 = 0.0389 \times 100 = 3.89\%$
Repeat percentage for artifacts:
    $7/1542 = 0.0045 \times 100 = 0.45\%$
Repeat percentage for all exposure errors:
    $60 + 68 = 128/1542 = 0.083 \times 100 = 8.3\%$

284–290. The answers are 284-B, 285-A, 286-C, 287-C, 288-A, 289-A, 290-B. *(Bushong, 5/e, pp 231–232. Carlton, pp 335–337. Carroll, 5/e, pp 372–373. NCRP No. 99, pp 79–81, 198.)* In addition to the radiographic unit itself, all ancillary equipment involved in the imaging process must be evaluated for identification of problems that may cause suboptimum images and require repeat exposures. In film-screen imaging systems, the areas to be monitored are cleanliness and general condition of screens and cassettes and the level of film-screen contact.

Cassettes are designed to hold the intensifying screens and provide protection of the film from white light. Modern cassettes are made of lightweight, radiolucent plastic. The curved design of the cassette, when open, promotes the elimination of air from within the cassette during closure and ensures complete contact between the film and screen surfaces. In addition, the screens are mounted on foam backing to further aid in adequate film-screen contact. Breakdown of this padding, the presence of air bubbles, or damage to the cassette frame or hinges can contribute to areas of poor film-screen contact. This will be evident on radiographic images as areas of blurriness or loss of recorded detail. Evaluation of film-screen contact should be performed at least annually or whenever poor contact is suspected. Evaluation requires the imaging of a patterned test object, such as a wire mesh, placed in contact with the cassette. The image is then viewed on a viewbox. Poor contact will be seen as localized areas of blurriness of greater density than the surrounding, sharp areas.

Monitoring should be done to eliminate the influence of artifacts on the radiographs. Artifacts arising from the imaging system are most commonly the result of dirt particles on the screen surface. Dirt on the cassette surface will also obstruct the exit beam and create unwanted images on the radiograph. Cassette fronts should be cleaned whenever something is spilled onto them or other dirt is noted. Screen surfaces should be routinely cleaned with an antistatic solution and nonabrasive cleaning pad, especially when numerous white specks are noted on images. The screens need to be allowed to air dry before refilling with film. Rough handling and the repeated action of loading and unloading cassettes with film can result in pitting of the screen surface or embedded dirt particles. Scanning the surface with an ultraviolet light will show such imperfections more readily. Screens with serious imperfections should be replaced.

Each screen type purchased and in use in a radiology department is selected according to its speed factor for the specific type of examinations to be performed. Medium- and fast-speed screens are constructed with a reflective layer that contributes to the white appearance of the screen. (Slow- or detail-speed screens have a dye added instead of the reflective layer, producing a yellow appearance.) Over time, the screens may discolor or become stained, changing their white appearance to yellow. This change will act to reduce light emissions from the screen and lower its speed factor. Screens of the same type of speed need to be compared with each other for loss of speed. This is done by making an exposure of a test object (penetrometer) with the same radiographic equipment, film from the same box, and the same processor. A specified area on each image is then measured with a densitometer. Density variations should not exceed 0.05. Fogged film can be the result of numerous problems, including improper storage, inadequate safelights, and structurally damaged cassettes.

291–295. The answers are 291-D, 292-C, 293-A, 294-D, 295-B. *(Bushong, 5/e, pp 325–328, 330. Carlton, pp 576–579. Carroll, 5/e, pp 414–417.)* The tomographic principle is based on the use of motion to create blurring of structures outside a specific plane of interest while the structures of interest are kept in focus. The tube and image receptor are the objects that move (except in autotomography, in which the patient moves) in opposite directions around a pivot point referred to as the fulcrum. The *fulcrum* may be stationary or variable (most common). It is also the location of the plane of interest, referred to as the *focal plane*. Any structures located at this level will be in focus. In order to image an entire structure in sections, there must be a means of changing the relationship between the anatomic structure and the fulcrum. The simplest method employs a variable fulcrum mechanism to adjust the fulcrum to various levels within the anatomic structure. Fixed fulcrum units require a means of moving the patient vertically to align the structures to be imaged with the fulcrum. The *angle or amplitude* is described as the path the tube travels during the tomographic motion. The term can be further subdivided to specify two paths of travel: the exposure angle and the tomographic angle. The tomographic angle is wider and refers to the entire distance the tube travels. The exposure angle is less than the tomographic angle and refers to the distance the tube moves while the actual x-ray exposure is being made. The proper sequence of tube motion and exposure should be as follows: the tube begins to move, exposure starts, exposure stops, the tube stops moving. Since the motion is in an arc, it is described in terms of an angle (wide to narrow). The width of the angle/amplitude determines the thickness of the section in focus and influences the quality of the blur produced. Wider angles will yield a thinner section in focus and vice versa. They will also create a better blurring effect of the structures outside the focal plane and will require increased exposure time in order to complete their travel. Angles of 10° or less are referred to as *zonograms* and are used for tomographic imaging of relatively thick anatomic structures, e.g., kidneys.

296–300. The answers are 296-A, 297-D, 298-C, 299-D, 300-A. *(Bushong, 5/e, pp 328–330. Carlton, pp 577, 581–583. Carroll, 5/e, pp 417–419. Curry, 4/e, pp 247–252.)* Linear tomography is the simplest type of motion available and can be adapted to a routine radiographic unit fairly easily. The amplitude can be varied with linear tomography, providing a wide range of section thicknesses to best image various body structures. Narrow angle linear motion will produce the thickest section and should be used to image large structures with low subject contrast, such as the kidneys during IVU procedures. The quality of the tomographic image is greatly dependent on how well the structures outside the focal plane are blurred. The factors that influence blur quality are the type of motion (the more complex, the better), the distance of the structures from the fulcrum and from the image receptor (the greater the distance, the better, for both of these), and the direction of the long axis of the structure relative to the direction the tube travels (the closer to 90°, the better). These conditions are best met by the hypocycloidal motion. This complex motion has a wide angle of 48° and thus produces very thin sections of about 1 mm, which makes it effective for imaging the small, bony structures of the inner auditory canals. Phantom artifacts, which do not represent any real anatomic structure, may be created by some tomography motions, especially the circular motion.

Production and Evaluation of the Image

STANDARD DEFINITIONS—RADIOGRAPHY EXAMINATION*

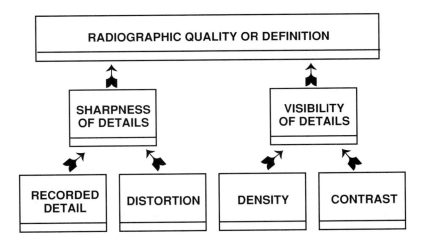

RECORDED DETAIL — is the sharpness of the structural lines as recorded in the radiographic image.

DISTORTION — is the misrepresentation of the size or shape of a structure recorded in the radiographic image.

Size Distortion or magnification is the enlargement of the recorded image as compared to the actual size of the structure.

Shape Distortion is the misrepresentation (elongated or fore-shortened) of the shape of the structure recorded as compared to the actual shape of the structure.

DENSITY — Radiographic density is the degree of blackening or opacity of an area in a radiograph due to the accumulation of black metallic silver following exposure and processing of a film.

$$\text{Density} = \text{Log}\frac{\text{incident light intensity}}{\text{transmitted light intensity}}$$

*©1990 The American Registry of Radiologic Technologists

CONTRAST — Radiographic contrast is defined as the visible differences between any two selected areas of density levels within the radiographic image.

           Contrast — Scale of Contrast refers to the number of densities visible (or the number of shades of gray).

           Long Scale is the term used when slight differences between densities are present (low contrast) but the total number of densities is increased.

           Short Scale is the term used when considerable or major differences between densities are present (high contrast) but the total number of densities is reduced.

FILM CONTRAST — is the inherent ability of the film emulsion to react to radiation and record a range of densities.

FILM LATITUDE — is the inherent ability of the film to record a long range of density levels on the radiograph.

           Film latitude and film contrast depend upon the sensitometric properties of the film and the processing conditions and is determined directly from the characteristic H and D curve.

EXPOSURE LATITUDE — is the range of exposure factors which will produce a diagnostic radiograph.

SUBJECT CONTRAST — is the difference in the quantity of radiation transmitted by a particular part as a result of the different absorption characteristics of the tissues and structures making up that part.

DIRECTIONS: Each numbered question or incomplete statement below contains lettered responses. Select the **one best** response.

301. Long-scale contrast would be most correctly defined as

    (A) increased difference between adjacent densities
    (B) narrow latitude
    (C) high contrast
    (D) many shades of gray

302. Which of the following pertain to long-scale radiographic contrast?
    1. It is produced by low kilovoltage
    2. It produces many shades of gray
    3. It produces small differences between adjacent densities

    (A) 1 & 2
    (B) 2 & 3
    (C) 1 & 3
    (D) 1, 2, & 3

303. What effect will beam penetrability have on radiographic contrast?

    (A) Increased kilovoltage will decrease contrast
    (B) Increased kilovoltage will increase contrast
    (C) Kilovoltage has no influence on contrast

304. The effect of scattered radiation in the exit beam will cause an increase in

    (A) recorded detail
    (B) density
    (C) contrast
    (D) magnification

305. The use of high kilovoltage peak techniques would result in:
    1. Lower patient dose
    2. Increased contrast
    3. Increased scatter fog

    (A) 1 & 2
    (B) 2 & 3
    (C) 1 & 3
    (D) 1, 2, & 3

306. What radiographic quality factor would be most affected by an excessive amount of geometric blur?

    (A) Radiographic density
    (B) Radiographic contrast
    (C) Recorded detail
    (D) Distortion

307. Which of the following test devices would provide a means of evaluating recorded detail of an image?

    (A) Densitometer
    (B) Resolution grid
    (C) Sensitometer
    (D) Pinhole camera

308. Which of the following factors will improve recorded detail?

    (A) Long OID
    (B) Long SID
    (C) Large focal spot
    (D) An angle of 30° on the x-ray tube

309. The ratio of SID to SOD is used to determine

    (A) density level
    (B) average gradient
    (C) geometric blur
    (D) magnification factor

310. What is the magnification factor for imaging conditions that include 12 mm focal spot, 40 inches SID, 5 inches OID, and 10° caudad tube tilt?

    (A) 0.15
    (B) 1.14
    (C) 5
    (D) 8

311. Which set of conditions will produce an image with the greatest magnification percentage?

    (A) 20 inches SID, 1 inch OID
    (B) 40 inches SID, 3 inches OID
    (C) 50 inches SID, 5 inches OID
    (D) 60 inches SID, 5 inches OID

312. What is the controlling factor of radiographic density?

    (A) Kilovoltage
    (B) Milliampere-seconds
    (C) SID
    (D) Focal-spot size

313. Which of the following has a *direct* effect on radiographic density?

    (A) Processing temperature
    (B) SID
    (C) Collimation
    (D) Grids

314. Which of the following factors would influence the quality of the x-ray beam?

    (A) Kilovoltage and milliampere-seconds
    (B) Focal-spot size and filtration
    (C) SID and milliampere-seconds
    (D) Kilovoltage and filtration

315. All the following factors will affect the quantity of x-rays in the primary beam EXCEPT

    (A) kilovoltage
    (B) focal-spot size
    (C) milliampere-seconds
    (D) filtration

316. The role of compensating filters is to

    (A) increase contrast
    (B) provide uniform penetration of varied anatomic structures
    (C) reduce patient exposure to unnecessary radiation
    (D) ensure that only the part of interest is exposed to radiation

317. Radiographic density will increase by varying

    (A) kilovolts from 80 to 92
    (B) SID from 40 to 56 inches
    (C) focal-spot size from large to small
    (D) milliampere-seconds from 25 to 12

318. What is the relationship between milliampere-seconds and density?

    (A) Direct, but not proportionate
    (B) Inverse, but not proportionate
    (C) Directly proportionate
    (D) Inversely proportionate

319. What is the relationship between kilovoltage and radiographic density?

    (A) Direct, but not proportionate
    (B) Inverse, but not proportionate
    (C) Directly proportionate
    (D) Inversely proportionate

320. Which of the following combinations of exposure factors will produce approximately the same density as 32 mAs, 70 kV?

    (A) 64 mAs, 80 kV
    (B) 64 mAs, 60 kV
    (C) 32 mAs, 60 kV
    (D) 16 mAs, 60 kV

321. Which combinations of technical factors would provide an image with higher contrast than that produced by 12 mAs and 92 kV, but maintain the original density?

    (A) 25 mAs, 92 kV
    (B) 50 mAs, 78 kV
    (C) 50 mAs, 66 kV
    (D) 12 mAs, 78 kV

322. The exposure factors of 300 mA, 0.017 s, and 79 kV would produce a milliampere-second value of

    (A) 5
    (B) 50
    (C) 500
    (D) 5000

323. How much of an adjustment in milliampere-seconds must be made in order to perceive a change in radiographic density?

    (A) 15 percent
    (B) 30 percent
    (C) 50 percent
    (D) 70 percent

324. A radiographic image is underexposed, but the object was sufficiently penetrated. The correct change in technical factors would be to

(A) increase kilovoltage
(B) decrease SID
(C) increase processing temperature
(D) increase milliampere-seconds

325. The controlling factors of magnification are

(A) angulation of the central ray and SID
(B) OID and focal-spot size
(C) focal-spot size and angulation of the central ray
(D) SID and OID

326. If a linear structure is positioned with its long axis parallel to the plane of the image receptor and the central ray is angled 30° cephalad, what radiographic effect will occur?

(A) Increased density
(B) Increased magnification
(C) Elongation of the part
(D) Foreshortening of the part

327. What is the optimum relationship between the central ray, the body part of interest, and the image receptor in order to produce minimal shape distortion on a radiograph?

(A) Part perpendicular to image receptor, with central ray parallel to image receptor
(B) Central ray, part, and image receptor all parallel to each other
(C) Part parallel to image receptor, with central ray perpendicular to part
(D) Central ray and image receptor parallel to each other, with part perpendicular to central ray

328. The definition of *grid radius* is the

(A) number of lead strips per inch (or centimeter)
(B) height of the lead strips to the distance between them
(C) height of the lead strips to the thickness of the lead strips
(D) SID at which a grid may be used

329. The correct definition of *grid ratio* is the

(A) number of lead strips per inch (or centimeter)
(B) height of the lead strips to the distance between them
(C) height of the lead strips to the thickness of the lead strips
(D) SID at which a grid may be used

330. *Grid frequency* is defined as

(A) number of lead strips per inch (or centimeter)
(B) height of the lead strips to the distance between them
(C) height of the lead strips to the thickness of the lead strips
(D) SID at which a grid may be used

331. The grid type with the widest range of grid radius is the

(A) 10:1 crossed, focused
(B) 8:1 linear, focused
(C) 16:1 rhombic, focused
(D) 10:1 linear, parallel

332. What effect will the use of a grid versus no grid have on radiographic quality?

(A) Increase in density and contrast
(B) Decrease in density and contrast
(C) Increase in density and decrease in contrast
(D) Decrease in density and increase in contrast

333. The following original technical factors were used to produce a satisfactory radiograph: 500 mA, 0.012 s, 80 kV, 40 inches SID, 8:1 grid. What change in exposure factors would be needed to compensate for the use of a 16:1 grid?

    (A)   500 mA, 0.024 s, 90 kV
    (B)   500 mA, 0.008 s, 80 kV
    (C)   300 mA, 0.03 s, 80 kV
    (D)   300 mA, 0.013 s, 70 kV

334. Which grid ratio will provide the greatest contrast improvement?

    (A)   5:1
    (B)   8:1
    (C)   12:1
    (D)   16:1

335. The criteria for grid use include:
    1. High kilovoltage (>70)
    2. Thick body parts (>10 cm)
    3. Barium studies

    (A)   1 & 2
    (B)   2 & 3
    (C)   1 & 3
    (D)   1, 2, & 3

336. The improper use of a grid may result in the absorption of primary radiation and is known as grid

    (A)   selectivity
    (B)   clean up
    (C)   cutoff
    (D)   improvement

337. Which of the following types of grids would have the most positioning latitude?

    (A)   5:1 linear, parallel
    (B)   8:1 crossed, parallel
    (C)   16:1 crossed, focused
    (D)   10:1 linear, focused

338. A grid constructed with 200 lines per inch would be considered

    (A)   low frequency
    (B)   high frequency
    (C)   low ratio
    (D)   high ratio

339. In addition to the use of a grid, other techniques or devices that will increase radiographic contrast include:
    1. Collimation devices
    2. Air-gap technique
    3. Compensating filters

    (A)   1 & 2
    (B)   2 & 3
    (C)   1 & 3
    (D)   1, 2, & 3

340. Materials used for the interspace in a grid have included:
    1. Lead
    2. Cardboard
    3. Aluminum

    (A)   1 only
    (B)   2 & 3
    (C)   1 & 3
    (D)   1, 2, & 3

341. What is the primary purpose for using intensifying screens in film-screen radiography?

    (A)   Improve recorded detail
    (B)   Increase image contrast
    (C)   Decrease patient dose
    (D)   Decrease processing time

342. A screen's *spectral emission* refers to

    (A)   the quantity of light a phosphor will produce
    (B)   the color of light a phosphor will produce
    (C)   screen lag or afterglow
    (D)   the range of x-ray energies to which the phosphor is sensitive

343. Changing from an intensifying screen with a relative speed of 50 to one with a relative speed of 200 will result in an increase in

    (A)   contrast
    (B)   recorded detail
    (C)   density
    (D)   magnification

344. Recorded detail will decrease when using intensifying screens constructed with a

(A) small phosphor size
(B) thin active layer
(C) reflective layer
(D) light-absorbing dye

345. Those characteristics that make rare-earth phosphors more efficient for intensifying screen purposes than calcium tungstate include:
1. Better spectral matching
2. Higher absorption efficiency
3. Higher conversion efficiency

(A) 1 & 2
(B) 2 & 3
(C) 1 & 3
(D) 1, 2, 3

346. The construction of intensifying screens commonly includes

(A) silver halide crystals, gelatin, polyester base, reflective layer
(B) polyester base, phosphor crystals, reflective layer, protective coating
(C) cardboard base, silver halide crystals, adhesive, supercoating
(D) aluminum base, phosphor crystals, light absorbing dye, supercoating

347. What is the relationship between relative screen speed and radiographic density?

(A) Inversely proportional
(B) Directly proportional
(C) Inverse, but not proportional
(D) Direct, but not proportional

348. Which of the following expresses the relationship between relative screen speed (RS) and milliampere-seconds in order to produce equal film density?

(A) $mAs_o / mAs_n = SID_o / SID_n$
(B) $mAs_o / mAs_n = SID_n / SID_o$
(C) $mAs_o / mAs_n = RS_o / RS_n$
(D) $mAs_o / mAs_n = RS_n / RS_o$

349. Which of the following will produce the greatest film density?

(A) 200 RS screen, 400 mA, 0.012 s, 70 kV
(B) 400 RS screen, 400 mA, 12.5 ms, 70 kV
(C) 200 RS screen, 800 mA, 0.006 s, 70 kV
(D) 400 RS screen, 600 mA, 6 ms, 70 kV

350. A radiographic exam was optimally performed using technical factors of 12 mAs, 80 kV, 40 inches SID, 8:1 grid, and 200 RS screen. What new factors would be needed to maintain density if the screen was changed to 600 RS?

(A) 4 mAs, 80 kV, 40 inches SID, 8:1 grid
(B) 12 mAs, 80 kV, 36 inches SID, 8:1 grid
(C) 12 mAs, 70 kV, 40 inches SID, 8:1 grid
(D) 12 mAs, 80 kV, 40 inches SID, 5:1 grid

351. What new milliampere-second value would be needed to produce the same density results if an original 32 mAs was used with a 50 RS screen and screens were changed to 400 RS?

(A) 4 mAs
(B) 40 mAs
(C) 175 mAs
(D) 256 mAs

352. What effect, if any, does kilovoltage have on screen speed?

(A) An increase in kilovoltage will increase screen speed
(B) An increase in kilovoltage will decrease screen speed
(C) Screen speed is not influenced by kilovoltage selection

353. The spectral emission of calcium tungstate phosphors is in what range?

(A) Yellow-green
(B) Blue-ultraviolet
(C) Blue-green
(D) Yellow-amber

354. Which of the following light photons has the highest energy level?

(A) Yellow
(B) Red
(C) Green
(D) Blue

355. The layer of screen construction responsible for light emission is the

    (A) base
    (B) reflective
    (C) phosphor
    (D) protective

356. Which of the following are true rare-earth phosphors?

    (A) Barium lead sulfate and gadolinium oxysulfide
    (B) Yttrium tantalate and lanthanum oxybromide
    (C) Yttrium tantalate and barium lead sulfate
    (D) Gadolinium oxysulfide and lanthanum oxybromide

357. What is the primary advantage of using rare-earth phosphors in intensifying screens instead of calcium tungstate?

    (A) They are less expensive to manufacture
    (B) They produce light emission to which film is naturally sensitive
    (C) They produce less distortion of structures imaged
    (D) They require less exposure for an equal amount and thickness of phosphor layer

358. The radiographic image is actually formed by which film component?

    (A) Phosphor crystals
    (B) Silver halide crystals
    (C) Reflective layer
    (D) Antihalation layer

359. The best recorded detail will be provided by screens with a relative speed of

    (A) 800
    (B) 400
    (C) 200
    (D) 100

360. What effect will quantum mottle have on the quality of the radiographic image?

    (A) Better recorded detail
    (B) Uneven densities
    (C) Improved resolution
    (D) Increased magnification

361. Quantum mottle can be reduced by the use of

    (A) screens of faster speed
    (B) higher kilovoltage
    (C) increased milliampere-seconds
    (D) smaller focal spot

362. Modern radiographic film has a base layer composed of

    (A) glass
    (B) polyester
    (C) cellulose acetate
    (D) silver bromide

363. Which of the following are important qualities for the base material of radiographic film?

    (A) Opacity
    (B) Translucence
    (C) Ability to swell and then shrink during processing
    (D) Ability to darken in response to x-ray or light exposure and processing

364. Which components make up the emulsion of x-ray film?

    (A) Silver halide crystals in a polymer matrix
    (B) Gadolinium phosphor crystals in gelatin
    (C) Silver halide crystals in gelatin
    (D) Gadolinium phosphor crystals in a polymer matrix

365. Which of the following is an important quality for the gelatin of film emulsions?

    (A) Rigidity
    (B) Ability to swell and shrink during processing
    (C) A chemical effect on silver halide crystals
    (D) Ability to darken in response to x-ray or light exposure and processing

366. What specific elements are used in the construction of the photosensitive crystals of radiographic film?
    1. Silver
    2. Bromine
    3. Iodine

    (A) 1 & 2
    (B) 2 & 3
    (C) 1 & 3
    (D) 1, 2, & 3

367. How do the silver halide elements form the crystal lattice?

    (A) Ionic bonds between the silver and bromide atoms with sulfur particles on the surface
    (B) Covalent bonds between the silver and bromide atoms with sulfur particles on the surface
    (C) Ionic bonds between the silver and sulfur atoms with bromine particles on the surface
    (D) Covalent bonds between the silver and sulfur atoms with bromine particles on the surface

368. The low-level density that is present on all radiographic film, even that which has not been exposed to light or x-rays, is referred to as

    (A) scatter fog density
    (B) fog density
    (C) base density
    (D) base plus fog density

369. The majority of medical radiographic film currently used is

    (A) direct exposure film
    (B) screen film
    (C) video film
    (D) subtraction film

370. In order to obtain the maximum efficiency from a single emulsion, single intensifying screen combination, what must be remembered?

    (A) Single emulsion film must be matched with a screen emitting red light
    (B) The emulsion surface of the film must be against the screen surface
    (C) This system must not be used in the bucky
    (D) High kilovoltage exposures must be used

371. Blue-sensitive film may be effectively handled using safe lights that emit which of the following colors of light?
    1. Red
    2. Amber
    3. Green

    (A) 1 only
    (B) 2 only
    (C) 1 & 2
    (D) 2 & 3

372. Appropriate safelight colors when handling orthochromatic film include:
    1. Red
    2. Amber
    3. Green

    (A) 1 only
    (B) 2 only
    (C) 1 & 2
    (D) 2 & 3

373. Which of the following conditions must be met to ensure proper storage of radiographic film?

    (A) Humidity >80 percent, temperature 60 to 80°F, protection from electromagnetic radiation
    (B) Humidity <40 percent, temperature <70°F, protection from heat and moisture
    (C) Humidity 60 to 80 percent, temperature >70°F, protection from fumes and high frequencies
    (D) Humidity 40 to 60 percent, temperature <70°F, protection from electromagnetic radiation

374. Safelight fog is of most concern when

(A) loading cassettes with freshly opened, unexposed film
(B) handling unexposed film nearing its expiration date
(C) unloading cassettes of exposed film for processing
(D) handling film as it comes out of the processor

375. An efficient darkroom facility should have:
1. Uncluttered countertops
2. Dark colored walls
3. Safelights positioned 3 feet from work area

(A) 1 & 2
(B) 2 & 3
(C) 1 & 3
(D) 1, 2, & 3

376. Which of the following may be sources of fogging in a darkroom?
1. White light leaks around doors
2. Safelights
3. Increased environmental temperature

(A) 1 & 2
(B) 2 & 3
(C) 1 & 3
(D) 1, 2, & 3

377. Film fogging in the darkroom may be caused by which conditions?

(A) Safelight mounted over processor rather than work area
(B) Cracks around doors, passboxes, or processor
(C) Red safelight with blue-sensitive film
(D) Use of interlocking passboxes

378. What is meant by *daylight processing*?

(A) Solar-operated processors
(B) Ability to load and unload cassettes within a darkroon
(C) Ability to load and unload cassettes without a darkroom
(D) Use of light-resistant film

379. What identification information should be included on all radiographic images?

(A) Patient's name, address, exam type, and date
(B) Patient's social security number, date of birth, exam type, and date
(C) Patient's name, x-ray number, radiologist's name, exam type, and date
(D) Patient's name, age, x-ray number, exam type, and date

380. When should "R" or "L" lead markers be used as part of the radiographic imaging process?

(A) For exams of the extremities only
(B) When ordered to do so by the radiologist
(C) For exams of the extremities and skull only
(D) For all exams

381. Which phase of chemical processing is responsible for converting the latent image to the manifest image?

(A) Development
(B) Fixing
(C) Washing
(D) Drying

382. The role of the development phase of film processing is to

(A) sensitize the silver halide crystals to radiation exposure
(B) convert exposed silver halide crystals to black metallic silver
(C) remove unexposed silver halide crystals from the film
(D) make up for insufficient x-ray or light exposure to the film

383. Possible sources of chemical fog include:
1. Increased developer temperature
2. Decreased development time
3. Increased developer strength

(A) 1 & 2
(B) 2 & 3
(C) 1 & 3
(D) 1, 2, & 3

384. Which of the following is a reducing agent?

(A) Glutaraldehyde
(B) Sodium carbonate
(C) Hydroquinone
(D) Potassium bromide

385. What role does the activator of the developer play?

(A) Reduces exposed silver halide crystals
(B) Prohibits developing agents from acting on unexposed silver halide crystals
(C) Limits the amount of swelling of emulsion
(D) Maintains an alkali pH level and softens the emulsion

386. What chemistry problem may lead to films jamming in an automatic processor?

(A) Insufficient developer replenishment
(B) Overfixation
(C) Insufficient washing
(D) Overdevelopment

387. What role does washing play during film processing?

(A) It clears unexposed silver halide crystals from film
(B) It stops the developer action prior to fixing
(C) It removes excess chemicals from the film
(D) It softens the film emulsion prior to development

388. What role does ammonium thiosulfate have in radiographic processing?

(A) Developing agent
(B) Clearing agent
(C) Preservative for developer and fixer
(D) Hardener of the image following development

389. What is the primary purpose of the fixing phase of chemical processing?

(A) To convert exposed silver to black metallic silver and soften emulsion
(B) To clear unexposed silver crystals and shrink and harden emulsion
(C) To remove retained chemicals from film
(D) To control the amount of swelling of the emulsion

390. The role of the activator in the fixing phase of processing is to

(A) maintain alkaline pH (10 to 11.5)
(B) maintain acidic pH (4 to 4.5)
(C) maintain neutral pH
(D) stop the clearing action

391. Which systems contribute to chemical agitation during processing?
    1. Transport
    2. Replenishment
    3. Recirculation

(A) 1 & 2
(B) 2 & 3
(C) 1 & 3
(D) 1, 2, & 3

392. Underdevelopment of a radiograph may be due to

(A) developer temperature above optimum level
(B) transport system operating too slowly
(C) replenishment rates too low
(D) wash water temperature too high

393. Why is the method in which a film is fed into a processor of concern in maintaining processing efficiency?

(A) The replenishment system is activated as each film is fed into the processor
(B) The manner in which the film is fed into the processor determines the overall development time
(C) The temperature control system is regulated by how films are fed into the processor
(D) Proper mixing of the chemicals depends on how the film is fed into the processor

394. What type of film is used for recording images from the cathode ray tube (CRT) of a computer-assisted imaging system?

(A) Direct exposure film
(B) Screen film
(C) Video film
(D) Subtraction film

395. How does direct exposure film differ from screen type film?

(A) It is more sensitive to light than x-rays
(B) It is more sensitive to x-rays than light
(C) It has a thinner emulsion
(D) It is easier to develop in automatic processors

396. What method of monitoring is recommended to ensure optimum operation of the automatic film processor?

(A) Dosimetry
(B) Densitometry
(C) Sensitometry
(D) Troubleshooting

397. How frequently should the operation conditions of the processor be monitored?

(A) Daily
(B) Twice a week
(C) Weekly
(D) Biweekly

398. The basic material and equipment that should be available for monitoring the processor include

(A) chemicals, exposed films, dosimeters
(B) sensitometer, densitometer, step wedge, magnifying glass
(C) dosimeter, step wedge, supply of test film, thermometer
(D) supply of test film, thermometer, densitometer, sensitometer

399. Which of the following are examples of artifacts caused by the automatic processor?

(A) Crescent marks, guide shoe marks, static
(B) Pi lines, guide shoe marks, emulsion pickoff
(C) Chemical stain, crescent marks, emulsion pickoff
(D) Static, pi lines, chemical stain

400. Why is it recommended for unexposed film to be stored *on end* rather then *flat* prior to being loaded into the film bin?

(A) Saves space so that more boxes can be stored
(B) Reduces the occurrence of static artifacts
(C) Reduces the occurrence of pressure artifacts
(D) Allows for better circulation of cool air around the film

401. If a film is still tacky to the touch when it comes out of the processor, what is the most likely cause?

(A) Low dryer temperature
(B) Insufficient developer replenishment
(C) Insufficient fixer replenishment
(D) Excessive wash time

402. The dryer temperature should be a minimum of about

(A) 85° F
(B) 94° F
(C) 108° F
(D) 120° F

403. Each of the following are correct actions to be followed when feeding films into the processor EXCEPT

(A) use the edge of the feed tray to guide the film straight into the processor
(B) use alternate sides of the feed tray when processing multiple films
(C) pull film back out of the processor if it is a little crooked
(D) check the feed tray for spills and debris

404. According to the inverse square law, what is the relationship of radiographic density to changes in SID?

(A) Inversely proportional
(B) Directly proportional
(C) Inversely proportional to the square of the SID
(D) Directly proportional to the square of the SID

405. All the following are influenced by changes in SID EXCEPT

(A) recorded detail
(B) distortion
(C) density
(D) contrast

406. The factor that influences recorded detail (sharpness) *only* is

(A) OID
(B) SID
(C) image receptor speed
(D) focal-spot size

407. A radiographic accessory device that will modify the primary beam's intensity pattern in order to provide more uniform exposure of an anatomic structure is the

(A) collimator
(B) grid
(C) wedge filter
(D) shadow shield

408. Proper collimation will result in an increase in

(A) density
(B) contrast
(C) recorded detail
(D) distortion

409. How does the use of proper collimation affect image quality?

(A) Prevents radiation from scattering away from the image receptor
(B) Focuses the primary beam on the area of interest
(C) Hardens the beam
(D) Decreases the likelihood of Compton interactions

410. If an optimum image of the abdomen demonstrated a suspicious area requiring a well-collimated image, what change in technique should be made to maintain image quality?

(A) Increased milliampere-seconds
(B) Decreased kilovoltage
(C) Increased grid ratio
(D) Decreased SID

411. For which of the following exams would a high–kilovoltage peak technique be advantageous?

(A) Adult chest radiography
(B) Pediatric abdominal radiography
(C) IVU exams
(D) Extremity radiography of the elderly

412. Each of the following technical factors would be included on a technique chart EXCEPT

(A) image receptor type/speed
(B) grid ratio
(C) SID
(D) patient's age range

413. Which set of technical factors will produce an image with the highest contrast?

	mAs	kV	SID	Grid
(A)	20	82	40"	5:1
(B)	24	72	40"	8:1
(C)	18	92	40"	10:1
(D)	24	66	40"	10:1

414. Which set of technical factors will produce the LEAST amount of radiographic contrast?

	mAs	kV	Grid	Filtration	Screen speed
(A)	15	96	12:1	3.0 mm	200
(B)	18	82	12:1	3.0 mm	400
(C)	22	66	8:1	2.0 mm	200
(D)	25	72	8:1	2.0 mm	400

415. When using the automatic exposure control, what step may be eliminated?

(A) Kilovoltage selection
(B) Milliampere-second selection
(C) Central ray alignment
(D) Collimation

416. The successful use of the AEC requires:
1. Proper positioning and centering
2. Standardized image receptor speed
3. Close collimation

(A) 1 & 2
(B) 2 & 3
(C) 1 & 3
(D) 1, 2, & 3

417. Proper use of the AEC for a typical PA chest radiograph requires the selection of

    (A) the middle sensing chamber only
    (B) one or two side sensing chambers only
    (C) all three sensing chambers
    (D) manual technique only

418. Which of the following expressions is used to determine optical density on a finished radiograph?

    (A) 1/R

    (B) $\dfrac{D_2 - D_1}{LRE_2 - LRE_1}$

    (C) $\log = I_o/I_t$

    (D) SID/SOD

419. The chart shown below may be used to provide information on which of the following characteristics of film?
            1. Spectral sensitivity
            2. Film speed
            3. Base-plus-fog density

    (A) 1 & 2
    (B) 2 & 3
    (C) 1 & 3
    (D) 1, 2, & 3

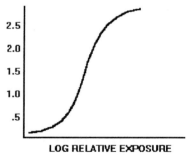
LOG RELATIVE EXPOSURE

420. Film contrast is inversely proportional to

    (A) mottle
    (B) latitude
    (C) speed
    (D) grain size

421. The shape of an H&D curve will be influenced by

    (A) screen speed
    (B) development conditions
    (C) quantum mottle
    (D) film speed

422. A technique chart suggests using 80 kV, 400 mA, 1/60 s, and 100 cm SID for an exam. The result will be

    (A) 2 mAs
    (B) 7 mAs
    (C) 20 mAs
    (D) 70 mAs

423. Damage to intensifying screens or the cassette may cause which of the following artifacts?
            1. High-density crescent marks
            2. Regularly repeating high-density marks
            3. Random low-density specks
            4. Localized areas of blur

    (A) 1 & 2
    (B) 2 & 3
    (C) 3 & 4
    (D) 1 & 4

424. Which action will reduce the formation of artifacts?

    (A) Cleaning of screen
    (B) Monitoring of focal-spot size
    (C) Flat storage of unopened boxes of film
    (D) Use of pillows to support the anatomic area of interest

425. The components of the transport system of the automatic film processor include:
            1. Racks of rollers
            2. Pumps
            3. Drive mechanism

    (A) 1 & 2
    (B) 2 & 3
    (C) 1 & 3
    (D) 1, 2, & 3

426. If development time is purposefully increased, what change must be made to maintain optimum image quality?

    (A) Increase fixer time
    (B) Decrease fixer time
    (C) Increase SID
    (D) Decrease milliampere-seconds

427. What system in the processor determines how long the film is in each section of the processor (developer, fixer, wash, and dryer)?

(A) Replenishment
(B) Transport
(C) Circulation
(D) Temperature control

428. How do the temperatures of the developer, fixer, and wash water compare?

(A) Fixer temperature is higher than developer and lower than wash water temperatures
(B) Developer temperature is higher than fixer and wash water temperatures
(C) Wash water temperature is higher than developer and fixer temperatures
(D) Developer temperature is higher than fixer and lower than wash water temperatures

429. For what reason should the rollers of an automatic processor transport system be periodically cleaned?

(A) To keep rollers smooth and slippery, thereby improving the movement of films
(B) To remove built-up debris, thereby reducing artifact formation
(C) To improve the speed at which the roller turns, thereby decreasing processing time
(D) To decrease excessive oxidation, thereby increasing the life of the chemicals

430. What will result if orthochromatic film is used with calcium tungstate screens?

(A) Optimum image quality
(B) Loss of contrast
(C) Loss of speed
(D) Increased density

431. Changing from a double film and screen combination to a single film and screen combination will require an increase in

(A) kilovoltage
(B) milliampere-seconds
(C) SID
(D) focal-spot size

432. Physical differences between orthochromatic and standard silver halide films include:
    1. Orthochromatic film has a reflective layer
    2. Orthochromatic film is treated with a light absorbing dye
    3. Orthochromatic film is *not* sensitized with sulfur

(A) 1 only
(B) 2 only
(C) 1 & 3
(D) 2 & 3

433. An increase in OID will cause an increase in

(A) density
(B) magnification
(C) recorded detail
(D) distortion

434. An unavoidable OID may be compensated for by

(A) increasing focal-spot size
(B) decreasing kilovoltage
(C) increasing SID
(D) decreasing milliampere-seconds

435. A change in screen speed from 50 to 200 and in SID from 40 to 52 inches will require the milliampere-second to be adjusted from 48 to

(A) 15
(B) 20
(C) 60
(D) 150

436. A change in technical factors from 80 to 106 kV and from a 5:1 to a 12:1 grid will require a change from 24 mAs to

(A) 5 mAs
(B) 10 mAs
(C) 15 mAs
(D) 30 mAs

437. Angling of the x-ray beam will have a most noticeable effect on

(A) radiographic density
(B) radiographic contrast
(C) magnification
(D) true distortion

438. *Unequal magnification* of the object during the imaging process best describes

   (A)   contrast
   (B)   true distortion
   (C)   absorption blur
   (D)   geometric blur

439. A linear object is placed at an angle to the image receptor. If the central ray is directed perpendicular to the image receptor, the image of the object will be

   (A)   magnified
   (B)   foreshortened
   (C)   elongated
   (D)   blurred

440. What effect will tight collimation have on the quantity and quality of the beam reaching the patient?

   (A)   Decrease in quantity and quality
   (B)   Increase in quantity and quality
   (C)   Decrease in quantity and no effect on quality
   (D)   Decrease in quality and no effect on quantity

441. Patient motion can be controlled by

   (A)   decreasing exposure time
   (B)   increasing kilovoltage
   (C)   increasing SID
   (D)   decreasing milliampere-seconds

442. If a radiograph of an extremity demonstrates motion of the part of interest when using technical factors of 200 mA, 0.1 s, 70 kV, and 40 inches SID, improved results may be gained by using which alternate set of technical factors?

   (A)   200 mA, 0.05 s, 80 kV, 40 inches SID
   (B)   200 mA, 0.05 s, 70 kV, 28 inches SID
   (C)   400 mA, 0.025 s, 80 kV, 40 inches SID
   (D)   600 mA, 0.033 s, 70 kV, 40 inches SID

443. A radiographic exam of the chest (PA projection) is performed on a small, elderly patient, using the usual factors of 400 mA, 100 kV, 72 inches SID, a wide-latitude imaging system, and the left sensing chamber of the AEC. This produces an image with excessive density. The best method for correcting this problem would be to select

   (A)   a lower milliamperage
   (B)   a lower kilovoltage
   (C)   a longer SID
   (D)   the center sensing chamber

444. A radiographic exam of the supine abdomen (without contrast media) is obtained using all three sensing chambers of the AEC, 400 mA, 75 kV, 40 inches SID, and a 400 speed imaging system. If the resulting image is underexposed, the most probable cause would be that the

   (A)   exposure time was limited by the minimum response time of the unit
   (B)   backup time was set too short
   (C)   density selection was set on +2
   (D)   milliamperage was set too low

445. A radiographic exam of the shoulder is performed using the center chamber of the AEC, 400 mA, 70 kV, −1 density, and 40 inches SID with the collimator set at just smaller than a 10 by 12 inch image receptor. If the image demonstrates underexposure, the best correction factor would be to

   (A)   increase kilovoltage
   (B)   increase milliamperage
   (C)   increase collimation
   (D)   use a side chamber instead of the center chamber

446. All the following will influence magnification EXCEPT

   (A)   SID
   (B)   OID
   (C)   SOD
   (D)   focal-spot size

447. A radiographic exam of a stomach filled with barium is performed using the center chamber of the AEC, 400 mA, 110 kV, and 40 inches SID. If a large quantity of barium is positioned over the activated sensing chamber, the image will most likely show

(A) patient motion
(B) overexposure
(C) underexposure
(D) no exposure

448. The density controls of the AEC may be used as an acceptable means of compensating for

(A) temporary problems with the unit's exposure output
(B) difficulties in accurate positioning of the part of interest
(C) an inability to position sufficient tissue structures over the activated chamber(s)
(D) variations in patient thicknesses

449. While using the AEC, the need for an exposure time that is shorter than the unit's minimum response time is likely to occur in all the following situations EXCEPT

(A) the selected milliamperage is too high
(B) the selected kilovoltage is too high
(C) a very small patient is radiographed
(D) very tight collimation is used

450. When using the AEC for a radiographic exam of the lumbar spine in the RPO projection, which sensing chamber or combination of chambers should be used?
    1. Right side
    2. Left side
    3. Center

(A) 1 only
(B) 1 & 2
(C) 1 & 3
(D) 3 only

451. Which error would produce an underexposed image?

(A) An increase in developer concentration in the processor
(B) A SID shorter than stated on the technique chart
(C) Use of a 200 speed image receptor instead of a detail system
(D) A field size as large as the image receptor

452. What condition is most likely to occur as a result of insufficient washing during film processing?

(A) Loss of density and contrast
(B) Reduced archival quality
(C) Fogged areas
(D) Softening of emulsion

453. How frequently should the tanks of a processor be emptied and cleaned?

(A) Weekly
(B) Monthly
(C) Quarterly
(D) Yearly

454. Storage conditions for processing chemicals require temperatures

(A) greater than 70°F and about 60 percent humidity
(B) less than 50°F and about 40 percent humidity
(C) less than 70°F and about 60 percent humidity
(D) greater than 50°F and about 40 percent humidity

455. All the following processor maintenance actions should be performed on a daily basis EXCEPT

(A) cleaning of the feed tray
(B) cleaning of the deep roller racks
(C) cleaning of the crossover rollers
(D) checking of the developer temperature

456. Exhausted developer may cause all the following problems EXCEPT

   (A)   film jams during transport
   (B)   increased image contrast
   (C)   tacky finished film
   (D)   chemical fog

457. Exhausted fixer may cause all the following problems EXCEPT

   (A)   tacky finished films
   (B)   milky appearance of the image
   (C)   continued darkening of the film during storage
   (D)   brittle film

458. Which situation will result in the most serious contamination of processor solutions?

   (A)   Fixer spilled into developer
   (B)   Developer spilled into fixer
   (C)   Fixer spilled into wash water
   (D)   Developer spilled into wash water

459. The proper pH level for the developer solution is

   (A)   acidic
   (B)   alkali
   (C)   neutral

460. The quality of the image demonstrated below would be improved by

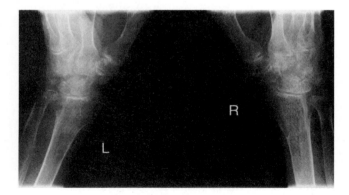

   (A)   increased milliampere-seconds
   (B)   increased kilovoltage
   (C)   decreased milliampere-seconds
   (D)   decreased kilovoltage

461. What type of plus density artifact is evident on the image below?

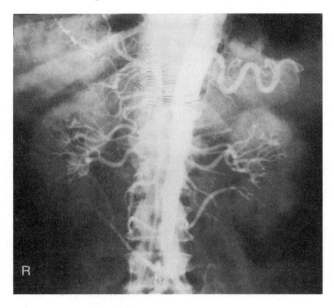

   (A)   Pressure mark
   (B)   Fingernail mark
   (C)   Guide shoe mark
   (D)   Static mark

462. What is the most likely cause of the artifact evident on the image in the previous question?

   (A)   Damaged roller in the processor transport system
   (B)   Misaligned roller in the processor
   (C)   Handling film in a cold, dry environment
   (D)   Handling film in a hot, humid environment

463. Artifacts that appear as a minus density are caused by what action?

   (A)   Increased sensitization of the film due to deposits on a roller
   (B)   Creasing of the film during handling
   (C)   Static discharges while the film is being handled
   (D)   Scratching away of the emulsion

Questions 464–466

For each item, select the set of technical factors that will provide the greatest radiographic density.

464.

		mA	Time	kV	SID
	(A)	600	0.017	75	40″
	(B)	400	0.05	86	46″
	(C)	400	0.025	75	40″
	(D)	200	0.05	75	40″

465.

		mAs	kV	SID	Grid ratio
	(A)	32	74	40″	10:1
	(B)	10	64	40″	no grid
	(C)	18	74	40″	8:1
	(D)	24	84	72″	10:1

466.

		mAs	kV	SID	Screen speed
	(A)	10	70	40″	400
	(B)	20	60	40″	600
	(C)	30	80	48″	200
	(D)	40	70	48″	200

Questions 467–469

For each item, select the group of technical factors that will provide the LEAST radiographic density

467.

		mA	Time	kV	Grid
	(A)	200	50 ms	72	10:1
	(B)	400	10 ms	72	10:1
	(C)	600	5 ms	82	12:1
	(D)	800	5 ms	82	12:1

468.

		mAs	kV	SID	Grid
	(A)	15	66	32″	5:1
	(B)	18	70	40″	8:1
	(C)	18	80	40″	12:1
	(D)	12	92	48″	16:1

469.

		mAs	kV	SID	Grid ratio	Screen speed
	(A)	32	70	100 cm	10:1	100
	(B)	24	80	100 cm	10:1	200
	(C)	18	92	180 cm	16:1	400
	(D)	12	106	180 cm	16:1	600

Questions 470–473

Use the H&D curves below to answer each question.

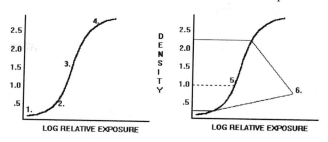

470. The *body* of the curve is represented by number

(A) 1
(B) 2
(C) 3
(D) 4

471. Film contrast is determined by calculating the numerical value of which part of the curve?

(A) 2
(B) 4
(C) 5
(D) 6

472. The speed of a film would be determined at the point numbered

(A) 1
(B) 3
(C) 5
(D) 6

473. The area on the curve that represents maximum densities is number

(A) 2
(B) 4
(C) 5
(D) 6

Questions 474–475

Find the set of technical factors that will result in the best recorded detail.

474.

	mAs	kV	SID	OID	Focal spot	Receptor speed
(A)	25	70	40″	4″	0.6 mm	200
(B)	12	80	72″	4″	0.6 mm	100
(C)	15	70	72″	8″	0.6 mm	200
(D)	20	80	40″	8″	1.2 mm	100

475.

	mAs	kV	SID (cm)	OID (cm)	Focal spot	Receptor speed
(A)	8	62	80	10	1.2 mm	50
(B)	10	68	100	12	1.2 mm	100
(C)	12	74	100	20	0.6 mm	100
(D)	15	78	120	20	0.3 mm	100

Questions 476-477

Determine which set of technical factors will result in the *most* geometric blur.

476.

	mAs	kV	SID	OID	Focal spot	Receptor speed
(A)	25	70	40″	6″	1.2 mm	100
(B)	18	76	72″	6″	0.6 mm	200
(C)	10	84	60″	4″	0.6 mm	100
(D)	15	90	72″	4″	1.2 mm	200

477.

	mAs	kV	SID	OID	Focal spot	Receptor speed
(A)	32	80	40″	2″	1.2 mm	200
(B)	24	85	32″	4″	1.2 mm	400
(C)	18	90	50″	4″	1.2 mm	200
(D)	15	100	60″	6″	1.2 mm	400

DIRECTIONS: Each group of questions below consists of lettered headings followed by a set of numbered items. For each numbered item select the **one** lettered heading with which it is **most** closely associated. Each lettered heading may be used **once, more than once, or not at all.**

Questions 478–479

Use the H & D chart to match each film to the correct curve or curves.

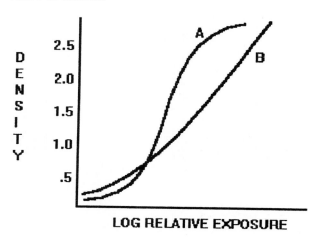

(A) Curve A
(B) Curve B
(C) Both
(D) Neither

478. Representation of low contrast film

479. Representation of fast speed film

Questions 480–484

Indicate how density will be influenced by each change in technical factors.

(A) Increase density
(B) Decrease density
(C) No effect on density

480. Grid type from 12:1 to 8:1 ratio

481. Relative speed of the imaging system used from 200 speed to 400 speed

482. Processing temperature from 95° F to 92° F.

483. Field size from 14 × 17 to 8 × 10

484. Focal-spot size from 1.2 mm to 0.6 mm

Questions 485–487

Match each description with the appropriate object in the diagram.

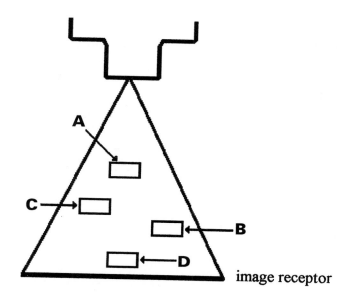

image receptor

(A) A
(B) B
(C) C
(D) D

485. Most magnification on the radiographic image

486. Greatest amount of shape distortion

487. Best recorded detail

Questions 488–491

Choose the correct chemical agent found in the radiographic processor to perform the function stated.

(A) Glutaraldehyde
(B) Ammonium thiosulfate
(C) Hydroquinone
(D) Potassium bromide
(E) Sodium sulfite

488. Inhibits development of unexposed silver halide crystals

489. Acts as the clearing agent

490. Acts as a hardener in the developer

491. Is one of two reducing agents used in the developer solution

Questions 492–496

For each chemical agent, select the function it performs in the processing of an image.

(A) Acts to shrink and harden film emulsion during fixation
(B) Maintains the desired pH level of the fixer
(C) Maintains the desired pH level of the developer
(D) Preserves the chemistry of both developer and fixer
(E) Reduces exposed silver halide crystals, producing the gray shades of the image

492. Sodium carbonate

493. Phenidone

494. Acetic acid

495. Potassium alum

496. Sodium sulfite

Questions 497–499

Use the step wedge images below to answer *True* or *False* to each question.

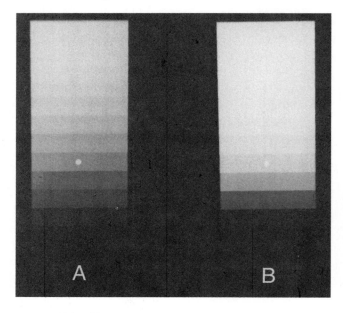

(A) True
(B) False

497. Image A is an example of high contrast

498. Image A is an example of short-scale contrast

499. Image B was produced using higher kilovoltage than for image A

Questions 500–503

For each question regarding technique charts, answer *True* or *False*.

(A) True
(B) False

500. Fixed kilovoltage peak charts use a constant milliampere-second value for various thicknesses of a specific structure

501. Fixed kilovoltage peak charts tend to produce images with a longer scale of contrast than variable charts

502. Variable kilovoltage peak charts group patient sizes into categories of small, medium, or large

503. Variable kilovoltage peak charts require milliampere-second adjustments for the various changes in part thickness

Questions 504–509

Note whether a change in each of the factors below will influence density, contrast, both, or neither.

(A) Density
(B) Contrast
(C) Both
(D) Neither

504. Alignment between the x-ray tube, the part to be imaged, and the image receptor

505. SID

506. Development conditions

507. Beam filtration

508. Grid ratio

509. Image receptor speed

Questions 510–514

For each change or condition, indicate the best adjustment in exposure factors.

(A) Increase milliampere-seconds only
(B) Decrease milliampere-seconds only
(C) Increase milliampere-seconds; decrease kilovoltage
(D) Decrease milliampere-seconds; increase kilovoltage

510. Addition of barium sulfate contrast medium

511. Insufficient radiographic density

512. Decrease in SID

513. Increase in grid ratio

514. Decrease in part thickness

Questions 515–520

Use the answers provided to indicate the most probable source for each type of radiographic artifact listed.

(A) Film handling or storage
(B) Processor transport system
(C) Processor chemistry
(D) Effects related to cassette or screen
(E) Patient effects

515. Random, small, white specks on the image

516. High- or low-density marks, usually in a fairly linear form

517. Brown or grayish-white stain across the image in the finished radiograph

518. Generalized blurring of the entire image

519. High-density artifacts resembling lightning or trees on the image

520. Loss of contrast due to elevated base-plus-fog densities on the finished image

Questions 521–526

Indicate whether the stated pathologic condition is additive (characterized by an increase in absorption factors) or destructive (characterized by a decrease in absorption factors).

(A) Additive
(B) Destructive

521. Ascites

522. Emphysema

523. Bowel obstruction

524. Osteoporosis

525. Cirrhosis

526. Hydropneumothorax

Questions 527–531

Indicate the correct change in exposure factors needed to compensate for each anatomic or pathologic condition.

(A)   Increase milliampere-seconds
(B)   Decrease milliampere-seconds
(C)   Increase kilovoltage
(D)   Decrease kilovoltage

527.   Paget's disease

528.   Callus formation

529.   Soft tissue imaging

530.   Atrophy of a limb

531.   Pneumonia

Questions 532–536

Indicate which radiographic quality factors would be influenced by each stated change in technical factors.
1. Recorded detail (sharpness)
2. Magnification
3. Shape distortion

(A)   1 only
(B)   2 only
(C)   3 only
(D)   1 & 2
(E)   1, 2, & 3

532.   Decrease SID from 40 to 72 inches

533.   Change central ray direction from perpendicular to 30° caudad.

534.   Alter focal-spot size from large to small

535.   Increase OID to 20 inches while decreasing focal-spot size to 0.3 mm or less

536.   Increase central ray angle from 10° to 30° while decreasing SID from 40 to 30 inches

Questions 537–541

Indicate the type of radiation each statement is describing.

(A)   Primary radiation
(B)   Secondary radiation
(C)   Scattered radiation
(D)   Leakage radiation
(E)   Exit (remnant) radiation

537.   The radiation available to expose the image receptor

538.   The end result of Compton interactions between x-ray photons and matter

539.   The radiation that exits the tube via the window

540.   The radiation that results during photoelectric interactions between x-ray photons and matter

541.   The radiation composed of primary and scattered radiation components

Questions 542–544

Use the answers provided to indicate the effects on radiographic quality caused by the processing conditions stated.
1. Increased contrast
2. Increased density
3. Decreased contrast
4. Decreased density

(A)   1 & 2
(B)   2 & 3
(C)   3 & 4
(D)   1 & 4

542.   An increase in developer replenishment rate

543.   A decrease in developer activity due to improper mixing (too much water)

544.   Extended processing achieved by increasing developer time and using a less concentrated developer

Questions 545–550

Use the list of answers provided to indicate how frequently the stated processor maintenance action should be performed.

    (A) Daily
    (B) Weekly
    (C) Monthly
    (D) Quarterly

545. Check the replenishment rates for developer and fixer

546. Empty and wash the developer, fixer, and wash tanks

547. Clean all deep racks (developer, fixer, wash, and dryer)

548. Clean crossover racks

549. Drain chemical and replace with fresh chemicals

550. Clean replenishment tanks

Production and Evaluation of the Image

Answers

301. The answer is D. *(Bushong, 5/e, pp 308–310. Carlton, p 381. Carroll, 5/e, pp 38–40. Selman, 8/e, pp 337–338.)* Radiographic contrast is defined as the differences in radiographic density on a processed image. This important radiographic quality factor is influenced by numerous patient, exposure, and processing factors. These many influencing variables produce a range or scale of contrast, either long or short. Optimum radiographic quality demands sufficient contrast to best demonstrate the structures of interest on each radiograph. In general, long-scale contrast is desirable because of the many shades of gray available to form an image. However, long-scale contrast also produces a small difference in adjacent densities, which limits the visibility of the density variations. Each department should set its own optimum levels of radiographic quality based on the department's imaging equipment and radiologists' preferences.

302. The answer is B (2, 3). *(Bushong, 5/e, pp 308–310. Carlton, pp 384–385. Carroll, 5/e, p 87. Selman, 8/e, pp 337–340.)* The scale of radiographic contrast is chiefly controlled by the penetrability of the x-ray beam (regulated by the kilovoltage selection). Increased kilovoltage creates a high-energy beam, which is more likely to penetrate the object irradiated and less likely to undergo x-ray/matter interactions of any kind. The end result is low differential absorption and an exit beam composed of photons of similar energies. This exit beam will be recorded as many shades of gray with minimal difference in densities between adjacent structures. In summary, long-scale contrast may be defined as having many shades of gray with minimal density differences and is produced by high kilovoltage. Other factors influencing the scale of contrast include the patient (makeup of the body part irradiated) and processing of the radiographic image (which should be optimized and, therefore, not a factor).

303. The answer is A. *(Bushong, 5/e, p 309. Carlton, pp 384–385. Carroll, 5/e, p 87. Selman, 8/e, pp 339–340.)* The penetrability of the beam, which is controlled by kilovoltage selection, determines the likelihood of x-ray/matter interactions. At higher kilovoltage settings, the beam will have shorter wavelength, be more penetrating, and be less likely to undergo photoelectric or Compton interactions. This will result in decreased differential absorption of the beam's energy by the irradiated matter and produce a long-scale, lower contrast radiographic image. Higher kilovoltage also produces scattered radiation of higher energy, which is more likely to reach the recording medium and again lower radiographic contrast. Although numerous other factors contribute to the overall contrast of an image, variation of the kilovoltage selection is necessary to optimally penetrate the part of interest and is controlled by the radiographer.

304. The answer is B. *(Bushong, 5/e, pp 247–248. Carlton, pp 384–385. Carroll, 5/e, p 87. Selman, 8/e, p 341.)* Scattered radiation is a source of fog, which is defined as "unwanted density." Since scattered radiation is nondirectional, it will influence the entire image by increasing overall density and decreasing contrast. This effect lowers overall radiographic quality and should be controlled for by using optimum kilovoltage, collimation, grids, and optimum processing conditions. Recorded detail and magnification are geometric factors of image quality and thus are not influenced by scattered radiation.

305. The answer is C (1, 3). *(Bushong, 5/e, pp 316–317. Carlton, pp 384–385. Carroll, 5/e, p 87. Selman, 8/e, p 531.)* The use of high kilovoltage peak techniques has the advantage of reducing patient dose and the disadvantages of lower contrast and increased scatter fog in the exit beam. The reduction in patient dose is achieved by the increased penetration of the x-ray beam at higher energies. Less x-ray/matter interaction will occur and thus less biologic disruption. High kilovoltage techniques also allow the use of lower milliampere-second values, further contributing to decreased patient dose. On the disadvantage side of this issue, the increased penetration associated with high kilovoltage results in longer scale and lower contrast, which may be further reduced by the more energetic scattered radiation recorded on the image.

306. The answer is C. *(Bushong, 5/e, p 311. Carlton, pp 398–399. Carroll, 5/e, pp 29–32. Selman, 8/e, pp 318–319.)* The list of terms used to describe structural sharpness on a radiographic image is quite long and can be confusing to any radiographer or student. The ARRT has settled on the term *recorded detail* to refer to this aspect of radiographic image quality. Specifically, recorded detail is the ability to visualize the abruptness of edges or the sharpness of structural lines of the elements of the object imaged. Blur is evident when the edges of a structure spread out and result in an inability to visualize where one structure ends and another begins. This factor contributes to poor recorded detail and may arise from patient, screens, or geometric factors within the imaging chain. Optimum image quality requires the radiographer to minimize those factors that would cause excessive blur.

307. The answer is B. *(Bushong, 5/e, p 223. Carlton, pp 398–399. Carroll, 5/e, p 48. Selman, 8/e, pp 325–326.)* The resolution grid, also known as a *line pair phantom,* may be used to evaluate the recorded detail of an imaging system. This device is constructed of lead foil arranged in linear groupings. Each group has several lead "lines," which decrease in thickness from one grouping to the next. When radiographed, an image of black and white lines of the varying groupings is produced. On close evaluation, the lines will become more difficult to distinguish as separate lines within a group as the thicknesses get smaller. The thicknesses of these lines are calibrated to correspond to the various small-sized structures that must be imaged as separate and true objects. The smaller the line grouping (line pairs) visible, the better the recorded detail. The densitometer is used to quantify the amount of blackening on a radiograph. The sensitometer is used to provide a reproducible level of exposure to a film for evaluation of the processor or the film itself. The pinhole camera is used to determine the size of the effective focal spot.

308. The answer is B. *(Bushong 5/e, pp 286–287. Carlton, pp 398–399. Carroll, 5/e, pp 48, 263–264. Selman, 8/e, pp 319–321.)* The geometric factors that will improve recorded detail (by minimizing blur) are a long SID, a minimal OID, and a small focal spot size. SID is generally maintained at 40 or 72 inches for all radiographic procedures. This distance has been determined as adequate to utilize the most vertical photons of the x-ray beam and thereby reduce the blur effect that occurs when the more divergent rays are utilized, as when a short SID is employed. OID should always be kept as minimal as possible by placing the part of interest as close to the image receptor as possible. Although the use of a bucky mechanism does impose an unavoidable OID, this is acceptable for the gain in image quality obtained by using the grid device. Positioning of the patient, in terms of PA versus AP, should be considered also to place the object of interest as close to the image receptor as possible. The use of a small focal spot produces an x-ray beam with less divergent angles on the photons than does a large focal spot. However, the smaller area for electron bombardment on the target reduces the heat-loading capability of the tube and restricts the combinations of milliamperage, time, and kilovoltage that may be safely used. Angling the x-ray tube is used to create shape distortion. This in itself will not cause more or less blurring and therefore will not influence recorded detail.

309. The answer is D. *(Bushong, 5/e, p 280. Carlton, pp 417–418. Carroll, 5/e, pp 48, 254–257. Selman, 8/e, pp 348–349.)* Calculation of the SID/SOD ratio will indicate the amount of magnification present in the image. Further variations on this ratio can be made to determine the size of an object by modifying the ratio as follows: image size/object size = SID/SOD. Density is mathematically expressed as the $\log_{10}$ of the light available/light transmitted. Average gradient is calculated as follows: $D_2 - D_1 / LRE_2 - LRE_1$. The amount of geometric blur (penumbra) can also be determined by using focal spot size × OID/SID.

310. The answer is B.   *(Bushong, 5/e, p 280. Carlton, pp 417–418. Carroll, 5/e, pp 48, 254–257. Selman, 8/e, pp 348–350.)*   Magnification factor is calculated as SID/SOD. Therefore, to solve this problem only the SID and OID values need to be considered. SOD is the difference between SID and OID: 40 − 5 = 35 inches SOD. The magnification factor is 40/35 = 1.14. A very common error made by students is to use the OID value instead of finding the SOD value.

311. The answer is C.   *(Bushong, 5/e, p 280. Carlton, pp 417–418. Carroll, 5/e, pp 48, 254–257. Selman, 8/e, pp 348–350.)*   Magnification percentage is determined by the following equation: SID/SOD − 1 × 100. The magnification percentage for each of the answer options is:

(A)   20/19 = 1.05 − 1 = 0.05 × 100 = 5%
(B)   40/37 = 1.08 − 1 = 0.08 × 100 = 8%
(C)   50/45 = 1.11 − 1 = 0.11 × 100 = 11%
(D)   60/55 = 1.09 − 1 = 0.09 × 100 = 9%

This answer can also be determined nonmathematically by evaluating each set of conditions for the one with the most OID for the least SID.

312. The answer is B.   *(Bushong, 5/e, p 307. Carlton, pp 362–366. Carroll, 5/e, pp 79–81. Selman, 8/e, pp 332–333.)*   Radiographic density is primarily controlled by the milliampere-seconds selected. Density is the result of x-ray exposure and chemical processing. The milliampere-seconds selection directly determines the quantity of x-rays produced, thereby controlling the level of exposure to the patient and recording medium. The relationship between milliampere-second selection and density is directly proportional, all other factors remaining constant. Both kilovoltage and SID have a primary influence on density that must be considered whenever a variation of the usual technique is made. The effect of kilovoltage is direct, but not proportional. The effect of SID is inversely proportional to the square of the distance. Focal-spot size has no effect on density.

313. The answer is A.   *(Bushong, 5/e, pp 295, 308. Carlton, pp 366–375. Carroll, 5/e, pp 277–281.)*   *Direct effect* means that as one variable changes, another variable will change in the same direction, i.e., both increase or both decrease. All the answer options influence radiographic density, but only processing temperature varies in the same direction. An increase in temperature will increase radiographic density by the effect of temperature on chemical activity. An increase in SID will decrease radiographic density according to the inverse square law. An increase in collimation means the field size becomes smaller. This reduces the number of photons in the beam and the amount of tissue exposed, decreasing both primary and scattered rays in the exit beam and thus decreasing the amount of exposure to the recording medium. Grids absorb scattered rays from the exit beam before they are recorded. The reduction in scattered radiation means less fogging and less density on the radiograph.

314. The answer is D.   *(Bushong, 5/e, pp 294–295, 297, 301. Carroll, 5/e, pp 85–86, 125. Thompson, pp 225–226.)*   The quality of the x-ray beam refers to the average energy of the beam as determined by the wavelengths of each photon. This characteristic of the beam is also an indicator of the penetrability of the beam. There are four factors that may alter the quality of the x-ray beam: kilovoltage, target material, type of voltage waveform (generator type), and filtration. The first three factors all affect the energy of the beam at its origin. However, for a specific radiographic unit, only kilovoltage selection is variable; target material and generator type are fixed for that unit. The effect of kilovoltage on photon/beam energy is direct; increases in kilovoltage will increase the maximum energy a photon may attain and increase average beam energy. Filtration alters the average beam energy by absorbing low-energy photons as they leave the x-ray tube. Filtration devices are positioned before the patient in order to limit unnecessary exposure. As the low-energy photons are removed from the primary beam, average beam energy is increased and the beam is more penetrating.

315. The answer is B. *(Bushong, 5/e, pp 297–301. Carroll, 5/e, pp 85–86, 125. Thompson, pp 225–226.)* The quantity of photons in the x-ray beam for a given exposure is determined by milliampere-seconds, kilovoltage, filtration, target material, and the type of voltage waveform. Focal-spot size defines the area on the target that is bombarded during x-ray production; however, the number of electrons emitted during thermionic emission determines the number of x-rays produced. Thermionic emission is directly proportional to the heating of the filament, which is controlled through milliamperage selection. Focal-spot size influences one radiographic quality factor only: recorded detail (sharpness of structural lines). Increases in kilovoltage provide more energetic electrons, which are more likely to undergo multiple x-ray/target interactions and produce more x-rays. Targets made of elements of high atomic number produce an increased amount of bremsstrahlung ("brems") radiation. Three-phase and high-frequency generators are more efficient at producing x-rays because of the nearly constant supply of voltage across the terminals.

316. The answer is B. *(Bushong, 5/e, pp 168–170. Carlton, pp 177–178. Carroll, 5/e, pp 127–128. Selman, 8/e, pp 396–398.)* Compensating filters are accessory devices for use by the radiographer as the need arises. Their purpose is to provide more uniform exposure to a body part that is asymmetric in its structure. Most commonly, compensating filters are designed in a wedge or trough shape, with areas of increased and decreased thicknesses. The device is placed in the accessory tray at the bottom of the collimator and positioned with its thick area overlying the thinner anatomic structures and its thin area over the thicker anatomic structures. The radiographic result is a more evenly exposed subject matter. Overall, compensating filters may lower contrast by causing a uniform level of differential absorption. Patient dose will not necessarily decrease because of a required increase in exposure factors needed to compensate for the thickness of the filter device.

317. The answer is A. *(Bushong, 5/e, pp 301, 308. Carlton, pp 183–192. Carroll, 5/e, pp 217–221.)* Of the options listed, only the increase in kilovoltage will increase radiographic density. The increase in SID will decrease density, according to the inverse square law. The change from a large to a small focal spot will influence the recorded detail of the image. While milliampere-seconds is the controlling factor of density, its relationship is directly proportional; therefore, the decrease in milliampere-seconds will cause radiographic density to decrease.

318. The answer is C. *(Bushong, 5/e, p 307. Carlton, pp 368–369. Carroll, 5/e, p 221.)* Milliampere-seconds is the controlling factor of radiographic density. The relationship is directly proportional; that is, as one increases, the other increases at the same rate. If one selected a milliampere-second value of 12 and produced a radiographic density measuring 1.2_D and then increased the milliampere-seconds to 24, the new density would be about 2.4_D, assuming all other technical factors remained the same between the two exposures. This effect is the result of the influence of milliampere-seconds on filament heating and subsequent electron emission, x-ray production, and number of photons in the exit beam.

319. The answer is A. *(Bushong, 5/e, p 307. Carlton, pp 366–368. Carroll, 5/e, pp 95–104.)* The influence of kilovoltage on density is derived from the variation in penetrability as well as quantity of x-rays as kilovoltage is varied. For this reason, the relationship between kilovoltage and density is direct (or linear), but not proportionate. Increases in kilovoltage will produce more x-rays and more photons of higher energy, which will better penetrate the object and contribute to the exit beam. This increased number of photons in the exit beam will increase exposure to the recording medium and increase density. Slight changes in kilovoltage will more greatly affect density than similar changes in milliampere-seconds. A 15 percent increase in kilovoltage will produce the same density increase as a 100 percent increase in milliampere-seconds.

320. The answer is B. *(Bushong, 5/e, p 307. Carlton, pp 366–368. Carroll, 5/e, pp 95–104.)* A change in kilovoltage by 15 percent is equivalent to an inverse change in milliampere-seconds by a factor of 2 in order to maintain radiographic density. The combinations of exposure factors in the answers would have the following effects: (A) increase the milliampere-seconds by 100 percent (2 times) and kilovoltage by 15 percent, which would quadruple the density from the original technique; (B) maintain milliampere-seconds and decrease kilovoltage by 15 percent, which would reduce density by half from the original technique; (C) increase milliampere-seconds by 100 percent (2 times) and decrease kilovoltage by 15 percent, which would produce about the same density as the original technique; and (D) decrease milliampere-seconds by 50 percent (1/2) and kilovoltage by 15 percent, which would reduce density to one-fourth the original value.

321. The answer is C. *(Bushong, 5/e, p 307. Carlton, pp 366–368. Carroll, 5/e, pp 95–104.)* If higher contrast is desired through a change in exposure factors, the kilovoltage must be decreased. At the same time, milliampere-seconds must be increased in order to maintain the density level. The combinations of exposure factors listed as answer options would have the following effects: (A) increased milliampere-seconds and no change in kilovoltage would result in doubling the density; (B) increased milliampere-seconds four times and decreased kilovoltage by 15 percent would result in double the original density level; (C) increased milliampere-seconds by four times and decreased kilovoltage by two sets of 15 percent would increase contrast and maintain the original density; and (D) no change in milliampere-seconds and lower kilovoltage by 15 percent would produce an underexposed image with insufficient density.

322. The answer is A. *(Bushong, 5/e, p 299. Carlton, pp 183–186. Carroll, 5/e, pp 69–79.)* Milliampere-seconds is the product of milliamperage and exposure time expressed in seconds. Radiographic units will have a range of fixed milliampere stations available and a wider range of exposure times. Exposure times may be stated in fractions, decimals, or millisecond form. The radiographer must be capable of determining milliampere-second values using any of the three methods for expressing exposure time. For this example, the 300 mA must be multiplied by the 0.017 s exposure time to produce 5 mAs. When multiplying numbers in decimal form, take careful note of the correct placement of the decimal point.

323. The answer is B. *(Bushong, 5/e, p 307. Carroll, 5/e, pp 81–82.)* In order to perceive a density difference, a minimum change in milliampere-seconds of 30 percent is required. This variation should be used when only a slight decrease or increase in density is needed. Changes of less than this will effectively produce the same results as the initial image and unnecessarily expose the patient.

324. The answer is D. *(Bushong, 5/e, pp 306–308. Carlton, pp 183–186. Carroll, 5/e, pp 69–79.)* Each of the answers listed would increase the level of radiographic density. However, whenever density is the primary factor to be altered, the correction should be made in milliampere-seconds. If kilovoltage were increased, density would increase, yet contrast would decrease. Decreasing SID is never recommended as it will negatively influence patient dose (increase it) and the geometric integrity of the image (poor recorded detail and increased magnification). Processing conditions should be optimized for all radiographic images in order to minimize any negative influence they may have on image quality. Altering developing temperature is an unstable choice for this problem.

325. The answer is D. *(Bushong, 5/e, p 280. Carlton, pp 413–417. Carroll, 5/e, pp 254–257.)* Magnification is controlled by two factors: SID and OID. In order to minimize the amount of magnification produced, the SID should be kept as long as possible and the OID should be kept as short as possible. As the development of radiographic equipment has advanced, longer distances have become routine. Currently, the standard SID is a minimum of 40 inches, and there is a trend to increase this minimum in order to further improve image quality (less magnification and better recorded detail) as well as reduce patient dose. The increased SID will also compensate for the necessary OID of the bucky mechanism. The radiographer must remember to compensate for added OID, which may be due to patient or environmental limitations, by bringing the image receptor as close to the part as possible or by increasing the SID in order to maintain the desired SID/SOD ratio. Focal-spot size only influences recorded detail; it has no effect on magnification. Angulation of the central ray itself will not influence magnification, but will affect shape distortion of the object imaged. However, if the central ray angle is such as to cause a change in SID or the SID/SOD ratio, this would affect magnification. Whenever the central ray is angled, the change in SID must be noted and compensated for.

326. The answer is C. *(Bushong, 5/e, pp 282–286. Carlton, pp 418–419. Carroll, 5/e, pp 260–261.)* The angling of the central ray in any degree toward an object that is parallel to the image receptor will result in the object's appearing elongated on the radiographic image. This effect is often employed purposefully to project superimposed structures away from the part of interest, to open joint spaces, or to compensate for a curved structure. However, when elongation results from improper alignment of the beam with the part and image receptor, the effect is detrimental to optimum image quality. Angling the central ray may decrease density if the angled beam will traverse a larger quantity of tissue than it would in a perpendicular relationship with the part. Magnification would increase if the angled central ray altered the SID or SID/SOD ratio. Foreshortening of the structure on the radiographic image will occur if improper alignment of the beam, body part, and image receptor occurs, but not as was described in this situation.

327. The answer is C. *(Bushong, 5/e, p 312. Carlton, p 419. Carroll, 5/e, p 259.)* The optimum relationship between the central ray, the part of interest, and the image receptor should be such that the part and the image receptor are parallel to each other and the central ray is perpendicular to both. It must be remembered that the central ray is defined as the imaginary photon that exits the x-ray tube from the center of the focal spot and at a right angle with the bottom of the collimator surface. When there is no angle on the x-ray tube and the image receptor is parallel with the bottom of the collimator surface, the central ray will be projected perpendicular to the image receptor. Correct alignment of the part should be with its long axis parallel to the image receptor. The other answer options are all incorrect because they describe the relationship between the central ray and image receptor as parallel. This would result in an x-ray beam not directed toward the image receptor! In order to produce any type of image (desirable or not), the central ray must be directed in some manner toward the image receptor.

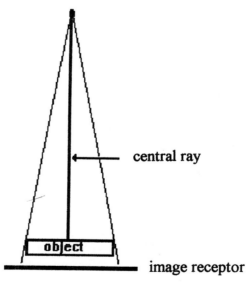

328. The answer is D. *(Bushong, 5/e, p 257. Carlton, pp 262–263. Carroll, 5/e, p 176. Curry, 4/e, pp 99–200. Thompson, p 327.)* Grid radius is the imaginary point at which the grid lines would converge if they were extended into space. The nonfocused (parallel) type of grid has an unlimited radius since its extended lines would never intersect (the lead strips are parallel to each other). However, the focused grid is constructed with the lead strips angled toward the center of the grid device with the central most strips perpendicular. This design is to complement the diverging rays of the x-ray beam and to reduce the occurrence of absorption of the primary beam. The convergence point of the lead strips defines the range of acceptable SIDs with which that particular grid can be used.

329. The answer is B.   *(Bushong, 5/e, p 250. Carlton, pp 262–263. Carroll, 5/e, p 176. Curry, 4/e, pp 99–200. Thompson, p 327.)*   The grid device is employed to absorb scattered radiation from the exit beam. To do so, it is constructed of thin lead strips alternating with radiolucent material. Both the lead and radiolucent strips are of specific thicknesses and are critically positioned to provide maximum absorption of scattered radiation with minimal absorption of primary radiation. Numerous factors, particularly grid ratio, contribute to the efficiency of the grid device. Grid ratio is defined as the height of the lead strips to the distance (thickness of the radiolucent strips) between them. The variations in grid ratio are generally accomplished by reducing the thickness of the interspace material and maintaining the height of the lead strips. For example, an 8:1 grid may have lead strips measuring 2.0 mm tall and interspace material measuring 0.25 mm wide, producing a ratio of 2:0.25 or 8:1 (2.0 divided by 0.25 = 8). If the thickness of the interspace material were decreased to 0.2 mm and the height of the lead strips maintained at 2.0 mm, the ratio would be increased to 10:1 (2.0 divided by 0.2 = 10).

330. The answer is A.   *(Bushong, 5/e, p 251. Carlton, p 264. Carroll, 5/e, p 179.)*   The design of a grid device is a pattern of alternating lead strips and radiolucent interspace material. In general, the interspace material is thicker than the lead strips. The efficiency of a grid is based on the lead content in the device. Two factors determine lead content: grid ratio and grid frequency. The number of lead strips per inch (or centimeter) is the definition of grid frequency. This factor has a direct effect on grid efficiency due to its role in determining lead content. There are two ways in which grid frequency can be altered. The first is to decrease the thickness of the interspace material in order to include more lead strips. This variation will also increase grid ratio due to the change in relationship between the height of the lead strips and the distance between them. The second method is to reduce the thickness of the lead strips in order to include more lead strips. This variation will not affect grid ratio since the height and distances are the same.

331. The answer is D.   *(Carlton, pp 265–266. Carroll, 5/e, pp 183–184. Thompson, pp 328–329.)*   Grid radius is defined as the distance at which imaginary extensions of the lead strips would converge to a single point. The radius is important in determining the correct SID to be used with a specific grid and is based on the position of the lead strips in relation to each other—specifically, parallel versus focused. The parallel grid is designed with its lead strips equidistant from each other. If an imaginary line was drawn from each lead strip, there would be no point of convergence. Parallel lines go on to infinity without intersecting. The focused grid is designed with its lead strips angled toward the center. This pattern attempts to mirror the pattern of the x-ray photons, which are perpendicular in the central beam and diverge away from center in the peripheral beam. If imaginary lines were drawn from these lead strips, there would be a point of convergence. This point identifies the optimum SID to be used with that grid. Therefore, the widest range of grid radius in the types of grids listed as answer options is found in the parallel grid, regardless of its lead strip pattern or ratio.

332. The answer is D.   *(Bushong, 5/e, pp 308–310. Carlton, pp 267–268. Carroll, 5/e, pp 176–177.)*   The use of a grid as part of the radiographic process is for improving contrast through the removal of scattered radiation from the exit beam. When scattered radiation is included in exposing the recording medium, a general haze or layer of fog (unwanted density) is added to the image. This fog hinders the ability to visualize density differences. The use of a grid also has an effect on radiographic density. Primarily, density is reduced by the removal of the scattered radiation. Although scatter fog is regarded as detrimental to image quality, it does contribute to image density. Also, the grid device is not able to differentiate between scattered and primary photons and will absorb a percentage of primary photons in the process. The grid is constructed on the principle that scattered rays are nondirectional, while primary rays travel in a straight line determined by their origin. Therefore, the lead strips are positioned to allow the primary rays to continue in their predictable path while absorbing the random scattered rays. The angled lead strips of the focused grid make that device more effective than the parallel lead strips of the nonfocused grid.

333. The answer is C.   *(Bushong, 5/e, pp 308, 310. Carlton, pp 267–268. Cullinan, 2/e, p 77.)*   The use of a grid will lower radiographic density enough to require a direct change in exposure (mAs) in order to maintain density levels when changing from one grid ratio to another or going from nongrid to grid techniques and vice versa. The correct exposure conversion factor is determined by the grid ratios involved. A wide range of conversion factors are offered by various authors. All radiographers should be aware of the actual conversion factors of the grids available in their work place. This author has based the conversion factors used in this text on the various sources available as well as practical experience in the laboratory setting. The conversion factors suggested are stated in the "Review of Mathematical Skills" section at the beginning of this book.

A change in grid ratio will have a most noticeable effect on radiographic density. In order to maintain the desired level of density, the exposure level must vary directly with the change in grid ratio; an increase in ratio requires an increase in milliampere-seconds. The original exposure was 6 mAs with the 8:1 grid. According to the grid conversion formula, the use of a 16:1 grid will require 9 mAs:

$$\frac{\text{mAs}_o}{\text{mAs}_n} = \frac{\text{grid conversion factor}_o}{\text{grid conversion factor}_n}$$
$$\frac{6}{x} = \frac{4}{6}$$
$$4x = 6 \times 6$$
$$4x = 36$$
$$x = 9$$

This milliampere-second value is provided by the product of 300 mA and 0.03 s. The kilovoltage should remain the same. Although an increase in kilovoltage will increase density, it may also decrease contrast, thereby nullifying the reason for use of the grid.

334. The answer is D. *(Bushong, 5/e, p 253. Carlton, pp 262–264. Carroll, 5/e, pp 176–177.)* Grid ratio is the primary indicator of how effective a grid device is in absorbing scatter from the exit beam. As grid ratio increases, lead content and scatter absorption increase. Therefore, the grid with the highest ratio (16:1) will provide the best contrast.

335. The answer is D (1, 2, 3). *(Bushong, 5/e, pp 234–238. Carlton, p 261. Carroll, 5/e, p 177.)* Grids should be employed when the likelihood of scattered radiation in the exit beam is increased. The factors that influence the production of scattered radiation and its effect on the radiographic image include beam energy (kVp), part thickness, and part density. At higher kilovoltage, the scattered radiation is more forward directed (toward the image receptor) and has higher energy, making it more likely to reach and expose the image receptor. The thicker the part irradiated, the greater the likelihood of x-ray/matter interactions, including scatter-producing Compton interactions. Likewise, tissues with high molecular density (more solid) increase the occurrence of x-ray/matter interactions. Barium studies are commonly performed in the high kilovoltage range (90 kV or more) of diagnostic radiology, making scatter production an issue to contend with.

336. The answer is C. *(Carlton, p 269. Carroll, 5/e, pp 182–183. Cullinan, 2/e, pp 82–84.)* Although the purpose of the grid is to absorb scattered radiation from the exit beam, some amount of primary radiation is absorbed also. The proper use of the grid is important to minimize the loss of primary radiation. Grid cutoff is the result of improper grid use and causes a noticeable loss of density across the image. Factors that contribute to grid cutoff include angling of the grid or x-ray tube so that they are not parallel to each other; off-centering of the tube with the grid; incorrect SID according to the grid radius; or use of a focused grid upside down. Positioning latitude (the amount of tolerance or margin for error) varies with the grid pattern, type, and ratio. Parallel, linear grids with low ratios are most tolerant and frequently recommended for mobile imaging, especially emergency room situations. Crossed grids and high-ratio grids are the most restrictive and should be used where positioning and centering control is readily available.

337. The answer is A. *(Bushong, 5/e, pp 261–263. Thompson, p 329.)* The greatest amount of positioning latitude is offered by the linear, parallel type of grid of a low ratio. The linear pattern allows some central ray angulation in the same direction as the lead strips without grid cutoff. The parallel type allows the grid to be used right side up or upside down since the lead strips are parallel to each other. This also increases the range of SIDs over which the grid may be used, but still will cause cutoff, especially at a short SID. The low ratio allows a more divergent photon to be transmitted through the grid, including scattered rays, which will reduce cleanup, but will also decrease the likelihood of primary absorption.

338. The answer is B. *(Bushong, 5/e, p 251. Carlton, p 264. Cullinan, 2/e, p 76.)* The number of lines per inch (or centimeter) in a grid is termed *grid frequency*. The average grid frequency is about 100 lines per inch. High-frequency grids (about 200 lines per inch) are constructed with thinner lead strips and are available for use in a stationary manner instead of requiring moving grid devices. Movement of the grid during radiographic exposure causes the lead lines to be blurred on the image, improving detail visibility. The mechanism required to move the grid creates an OID that may be unacceptable, as in mammography. The appearance of the lead lines is much less objectionable from a stationary high-frequency grid than the standard lead line image. The reduced OID improves recorded detail, which further compensates for tolerating the appearance of the lead lines. Grid ratio is defined as the ratio of the height of the lead strips to the distance between them.

339. The answer is A (1, 2). *(Bushong, 5/e, pp 263–264. Carlton, pp 226–227, 272–273. Carroll, 5/e, pp 132, 253. Cullinan, 2/e, pp 69, 85.)* Contrast is improved by the removal of scattered photons from the exit beam, which would cause a fogging effect on the radiographic image. Scatter production is controlled by the use of collimators, which limit the amount of tissue exposed, or by the air-gap technique. Grids are used to remove scattered radiation from the exit beam. In place of a grid, the air-gap technique may be employed. This requires a large OID (about 10 inches) and a longer SID (9 to 10 feet) in order to maintain the SID/SOD ratio and minimize magnification. The OID allows space for the nondirectional scattered photons to escape and thereby not reach the image receptor. The increased distance and exposure factors required to perform this technique limit its use. The reduction of the amount of tissue exposed through restriction of field size (collimation) and compression devices will reduce the number of x-ray/matter interactions, including scatter-producing Compton interactions. Compensating filters are used to modify beam intensity and more evenly expose subject matter that is inherently varied. This type of filter tends to lower image contrast by more uniform exposure of the part.

340. The answer is B (2, 3). *(Bushong, 5/e, p 251. Carroll, 5/e, p 179. Cullinan, 2/e, p 75. Curry, 4/e, p 99. Thompson, p 326.)* The interspace material used in the construction of grids must be radiolucent in comparison with the lead strips. The role of the interspace material is to allow the primary rays through to the image receptor, while the lead strips absorb the scattered rays. Both organic (cardboard, carbon fiber) and inorganic (aluminum) materials have been used. Cardboard interspace material is not currently recommended as it absorbs moisture and breaks down. Aluminum is very commonly used, particularly in grids designed for high-kilovoltage examinations. The increased ability to absorb radiation by the aluminum material makes it less desirable for use with low kilovoltage. Carbon or plastic fiber materials are currently the preferred materials for this purpose. Lead would not be a good interspace material as it is already used as the primary absorbing material.

341. The answer is C. *(Bushong, 5/e, p 217. Carlton, p 327. Carroll, 5/e, p 189. Curry, 4/e, p 118.)* The role of intensifying screens in the imaging process is to absorb the exit beam and emit a proportionate distribution of light, which will expose the radiographic film. The effect of this process is an amplification of x-ray exposure to the film, requiring less exposure for the desired results. Patient dose is decreased with this lower exposure requirement. Each photon absorbed produces hundreds (depending on the energy of the incident x-ray photon and the type of phosphor material) of light photons. The radiographic film is more sensitive to the energy of light than x-rays and thus the effect (radiographic density) is increased over direct x-ray exposure of film. Another advantage of using intensifying screens is the increase in radiographic contrast in comparison to direct exposure imaging. There are also disadvantages to using intensifying screens, such as the loss of recorded detail due to light diffusion, known as *screen blur*. Processing time is not altered by the use of screens.

342. The answer is B.   *(Bushong, 5/e, pp 226–227. Carlton, p 329. Cullinan, 2/e, pp 95–96, Curry, 4/e, pp 127–128.)*   The *spectral emission* of an intensifying screen refers to the color of light emitted by the phosphor. Spectral emission is important in determining the correct color sensitivity of a film to be used with a particular screen. The phosphors used in early screens, including calcium tungstate, emitted light in the blue/UV range. This emission was especially appropriate because of the natural sensitivity of standard radiographic film to blue/UV emissions. The development of rare-earth phosphors, some of which emit light in the green range, required special treatment of the standard film to enhance its sensitivity to green emissions.

343. The answer is C.   *(Bushong, 5/e, p 224. Carroll, 5/e, pp 202–203. Curry, 4/e, p 156.)*   When changing to an intensifying screen with a higher relative speed factor, radiographic density will be most directly affected. The relationship between screen speed and radiographic density is directly proportional. If the screen speed is increased by a factor of four, radiographic density will also increase four times, all other technical factors being the same. The increase in screen speed will cause a decrease in recorded detail, due to increased presence of screen blur (assuming the same type of phosphor is used). Magnification will not be affected by screen speed at all. Radiographic contrast noticeably improves when changing from a direct exposure imaging system to a film-screen combination. However, minimal, if any, change in contrast occurs between different speed screens.

344. The answer is C.   *(Bushong, 5/e, p 222. Carroll, 5/e, pp 199–200. Curry, 4/e, pp 122–123.)*   The relationship between relative screen speed and recorded detail on the radiographic image is an inverse one. Before the introduction of rare-earth phosphors, the standard methods for increasing screen speed also caused increased light diffusion and decreased recorded detail (sharpness). Generally, the gain in speed to reduce patient dose outweighed the associated loss of recorded detail. However, some radiographic exams require a high level of recorded detail, making the added exposure acceptable. Methods for improving recorded detail that pertain to screen construction are (1) use of small phosphor crystals, (2) use of a thin phosphor layer, and (3) the use of light-absorbing dyes to allow only the most forward-directed (toward the film) light photons to reach the film. Each of these methods produces less light diffusion (screen blur). The inclusion of a reflective layer ensures that all light is directed toward the film, thus increasing the speed of the screen and decreasing recorded detail.

345. The answer is B (2, 3).   *(Bushong, 5/e, pp 227–228. Carroll, 5/e, pp 193–194. Curry, 4/e, pp 124–130.)*   Until the introduction of rare-earth phosphors, the primary methods of increasing screen speed had been to increase phosphor size and quantity in screen construction. Since these factors also degrade recorded detail, there was a limit to screen speed. The major difference between calcium tungstate phosphors and rare-earth phosphors is the high absorption and conversion efficiencies of rare-earth phosphors. The emission of light photons is directly related to the amount of x-ray energy it absorbs. Absorption of photon energy is improved when it is equal to or slightly higher than the binding energy of the k-shell electrons of the phosphor elements; this is called *k-edge matching.* Rare-earth phosphors such as gadolinium and lanthanum have k-shell binding energies of 50 keV and 39 keV, respectively, while tungsten has k-shell binding energy of 70 keV. Since the average beam energy is about one-third of the peak energy, there is increased likelihood of photoelectric absorption between the average photon energy and the lower binding energies of the rare-earth elements. Screen efficiency is also improved by the ability to convert the x-ray energy to light energy. Rare-earth phosphors are able to produce more light photons per photon absorbed than are calcium tungstate phosphors. Spectral emissions of some rare-earth phosphors are in the green light range, which is not as efficient as the blue/UV emissions of calcium tungstate to which radiographic film is most sensitive.

346. The answer is B.   *(Bushong, 5/e, pp 217–219. Carlton, pp 327–328. Carroll, 5/e, pp 191–192. Curry, 4/e, p 119.)*   The typical construction of an intensifying screen includes a base layer, generally made of polyester; a reflective layer to direct light photons toward the film; a phosphor layer, where photons are absorbed and light emitted; and a protective coating of plastic to provide protection of the phosphor crystals and a cleaning surface to eliminate dust. Silver halide grains (crystals) provide the photographic effect and are combined with gelatin to form the film emulsion. Cardboard was initially used as a base material for screens, but would absorb moisture, causing problems with film-screen contact.

347. The answer is B. *(Bushong, 5/e, p 308. Carroll, 5/e, pp 192–193. Curry, 4/e, p 121.)* Using the intensification factor method of determining the effect of screens on exposure (and subsequently on density), a direct relationship is demonstrated between screen speed and density. The screen speed classification system assigns numerical values to indicate the speed of a screen relative to another screen. The relative speed factors indicate that the relationship between screen speed and density is directly proportional; e.g., as relative screen speed doubles, radiographic density will also double.

348. The answer is D. *(Carlton, pp 133–135. Carroll, 5/e, pp 195–196.)* Since the relationship between relative screen speed and density is directly proportional, any change in screen speed will require an *inverse* change in exposure (milliampere-seconds). This is mathematically expressed as $mAs_o/mAs_n = RS_n/RS_o$. Faster screen speed will provide the advantages of reduced patient dose, lower heat loading on the x-ray tube, and less chance of artifacts from patient motion.

349. The answer is B. *(Carlton, pp 514–515. Carroll, 5/e, pp 378–383.)* In order to solve problems of multiple-factor technique, one must first identify those factors that affect the radiographic quality factor of interest—in this case, density. All factors listed in the answer options will affect density; however, since the kilovoltage is the same for each, it can be eliminated as a factor. Next the milliampere-second values should be found. Finally, relative screen speed should be standardized for each option and the appropriate adjustment in the milliampere-second value made. Only the milliampere-second factors will remain as a variable and the highest one will produce the greatest density. The following is the solution:

    1. Initial mAs values are (A) 4.8, (B) 5, (C) 4.8, and (D) 3.6.

    2. Change all screens to 400 RS; mAs values for A and C will need to be converted. Since both have the same original mAs and RS values, the new mAs will be the same for each:

$$\frac{4.8}{x} = \frac{400}{200}$$
$$400x = 4.8 \times 200$$
$$400x = 960$$
$$x = 2.4 \, mAs$$

    3. Final new mAs values are (A) 2.4, **(B) 5**, (C) 2.5, and (D) 3.6

350. The answer is A. *(Carlton, pp 510–515. Carroll, 5/e, pp 378–383.)* The effect of increasing the relative screen speed will be to increase density. In order to maintain the original density, a decrease in exposure will be required. All the factors listed in the answer options will affect exposure; however, milliampere-seconds is the preferred factor to vary as it will only influence density and not other factors of radiographic image quality. Also the screen change requires a two-thirds decrease in exposure, which is only achieved by decreasing the mAs from 12 to 4. The decrease in kilovoltage is 15 percent, which will only halve density. The decrease in SID and in grid ratio will cause an increase in density.

351. The answer is A. *(Bushong, 5/e, p 221. Carlton, pp 510–515. Carroll, 5/e, pp 378–383.)* The relationship between relative screen speed and density is directly proportional, making the relationship between relative screen speed and milliampere-second selection inversely proportional. In order to maintain density, the solution to this problem is found as follows:

$$\frac{32}{x} = \frac{400}{50}$$
$$400x = 32 \times 50$$
$$400x = 1600$$
$$x = 4$$

352. The answer is A. *(Bushong, 5/e, p 222. Carroll, 5/e, pp 193–194. Curry, 4/e, pp 130–131.)* Absorption of x-ray photons by the phosphors causes excitation of the phosphor atoms due to the energy deposited. In the process of restabilization, the atom emits the excess energy in the form of light photons, each having the same energy value. As photon energy increases, more energy needs to be released, thus emitting a higher quantity of light. Screen speed is designated according to how much light it produces; the more light produced, the faster the screen. This response to kilovoltage is more dramatic with rare-earth phosphors than with calcium tungstate and at settings of 70 kVp or greater. It is a recommended that a fixed kilovoltage peak technique chart be established with rare-earth phosphors to minimize the influence of kilovoltage selection on screen speed and the associated fluctuations in radiographic density that may occur.

353. The answer is B. *(Bushong, 5/e, pp 221, 226. Curry, 4/e pp 127–130, 161.)* Spectral emission refers to the color of light produced during the luminescence process of phosphors. Calcium tungstate has been the standard phosphor since 1896, when Thomas Edison developed it and Michael Pupin combined it with film to form the first film-screen imaging system. It was so successful because of its emission of light in the blue-ultraviolet range to which the film was most sensitive (responsive). The availability of rare-earth phosphors in the early 1970s produced light with energies predominantly in the green range with some blue emissions. The result of combining blue-sensitive film with green-emitting phosphors was a less than optimum response. The film to be used with green-emitting screens must be sensitized during the manufacturing process. This is achieved by adding a layer of dye to enhance the absorption of light photons with energies in the green spectrum. Consequently, optimum results require that the film selection be suited to the screen type.

354. The answer is D. *(Bushong, 5/e, p 226. Curry, 4/e, pp 1–6, 130, 161.)* The electromagnetic (EM) spectrum organizes the various types of EM energies according to their energy, wavelength, and frequency. Examples of EM energies include x-rays, radio waves, and light waves. All types of EM radiation share some common properties: they all travel at the speed of light when in a vacuum, the smallest unit of EM energy is the photon, and all EM radiation has waveform characteristics (wavelength and frequency). Each type of EM radiation also has its own specific characteristics determined by its wavelength, energy, and frequency. The EM radiation that exists as visible light can be further differentiated into perceived colors based on differences in wavelength/energy. At the extremes of the color spectrum, the color red has the longest wavelength (700 nm) and lowest energy, while the color blue has a shorter wavelength (400 nm) and higher energy.

355. The answer is C. *(Bushong, 5/e, pp 217–220. Carlton, p 328. Carroll, 5/e, pp 191–192. Curry, p 119.)* The phosphor layer of an intensifying screen is also known as the *active* layer as it is the site of photon absorption and the resultant light emission. The remaining layers of screen construction play important roles in achieving the desired light emission. The base layer provides a supportive surface on which the phosphor matrix is coated. The reflective layer is commonly added to increase relative screen speed by directing all light photons toward the film. The protective layer is applied to the surface of the phosphor layer to guard against abrasion of the phosphors during use and cleaning of the screen.

356. The answer is D. *(Bushong, 5/e, p 227. Carlton, pp 329–330. Carroll, 5/e, p 193. Curry, 4/e, pp 124–125.)* True rare-earth phosphors are those made of elements assigned to the rare-earth section of the periodic table (elements 57 to 71). They acquired the term *rare earth* from the difficulty in extracting these elements from the earth and refining them. Gadolinium and lanthanum are true rare-earth elements with atomic numbers of 64 and 57, respectively, and are commonly used as phosphor material for modern intensifying screens. Although they are not true rare-earth elements, barium lead sulfate and yttrium tantalate phosphors provide some of the advantages of rare-earth phosphors. These include a higher absorption efficiency from the barium-based phosphor ($Z = 54$) and higher conversion efficiency (18 percent) with the yttrium-based phosphor ($Z = 39$) in comparison to calcium tungstate (conversion of 5 percent and $Z = 74$).

357. The answer is D. *(Bushong, 5/e, p 227. Carlton, pp 329–330. Curry, 4/e, pp 124–127.)* Rare-earth phosphors are more desirable in radiography than calcium tungstate because of the factor of greater intensification, which translates into less exposure required to obtain optimum images. This reduction in exposure lowers patient dose and extends tube life. As a result of the higher intensification, the active layer may be made thinner or with smaller phosphor crystals to obtain a speed equivalent to that of calcium tungstate and to improve recorded detail. Rare-earth phosphors cost more than calcium tungstate because of mining and refining processes. Also, some phosphors emit light centered in the green range rather than the blue to which film is naturally sensitive. Screen phosphors have no effect on distortion of structures imaged.

358. The answer is B. *(Bushong, 5/e, pp 191–192. Carlton, p 279. Carroll, 5/e, pp 205–206. Cullinan, 2/e, pp 96–97. Curry, 4/e, pp 138–139.)* The radiographic image is the result of exposure and chemical processing of the silver halide crystals in the film emulsion. Phosphor crystals and reflective layers are part of the construction of intensifying screens. Although screens have a direct influence on the radiographic image, the actual image is composed of the silver halide crystals. An antihalation layer may be added to the construction of film for the purpose of absorbing light reflected by the film base back to the emulsion. This layer is of particular importance in single-emulsion films, where the loss of recorded detail due to this halo effect is most significant.

359. The answer is D. *(Bushong, 5/e, p 224. Carlton, p 333. Curry, 4/e p 122.)* Assuming all other factors are the same, including phosphor type, recorded detail will vary inversely with screen speed. The limiting factor in developing faster-speed calcium tungstate screens is the amount of loss of recorded detail acceptable. The standard methods of increasing screen speed (large crystals, thick phosphor layer) cause increased light diffusion and a loss of recorded detail. The use of rare-earth phosphors provides increased speeds by higher conversion and absorption efficiencies, which do not increase light diffusion. The proper selection of screen type for each exam must take into consideration the balance of patient exposure and required level of recorded detail.

360. The answer is B. *(Bushong, 5/e, pp 227, 267. Carlton, pp 406–407. Carroll, 5/e, pp 82–83. Curry, 4/e, pp 202–204.)* Quantum mottle is a form of noise, or interference, of the radiographic image. It is defined as blotchy or uneven densities on the radiograph as a result of the natural fluctuation of photon distribution in the x-ray beam. Quantum mottle is affected by the number of photons in the x-ray beam. Slow-speed imaging systems require a high exposure (many photons), which makes it difficult to visualize the mottled effect. As imaging systems increase in speed and resolution (as with rare-earth systems), the reduction in number of photons makes this blotchy effect more visible, degrading image quality. Quantum mottle is particularly noticeable with rare-earth screens and is a limiting factor to further increases in screen speed.

361. The answer is C. *(Bushong, 5/e, p 267. Carlton, p 407. Carroll, 5/e, pp 82–83. Curry, 4/e, pp 202–204.)* Quantum mottle is the result of using very low milliampere-second values, which in turn produces only a few (relatively) photons in the x-ray beam to expose a specific area of film. This is a common occurrence as faster imaging systems and more efficient x-ray generators are available. The only means of reducing quantum mottle is an increase in the number of photons in the x-ray beam by using higher milliampere-seconds. This may require using a slower speed imaging system. Although kilovoltage selection influences quantity of photons, it also influences beam quality and image contrast, making it a less appropriate means of altering quantum mottle. The focal-spot size influences recorded detail only, not the quantity of photons in the beam.

362. The answer is B. *(Bushong, 5/e, p 190. Carlton, pp 277–278. Carroll, 5/e, p 205.)* Modern radiographic film has a film base made of polyester. This material satisfies the requirements of an optimum film base. It is durable to withstand rough handling without tearing, yet flexible enough to be transported through the automatic film processor. It has dimensional stability to withstand temperature variations and exposure to chemicals without losing its shape. The film base must be transparent and not contribute to the formation of the x-ray image, particularly in the form of artifacts. The majority of radiographic film has a blue tint added to the base material for the purpose of enhancing image contrast and reducing glare from the view boxes. However, this tint is uniform and lucent so as not to interfere with the image.

363. The answer is B.   *(Bushong, 5/e, p 190. Carlton, pp 277–278. Carroll, 5/e, p 205.)*   The important qualities of the material used as the base for radiographic film include the dimensional stability, durability, and lucency. Swelling and shrinking during processing are important qualities for the gelatin used in film emulsion. Darkening in response to x-ray or light exposure and processing is characteristic of the photosensitive elements in the film emulsion.

364. The answer is C.   *(Bushong, 5/e, p 191. Carlton, p 279. Carroll, 5/e, pp 205–206. Curry, 4/e, p 119, 138–140.)*   The emulsion of radiographic film is the site of the actual image formation. It is composed of photosensitive silver halide (bromide and iodide) crystals in gelatin. The gelatin acts as a suspension medium for the silver halide crystals so that they maintain a uniform dispersion on the film base. The gelatin is also able to swell during development and then shrink during fixing. The distribution of clumps of exposed and processed silver will form the actual radiographic image.

365. The answer is B.   *(Bushong, 5/e, p 191. Carlton, p 279. Carroll, 5/e, p 206. Curry, 4/e, p 139.)*   The combination of silver halide crystals and gelatin forms the emulsion used on radiographic film. This layer is important as it is the site of image formation. This occurs specifically within the silver halide crystals. However, the gelatin portion of the emulsion is extremely important to the ability to produce the image. Three important qualities of the gelatin are (1) ability to hold the silver halide crystals in place, even during processing; (2) ability to swell during development to allow the chemistry to act on all exposed crystals and then shrink during fixing to form a durable, long-lived image; and (3) absence of impurities that would contribute to the image in the form of artifacts or alter the silver halide crystals in any way.

366. The answer is D (1, 2, 3).   *(Bushong, 5/e, p 191. Carlton, p 279. Carroll, 5/e, p 206. Curry, 4/e, p 139.)*   The photosensitive element of the film emulsion is the silver halide crystal. The term *halide* refers to those elements in the seventh group of the periodic table. The specific halides commonly used in radiographic film emulsions are bromine and iodine. The majority of the silver halide crystals are silver bromide (90 to 99 percent) with silver iodide making up the remainder.

367. The answer is A.   *(Bushong, 5/e, p 192. Carlton, pp 280–282. Curry, 4/e, pp 139–140.)*   The crystal lattice of the silver halide elements is formed through the ionic bonding of the silver and bromide (or iodide) atoms with the addition of sulfur on the surface of the lattice to aid in the photosensitivity of the crystal. Ionic bonding is the joining together of atoms, one atom giving up an electron from its valence shell to another atom having almost a completely filled valence shell. In this case, silver has one electron in its outermost shell which it gives to bromine or iodine which each have seven electrons in their outermost shell. Atoms under these conditions are attracted to each other to form a union in which both atoms have eight electrons in the outermost shell according to the octet rule. However, if the bond is severed (as following irradiation), the atoms will be in ionic form. Silver will be a positive ion (it is missing an electron) and bromide or iodide will be a negative ion (they have an extra electron).

368. The answer is D.   *(Bushong, 5/e, p 271. Carlton, p 316. Carroll, 5/e, p 504.)*   All radiographic film will exhibit a low level of density following processing, even though it was not exposed to light or x-rays. This density is termed *base plus fog* density. The majority of medical radiographic film has a blue tint added to the base material of the film. This tint is used to enhance image contrast and improve viewing conditions by reducing glare from the illuminators. Although minimal, this tint provides a *base* density of about 0.05_D or more. Additionally, during processing there is a minimal level of chemical action on the film, even though it has not been sensitized by exposure, and this results in chemical fogging. This *fog* causes a density of about 0.05_D or higher for a combined minimum base plus fog density level of 0.1_D for freshly manufactured film. Base plus fog levels can increase with time or inappropriate storage conditions. Increased base plus fog levels will cause a loss of image contrast and for this reason must be monitored. Keeping base plus fog density to a minimum can be achieved by proper storage of film and rotation of film stock to avoid exceeding its expiration dates.

369. The answer is B. *(Bushong, 5/e, p 194. Carroll, 5/e, p 204. Curry, 4/e, pp 160–161.)* Screen film is most commonly used for radiography because of its increased sensitivity to the light emitted by intensifying screens rather than x-ray exposure. This increased sensitivity greatly reduces the amount of exposure needed to produce an optimum image and hence reduces patient dose. Screen film is manufactured as both single and double (duplitized) emulsion film; that is, the photosensitive emulsion is coated on one or both sides of the film base. The difference between single and double emulsion screen film is in its speed and ability to record fine details. Double emulsion film is combined with two screens, each of which emits light to expose its adjacent film emulsion. This increase in light provides a faster imaging system, but reduces recorded detail due to possible crossover exposure. The single emulsion film is combined with a single screen (film emulsion surface in contact with the screen) to provide better recorded detail with a forfeiture of speed. Direct exposure film is designed to be more sensitive to x-ray exposure and is not used with intensifying screens. Because of the increased amount of exposure required with this film type, it is rarely used in patient exams. Video and subtraction films are available for specific electronic imagers and special radiographic techniques.

370. The answer is B. *(Bushong, 5/e, p 343. Cullinan, 2/e, pp 93–94.)* Single emulsion and single screen systems must be combined with the emulsion surface of the film in contact with the screen surface. Generally, the screen is positioned on the inside back surface of the cassette, so that it is facing the x-ray source. The film is then placed emulsion side down onto the screen with its base surface against the inside front of the cassette. With this arrangement, the exit beam enters the cassette front, passes through the film (base to emulsion), and interacts with the screen, which then emits light directly toward the film emulsion. If the film is positioned with the film base against the screen, there will be a loss of density to the image due to light absorption by the antihalation coating commonly used on the nonemulsion side of this film type. Although single film and screen imaging systems are primarily used for table-top imaging of extremities, they are also used in the bucky for mammography.

371. The answer is C (1, 2). *(Bushong, 5/e, p 196. Carroll, 5/e, pp 491–492. Curry, 4/e, pp 161–162.)* The purpose of safelights in the darkroom is to provide sufficient illumination for handling film in the process of loading and unloading cassettes without fogging the film. The various types of film available in radiology have different spectral sensitivities to accommodate the light emissions of different screens. The optimum film-screen combination should consider the matching of spectral emission (screens) with spectral sensitivity (film). The blue/UV-sensitive films may be safely handled under red or amber safelights. Using the spectral chart for radiographic film below, it can be seen that the blue sensitivity curve does not intersect with either the amber or red regions of the spectrum. Should a green light be used, however, fogging would occur. It must be remembered that even a "safe" light will fog film if it is not correctly installed or if film is exposed to it for long periods of time. Therefore, evaluation of the safelights should be part of a darkroom quality control program, and film that has been found lying on the countertop should be discarded.

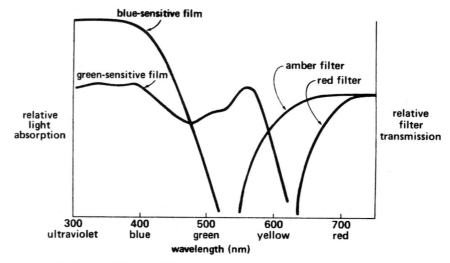

From Bushong, SC: *Radiographic Science for Technologists,* 5/e. St. Louis, Mosby—Year Book, 1993.

372. The answer is A (1 only). *(Bushong, 5/e, p 196. Carroll, 5/e, pp 205, 491–492. Curry, 4/e, pp 161–162.)* Orthochromatic film is designed to be sensitive to green light as well as blue light. This film type is used with green-emitting screens (rare-earth types). This range of light sensitivity makes the use of amber safelight inappropriate. Only red safelights should be used to ensure safe working conditions with orthochromatic film. Using the figure in the previous answer, it can be seen that the curve representing green-sensitive film crosses into the amber region, but does not reach the red zone of the spectrum.

373. The answer is D. *(Bushong, 5/e, pp 200–201. Carroll, 5/e, pp 486–488.)* Proper storage of radiographic film will ensure sufficient shelf life without increasing base plus fog density. Film should be stored in a cool, dry place protected against exposure from radiation or light. The environmental temperature should be not greater than 70° F for optimum shelf life. Longer shelf life can be obtained by refrigeration of the film. Humidity also must be controlled, at 40 to 60 percent. A too humid atmosphere will also increase fogging, which lowers film contrast and may cause film sheets to stick together. At the other extreme, very low humidity may cause an increase in static artifacts.

374. The answer is C. *(Carroll, 5/e, pp 490–492.)* Exposed radiographic film is more sensitive to safelight fog than is unexposed film. For this reason, it is important to properly unload cassettes of film for processing. This includes not piling up all exposed films on the countertop in order to process them in a continuous manner. Should the need arise to lay an exposed sheet of film on the countertop while waiting for processor availability, it should be placed away from direct exposure to the safelight.

375. The answer is C (1, 3). *(Carroll, 5/e, pp 488–492.)* Optimum radiographic quality at the lowest patient dose depends on all components of the imaging chain, including darkroom conditions. Poor darkroom conditions can lead to a loss of image contrast or the presence of unacceptable artifacts, which may require repeat exposure of the patient. The darkroom area must be designed and maintained to ensure proper storage and handling of radiographic film. This includes a clean work surface or countertop to minimize the dust, dirt, and debris that can damage image quality. Also, the safelights must provide the correct color and level of light intensity to be truly "safe" for the handling of film. Safelights should be mounted a minimum of 3 feet, preferably 4 feet, from the work surface and positioned to provide indirect lighting. The effect of safelighting can be enhanced by light colored walls in the darkroom, which will reflect the light and allow illumination of a larger area. Dark colored walls will absorb the light, minimizing the effectiveness of the safelights.

376. The answer is D. *(Bushong, 5/e, pp 200–202. Carroll, 5/e, pp 486–492.)* Film fogging can arise from numerous sources within a darkroom. These sources include heat, radiation, white light, humidity, fumes, and safelights. Proper storage conditions for film, whether it is in opened containers in the film bin or in sealed boxes, are vital to ensure optimum image quality for a minimum of patient exposure. The temperature of the film storage area (including darkrooms) should not be greater than 70° F. Humidity of the storage area must also be carefully maintained. High humidity and high temperature will cause increased base plus fog and a loss of contrast. Exposure to strong fumes may also increase base plus fog, requiring the darkroom to be well ventilated. The proximity of a darkroom to one or more radiographic rooms requires consideration of proper levels of shielding to prevent the film's exposure to radiation. Proper lighting of the darkroom needs to be considered in order to prevent fogging of film from the general white light leaks around doors, processors, and passboxes and from safelight exposure. Darkrooms should be monitored semiannually to evaluate the existence of film fogging.

377. The answer if B. *(Bushong, 5/e, pp 200–202. Carroll, 5/e, pp 486–492.)* The darkroom must provide a work area that will not negatively influence radiographic image quality. Film fogging is a primary cause of increased base plus fog on unexposed film, which will lead to a loss of image contrast. Fogging can be minimized by the correct replacement and use of safelights. The color light emitted by a safelight should not be in the sensitivity range of the film types being handled in a particular darkroom. Red safelights are safe for the widest variety of film types used in radiography. Mounting the safelights at a minimum distance of 3 feet above the processor feed tray or countertop will minimize inappropriate exposure of the films to safelight. White light sources may also contribute to film fogging and must be minimized. The use of interlocking passboxes, which does not allow the darkroom side of the passbox doors to be opened if either of the outside passbox doors are opened, will prevent white light from entering the darkroom. Blocking cracks around doors, passboxes, processors, or any other area of white light leakage will further reduce the chance of film fogging.

378. The answer is C. *(Bushong, 5/e, pp 214–215. Carroll, 5/e, pp 494–495.)* *Daylight processing* refers to the ability to load and unload cassettes into light-tight units, which automatically feed the exposed film into a processor and refill the cassette with unexposed film. This method does not require a darkroom facility and processing may be located more conveniently to the radiographic rooms. Special daylight cassettes, which are designed to work with the specific unloading and loading mechanism of each unit, must be available.

379. The answer is D. *(Ballinger, 7/e, p. 13. Carlton, p 288. Carroll, 5/e, p 494.)* All radiographic images must be properly marked with identification information pertaining to the patient and exam performed. This information should include the patient's name, age (date of birth), and x-ray or medical record number. It should also include data about the specific exam performed, the exam date, and the hospital or clinic where the exam was performed. This information is commonly printed on a card and will be transferred to a corner of the film reserved for patient identification. This is achieved by exposing the information card and the film to a white light "flash" prior to film development. The print on the card will absorb the light and produce white lettering on a black background. Identification cameras with windowed cassettes are most commonly used for this purpose. When the corner of the cassette with the window is placed into the camera containing the patient information card, the window is opened and a flash of white light makes the exposure. The window is then closed and the cassette may be removed from the camera. Other data that may also be added to a radiograph may include the name of the referring physician, the radiographer who performed the exam, and the radiographic room used. Additionally, for accuracy and legal purposes, right or left markers must be used at all times to properly indicate the side of the body imaged. This is commonly achieved by placing lead "R" or "L" markers on the cassette, without obstructing the area of interest. Often these lead markers will include the radiographer's initials or an identification number.

380. The answer is D. *(Ballinger, 7/e, p 13.)* Markers that indicate the side of the patient being radiographed should be included on all radiographic images. The finished radiograph will become part of the patient's medical record and has legal implications. Therefore, it is imperative that all images be marked correctly. Leaded "R" and "L" markers are positioned on the image receptor, within the field of exposure but not obstructing the area of interest.

381. The answer is A. *(Bushong, 5/e, p 205. Carlton, p 292. Carroll, 5/e, p 449.)* Development, the first phase of chemical processing, converts the latent (invisible) image to the manifest (visible) image. This is achieved through the process of oxidation and reduction via the developer chemicals, resulting in the deposit of black metallic silver where film crystals had been exposed to x-ray or light. The extent of the development process is a critical balance between the temperature of the developer, the developing time, and the strength of the developer chemistry. If any of these is out of proportion to the others, over- or underdevelopment may occur, resulting in suboptimum image quality.

382. The answer is B. *(Bushong, 5/e, p 205. Carlton, p 292. Carroll, 5/e, p 449.)* The development phase of chemical processing is responsible for speeding up the natural process of converting the exposed silver halide crystals to clumps of black metallic silver. Latent image centers are formed following exposure to x-ray or light and become the sites of chemical activity in the silver halide crystal. As part of latent image formation, the ionic bonds of the silver and halide atoms are broken and the excess electron acquired by the halide atoms is freed. As the freed electron drifts within the crystal, it ultimately will become trapped at a sensitivity speck, causing that area to take on its negative charge. Simultaneously, the positive silver ion is also drifting within the crystal and will become attracted to the negative area of the sensitivity speck. At this point the silver will take on a freed electron to neutralize its positive charge and create an atom of black metallic silver. As more silver is attracted and neutralized, the accumulation of black metallic silver will increase. Although this process will occur naturally, it is very slow. The developer chemistry speeds up this process by providing an ever present supply of electrons to be trapped and to form the clumps of black metallic silver more quickly. While variation in the development variables will influence radiographic density, optimum quality control is achieved by maintaining processing at optimum levels. The regulation of radiographic density must be done with proper levels of x-ray exposure. The removal of unexposed silver halide crystals is achieved during fixation.

383. The answer is D (1, 2, 3).   *(Bushong, 5/e, pp 208–209. Carlton, p 292. Carroll, 5/e, p 459.)*   Chemical fog results in the development of unexposed silver halide crystals. This may be caused by an increase in developer time, temperature, or chemical strength. This action will produce an increase in radiographic density and a loss of radiographic contrast. Chemical fog should be controlled for through daily monitoring of the processor, particularly the developer temperature and replenishment rates.

384. The answer is C.   *(Bushong, 5/e, p 206. Carlton, p 293. Carroll, 5/e, p 450.)*   The reducing agent is also known as the developing agent. This chemical component is responsible for the primary action of the developer, converting exposed silver halide crystals to black metallic silver. The term *reducer* is applied to describe the chemical action provided in order to speed up the development process. Reduction is the chemical process of acquiring of electrons. Through the chemical process of oxidation, the developing (reducing) agents give up numerous free electrons to the sensitivity specks, which are taken on by the silver ions, forming black metallic silver. The exposed silver is thus said to be "reduced" (converted to black metallic silver). There are two reducing agents commonly used in the developer for automatic processing. They are hydroquinone, for producing the black tones, and phenidone, which produces the gray shades. The remainder of the chemical components that compose the developer play supportive roles such as preservative, activator, restrainer, and hardener.

385. The answer is D.   *(Bushong, 5/e, p 206. Carlton, p 294. Carroll, 5/e, p. 451. Curry, 4/e, p 143.)*   The *activator* of the developer is responsible for maintaining the required pH level in the alkali range (10 to 11.5), which enhances the development action of the reducing agents. It also acts to soften the emulsion so that it can swell and allow the chemistry in to work on the deeper lying silver halide crystals. Sodium carbonate is the activator used commonly in automatic processors. The activator plays a necessary supportive role to the primary role of converting exposed silver in the development process. Other important supportive actions in the developer are those of *restrainer*, which prohibits developer action on unexposed crystals; *hardener*, which controls the amount of emulsion swelling in accordance with the transport system of the automatic processor; and *preservative*, for long chemical life.

386. The answer is A.   *(Bushong, 5/e, p 208. Carlton, p 295. Carroll, 5/e, p 452.)*   Film jams may occur as a result of insufficient developer chemistry. Replenishment systems are incorporated into automatic processing to maintain levels and activities of the developer and fixer solutions. Exhausted developer includes insufficient hardener (glutaraldehyde) to control the amount of emulsion swelling. This may cause the emulsion to become too thick for the tolerance allowed between the rollers, and the film may jam. Excessive swelling may also cause pieces of the emulsion to come off the film base and attach to the rollers, causing artifacts on future films. Overfixation of a radiograph may cause excessive hardening of the image, which may lead to cracking of the film in the future. Insufficient washing may not completely remove chemistry from the film, causing staining or yellowing of the image over time. Overdevelopment may occur from increased temperature, development time, or chemical strength and will cause excessive density and loss of contrast in the image, but it will not cause a transport problem in the processor.

387. The answer is C.   *(Bushong, 5/e, p 210. Carlton, p 297. Carroll, 5/e, p 449.)*   Washing of the film is the third of the four steps for radiographic processing. It follows the development and fixing phases. The purpose of washing is to remove the chemicals (developer and fixer, primarily) from the film, which will aid in its archival quality. Clean, continuously flowing water is used for the washing process. The agitation action provided by the flowing water and rollers of the transport system is necessary for optimum clearing of chemistry from the film. The removal of unexposed silver halide crystals is achieved by the clearing agent in the fixer. The acidic pH level of the fixer is responsible for neutralizing the action of the developing agents, once the film has moved into the fixer. The softening of the emulsion for development purposes is achieved by the activator of the developer.

388. The answer is B. *(Bushong, 5/e, p 209. Carlton, pp 296, 306. Carroll, 5/e, p 453.)* *Ammonium thiosulfate* is used as the clearing agent in the fixer. As a clearing agent, it is responsible for removing unexposed silver halide crystals from the developed radiograph. This action brings out the clear, unexposed areas of the image. Insufficient clearing will cause the image to darken over time. This is caused by the continued conversion of unexposed crystals. As with the developer, the fixer must be replenished as it is used up. Exhausted fixer will become so saturated with silver ions that it will be unable to take on any more. The heavy content of silver in the used fixer solution makes it necessary to reclaim the silver before it is dumped. The second major function carried out by the fixing process is the shrinking and hardening of the emulsion by the hardener, *potassium alum*. The reducing agents convert exposed crystals to black metallic silver. *Sodium sulfite* is the preservative in both the developer and fixer. It is included to provide a long life for the chemical activity.

389. The answer is B. *(Bushong, 5/e, p 209. Carlton, p 296. Carroll, 5/e, p 449.)* The fixing phase is the second of the four steps of radiographic processing. It has two primary roles: (1) to clear the film of unexposed silver halide; and (2) to shrink and harden the emulsion for long life. Two separate chemicals are used to complete these actions. The *clearing agent* is ammonium or sodium thiosulfate, which removes the unexposed silver. Omission of this step would result in the image darkening over time due to the retained silver halide crystals, which will become exposed to light once the film is processed. Remember, conversion of exposed silver halide to black metallic silver is a natural, albeit very slow, process. The second primary function is achieved by the use of the *hardener*, potassium alum, to shrink and harden the emulsion for safe handling and protection of the image against abrasions. The development phase is responsible for softening the emulsion and then converting the latent image to a manifest image. The amount of swelling is controlled by the hardener agents. The wash cycle is responsible for the removal of any retained chemicals following development and fixing, prior to the final stage, drying.

390. The answer is B. *(Bushong, 5/e, p 209. Carlton, p. 296. Carroll, 5/e, p 453.)* As in the developer, the activator maintains the desired pH level in the fixer—specifically in the acidic range. Acetic acid is commonly used as the activator. This component of the fixer acts as a stop bath for the development action when the film exits the developer and enters the fixer. The alkaline nature of the developer is neutralized by the acidic nature of the fixer. A primary role for the fixer is the clearing of the unexposed silver.

391. The answer is C. *(Bushong, 5/e, pp 210–213. Carlton, pp 297–303. Cullinan, 2/e, p 111.)* Agitation during processing is important to ensure thorough mixing of the chemicals. This action also promotes active contact between the chemicals and the film. In the automatic processor, the transport and recirculation systems contribute to the agitation. The rollers of the transport system are positioned in such a manner as to cause a wave motion of the film as it moves through the tank, rather than just moving straight down one side and up the other side of the roller rack. This wave motion sloshes the chemicals over the film surface. A recirculation system is incorporated in the developer, fixer, and wash cycles to keep the solutions constantly moving. In the developer and fixer tanks, a small amount of solution is removed from the bottom of the tank through lines and pumped back up to the top of the tank. This movement of solution helps to maintain well mixed chemicals and avoid temperature variations throughout the tank. In the wash tank, a constant flow of water is added to the tank and overflows at the top. This method provides a clean supply of wash water to remove excess chemicals from the film. The replenishment system is responsible for maintaining chemical levels and strength, which are depleted as films are processed.

392. The answer is C. *(Bushong, 5/e, p 213. Carlton, pp 300–302. Carroll, 5/e, p 477. Cullinan, 2/e, pp 242–243.)* *Underdevelopment* of a radiograph will occur for the following reasons: (1) developer temperature too low; (2) developing time too short; and (3) weak or exhausted developer chemicals. Developer temperature is regulated via a temperature control system. The optimum temperature for developer solution in rapid (90 s) processors is between 92 and 96° F, depending on the specific manufacturer of the chemicals. The transport system determines overall processing time by the speed at which the rollers turn and thus the amount of time the film spends in each tank in the processor. Underdevelopment may occur if the roller speed is too fast, reducing the amount of time the film spends in the developer tank. Chemical activity must be maintained at a constant working level. Proper mixing of the chemicals, initially and while in use (recirculation), and proper replenishment rates are important factors in maintaining the desired activity level for both the developer and fixer. Exhausted developer, generally due to low replenishment rates, will cause underdevelopment. The temperature of the wash water is maintained at about 5° below that of the developer. In some processors, an increase in wash water temperature may cause an increase in developer temperature.

393. The answer is A. *(Bushong, 5/e, p 213. Carlton pp 299–301. Carroll, 5/e, pp 473–474.)* The replenishment systems of most processors are activated by the opening of microswitches located on the entrance detector set of rollers. The opening of these switches occurs as each film is fed into the processor. In this manner, replenishment rates are set according to the length of film as it travels through the processor. Films should be positioned crosswise on the feed tray, so that replenishment occurs as the film travels its shortest distance. The feed trays for most processors are 17 inches wide in order to accommodate 14 by 17 inch films crosswise. (See diagram below: *A* demonstrates crosswise introduction of film into the processor; *B* demonstrates lengthwise introduction.) Small films such as 8 by 10 inch films should be fed in lengthwise, two films at a time. With each film aligned with its own feed guide (at the edge of the tray), they will cover 16 inches of the usual 17 inch tray width, without concern for crossover as they are transported. The recirculation system is responsible for maintaining proper mixing of the solutions. The overall processing time (dry to dry) is controlled by the rate at which the rollers turn, hence the speed at which the film moves through the processor. The temperature control system is a separate system for the regulation of developer temperature.

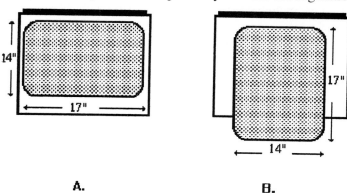

A.   **B.**

394. The answer is C. *(Bushong, 5/e, p 197. Carlton, p 286.)* The increasing availability of electronic imaging and computer-assisted imaging has altered the method of obtaining a permanent, hard copy of the radiographic images. Instead of having the exit beam recorded on radiographic film, radiation detectors are the receptors of the exit beam. These detectors are able to convert the radiation to an electronic signal for analysis and storage. The image is then displayed on a video monitor known as a cathode ray tube (CRT) for viewing and image manipulation. This image can be archived with a magnetic tape or disk system for future retrieval. However, most radiologists still prefer to view final images on film. To obtain these hard copy images, a multiformat camera containing video film is attached to the CRT and the images recorded from it. Video film is constructed with a single emulsion and its spectral sensitivity is matched with the spectral emission of the CRT.

395. The answer is B. *(Bushong, 5/e, pp 196–197. Carroll, 5/e, p 204. Cullinan, 2/e, p 93.)*   Direct exposure film is different from screen type film because it is made to be more sensitive to x-ray interaction than to the light from intensifying screens. To achieve this sensitivity, direct exposure film has a thicker emulsion (higher concentration of silver halide crystals) to increase absorption of the x-ray photons. The substantially lower penetrability of light photons would be unable to expose crystals in such a thick emulsion. This thicker emulsion makes direct exposure film a poor candidate for development in automatic processors. This is due to the increased amount of swelling of this emulsion type, which would lead to the film's being too thick for the roller interspaces and to subsequent jamming of the transport system.

396. The answer is C. *(Bushong, 5/e, p 443. Carroll, 5/e, pp 503, 506–509. Cullinan, 2/e, pp 244–245.)* Sensitometry is the monitoring system of the automatic film processor. It is recommended that this action occur on a daily basis, preferably in the morning before the bulk of the day's work has begun. This monitoring procedure provides a means of evaluating and adjusting, if necessary, the operation of the processor in order to eliminate processor error as a cause of unnecessary repeat exposures. This system employs the processing of a test film strip that has been exposed to a consistent level of exposure through the use of a sensitometer. Following development, the density scale is evaluated and compared with previous data pertaining to the operation of the processor. This system will indicate changes in base-plus-fog levels, film speed, and contrast levels. It will also demonstrate trends that will alert the radiographer to the potential of upcoming problems. In this manner, preventative maintenance can be performed before radiographic images have been affected and can reduce unexpected processor down time.

397. The answer is A. *(Bushong, 5/e, p 443. Cullinan, 2/e, p 244. Gray, p 38.)*   Processor sensitometry should be performed on a daily basis, preferably in the morning prior to the beginning of the day's work. In this manner, the operating conditions of the processor may be kept at optimum levels.

398. The answer is D. *(Bushong, 5/e, p 443. Cullinan, 2/e, pp 244–245. Gray, pp 45–47.)*   In order to perform film processor monitoring, daily sensitometry data should be obtained. The basic equipment needed to optimally carry out this task includes a densitometer, sensitometer, thermometer, and a supply of test film kept separate from the film used in reloading cassettes. On a daily basis, the temperature of the developer should be checked using a digital probe or metal stem thermometer and the crossover and feed tray cleaned. Once optimum temperature has been established, a test film that has been exposed to a sensitometer is processed. The sensitometer exposes the film to a repeatable level of light exposure through an optical step wedge, producing a gray scale upon processing. If a sensitometer is not available, the test film may be exposed to an aluminum step wedge using a radiographic unit. However, this method is less desirable due to the potential for a lack of reproducible exposures from day to day. The density steps on the test film are then evaluated with a densitometer to note any variation in fog, speed, or contrast from previous sensitometric evaluations. The densitometer should be used to determine density difference because the human eye does not have the same level of acuity and is influenced by the subjectivity of the individual viewer.

399. The answer is B. *(Bushong, 5/e, pp 443–445. Carroll, 5/e, pp 482–484. Cullinan, 2/e, p 94.)*   Artifacts are areas of plus or minus densities that are not representative of the object imaged. Due to the sensitive nature of radiographic film, artifacts may be caused by a variety of factors involved in the imaging chain, including handling and storage of film, exposure variables, and automatic processor errors. The types of artifacts most commonly caused by the processor are pi lines, guide shoe marks, emulsion pickoff, chemical stain, curtain effect, and wet pressure sensitization. Most of these effects are the result of problems with the transport system of the processor. Pi lines are regularly occurring marks of increased density that run *perpendicular* to the direction the film travels through the processor. The marks are the result of dirt or other deposits on the roller that cause a wet pressure sensitization (increased density) on the film with each revolution of the roller. Guide shoe marks are white or clear lines running *parallel* to the direction the film travels through the processor and are due to improperly seated guide shoes. The effect is caused by the tips of the guide shoe ribs as they come in contact with the film and scratch the emulsion from the film as it moves along. Emulsion pickoff is caused by dirt or other deposits on the rollers that remove a small bit of the softened emulsion when it comes in contact with the roller. These will appear as dust artifacts and are particularly bothersome with single emulsion film as is used for mammography. Chemical stain is a discoloration due to contamination or transport problems that cause films to overlap. These stains often appear as a *curtain effect* due to excess chemicals on the film that run along its surface. Careful monitoring and routine maintenance of the automatic processor will minimize these artifacts and the need for repeat images.

400. The answer is C. *(Bushong, 5/e, pp 443–445. Carroll, 5/e, pp 482–484. Cullinan, 2/e, p 94.)* Unopened boxes of film should be stored on end in the darkroom to avoid the occurrence of artifacts that result from pressure sensitization of the film. This type of artifact will appear as an area of increased density on the processed film. As with any artifact, these areas of increased density may impair visibility of vital anatomic structures, requiring repeat exposure to the patient. Unopened boxes of film should also be rotated (new film placed behind old film) in order to ensure use of the film before its expiration date. Film that has exceeded its shelf life may have an increased base-plus-fog level, making it unusable.

401. The answer is C. *(Carlton, p 300. Carroll, 5/e, p 480.)* Films that are still tacky when they exit the processor are most likely the result of insufficient fixing due to improper mixing of the fixer, exhausted fixer, or low replenishment rates for the fixer. The fixer is responsible for shrinking and hardening the emulsion following clearing of the unexposed silver crystals. Therefore, insufficient hardener in the fixer will leave the emulsion soft and tacky and easily damaged by the remainder of the processing cycle and handling of the film. Although low dryer temperature may cause insufficient drying of the film, the film will feel damp, but should not be tacky.

402. The answer is D. *(Carlton, p 300. Carroll, 5/e, p 480.)* The minimum dryer temperature is about 120° F. The dryer system consists of a large blower that takes room air past a set of heating elements and then forces the heated air into vented tubes. These tubes are positioned on either side of the film as it is transported through the dryer section. The heated air is directed across the surface of the film. Factors that may contribute to poor drying of a film include high humidity in the processing area, hot-air tubes installed backward so the opening is away from the film, excess water on film due to poor squeegee action prior to film entering the dryer, and insufficient fixing.

403. The answer is C. *(Carlton, pp 299–300. Carroll, 5/e, pp 483–484.)* Placing the edge of the film along the vertical edges of the feed tray will assist in guiding the film straight into the processor. However, it is important to remember to use both sides of the feed tray in processing successive films. This action will avoid uneven wearing of the rollers. Any spills or debris on the feed tray must be cleared away to prevent artifact formation on the radiograph. Wet spots of water or chemicals will adversely affect development of those areas and may contaminate the developer. Dirt and other debris may scratch the film surface. Once a portion of a film has entered the developer, it should not be pulled back. This action may sensitize the film where the entrance rollers were in contact with the film and cause dark ridges along the leading edge of the film. Also, developer may be splashed out onto the feed tray and the rest of the film, causing dark drip marks across the film. A little added pressure along the edge of the film should help to straighten it enough for safe transport.

404. The answer is C. *(Bushong, 5/e, p 300. Carroll, 5/e, pp 238–239. Selman, 8/e, pp 355–356.)* The inverse square law is used to explain the variation of radiation intensity to an object as SID changes. It states that as SID increases, the divergent rays will cover a larger area, causing intensity to decrease by a factor of the change of distance squared. For example, an x-ray source is located 20 inches from an object and delivers an exposure level of 120 mR; if the source was moved to 40 inches from the object (distance increased by a factor of 2) and the exposure factors remained the same, the exposure level would be decreased by a factor of 2^2, or 4 (the change in distance squared). The resulting exposure to the object would be one-fourth of the original 120 mR, or 30 mR. This fact demonstrates the need to compensate for changes in exposure output due to changes in SID by adjusting the milliampere-seconds (directly proportional to the distance squared).

405. The answer is D. *(Bushong, 5/e, pp 311, 330. Carroll, 5/e, pp 233, 246.)*   Although not a true exposure factor, SID influences the level of exposure to the image receptor as well as the accuracy with which the object is imaged. As stated in the inverse square law, changes in SID will inversely alter the radiation intensity. Since radiographic density is determined by exposure, any change in SID will have an inverse effect on density. Specifically, density is inversely proportional to the distance squared. For this reason, milliampere-seconds must be altered when SID is changed to compensate for the change in intensity and to maintain the optimum level of density. The radiographic quality factors of recorded detail and distortion are also influenced by SID. A long SID will create an x-ray beam in which the useful photons are less divergent, more vertical. The effect of this will be a reduction in geometric blur of the edges of the structures imaged. The long SID will also reduce the occurrence of magnification of the image, as long as the OID remains as minimal as possible. For these various reasons, SID should be kept at a constant level, which will produce optimum results. Since changes in SID have no influence on beam quality or scatter production there will be no effect on contrast.

406. The answer is D. *(Bushong, 5/e, p 295. Carroll, 5/e, p 221.)*   The technical factors involved in creating a radiographic image often influence more than one aspect of overall radiographic quality. Of these technical factors, the selection of a particular focal-spot size will only influence recorded detail, specifically geometric blur. Focal-spot size is not an electrical component, so it will not alter the beam's quantity or quality. Therefore, it has no influence on density or contrast. Also, the focal-spot size plays no role in the relationship of the object to be radiographed with the x-ray tube or image receptor; thus it has no influence on image distortion. Changes in SID or image receptors will alter density as well as recorded detail. Changes in OID will alter contrast, density, and recorded detail.

407. The answer is C. *(Bushong, 5/e, pp 168, 234, 249. Carroll, 5/e, p 127.)*   Compensating filters are accessory devices that may be employed to provide more uniform exposure of a specific body part. The most commonly used types of compensating filters are the wedge and trough, named for their shapes. Each filter shapes the pattern of beam intensities; its thick areas will attenuate much of the beam, producing an area of lower intensity, and its thin areas have the opposite effect. For example, the wedge filter has a thick end that tapers to a thin end. This device is positioned in the path of the primary beam with the thick end over the thin end of the anatomic structure and the thin end of the filter over the thick portion of the anatomy. The result is a more even exposure relative to the thickness of the anatomic structure. Such a device may be used when imaging the AP thoracic spine. The upper thoracic vertebrae are much thinner than the lower. Typically, the image is overexposed for the upper vertebrae as compared with the lower vertebrae. The wedge filter in this case would even out the exposure. The collimator only determines the size of the field of exposure. The grid device will absorb scattered rays from the exit beam; it has no effect on the primary beam. The shadow shield is a device that is attached to the collimator and can be positioned in the path of the primary beam to shield an area of the anatomy from exposure.

408. The answer is B. *(Bushong, 5/e, pp 234, 308, 310. Carlton, p 228. Carroll, 5/e, p 141.)*   The use of good collimation is important in keeping the patient's exposure as low as possible. The less tissue volume irradiated, the less scattered radiation produced. Therefore, collimation will reduce patient dose and increase radiographic contrast. When decreasing field size from a large area to a small area, the scatter reduction may be significant enough to lower radiographic density, requiring an increase in milliampere-seconds to maintain proper density level. Proper collimation limits the field size to the area of primary interest, and the field size should *never* be larger than the image receptor.

409. The answer is D. *(Bushong, 5/e, pp 235–238. Carlton, p 227. Carroll, 5/e, p 132.)*   The size of the field of exposure directly influences the number of x-ray/matter interactions likely to occur. This means that a smaller, more collimated field will reduce the production of scattered radiation, as well as photoelectric interactions. Less scatter in the exit beam will increase radiographic contrast. The collimator acts to restrict the beam size by eliminating the peripheral rays; it does not focus the photons toward the center of the beam. The collimator assembly does contribute to the sum of added filtration required for minimum filtration standards, but does not significantly harden the beam.

410. The answer is A. *(Bushong, 5/e, p 308. Carroll, 5/e, p 141.)* Changing field size from large (14 × 17 inches) to small will significantly reduce the number of scattered and primary photons in the exit beam, resulting in decreased image density. The best technical adjustment to maintain density is to increase the milliampere-seconds. Lowering the kilovoltage will further reduce image density. Increasing the kilovoltage will darken the image, but also may lower the contrast. A change in grid ratio would have an indirect effect on radiographic density, as will changes in SID. However, these factors will also alter image contrast, recorded detail, and distortion, thus potentially causing further image problems. When the image requires more or less radiographic density, a change in milliampere-seconds is the purest solution.

411. The answer is A. *(Bushong, 5/e, pp 308–310, 316–317. Carroll, 5/e, pp 100–101.)* High kilovoltage produces a highly penetrating beam that results in low differential absorption and low image contrast. However, it also reduces patient's exposure by requiring less milliampere-seconds. The naturally low subject contrast of the chest is one area in which use of high-kilovoltage techniques can be advantageous. The more energetic beam reduces the high subject contrast of the chest, improving visibility of soft tissue structures in the thorax and minimizing the distraction caused by the bony structures. While high kilovoltage would be desirable to reduce dose in pediatric patients, the overpenetration of their small structures would not contribute to optimal images. IVU exams employ water-soluble iodinated contrast media, which can be overpenetrated by high-kilovoltage techniques. Elderly patients most commonly present with demineralization of their bones. Therefore, low kilovoltage would be better to enhance contrast when radiographing their extremities.

412. The answer is D. *(Bushong, 5/e, pp 312–314. Carroll, 5/e, pp 319–320.)* Technique charts are designed to provide acceptable combinations of technical factors to produce optimum image results with the specific radiographic and accessory equipment of an imaging department. In addition to the exposure factors (milliampere-seconds, kilovolts), these charts should also include the type and speed of imaging system preferred, the correct SID, the grid ratio if one is to be used, and the specific factors relating to the automatic exposure control. In regard to patient information, the most reliable factor to consider between various patients is the thickness of the part to be imaged. Technique charts can be designed as either fixed- or variable-kilovoltage types. Both types alter the kilovolts/milliampere-seconds for variations in part size by listing appropriate factors for either specific part thicknesses (variable kilovoltage) or thickness ranges such as "small, medium, large" (fixed kilovoltage). Technique charts must be continually updated as changes in available equipment are made.

413. The answer is D. *(Bushong, 5/e, pp 308–310. Carroll, 5/e, pp 379, 381.)* Radiographic contrast is determined by beam quality, patient factors, and scatter control. Of the factors listed as possible influencing variables, only kilovoltage and grid ratio matter. Kilovoltage regulates the penetrability of the beam, and grid ratio indicates the ability to remove scatter from the exit beam. Low kilovoltage will produce higher contrast than high kilovoltage, and high grid ratio will clean up more scatter than low grid ratio. The influence of milliampere-seconds and SID on contrast is only in situations of extreme over- or underexposure. Changes in milliampere-seconds and SID primarily affect beam quantity, thus radiographic density. The answer for this problem is based on selecting the combination with the lowest kilovoltage and highest grid ratio. No mathematical computations are needed.

414. The answer is A. *(Bushong, 5/e, pp 308–310. Carroll, 5/e, pp 379, 381.)* The primary technical factors controlling and influencing contrast are beam quality and scatter control devices. Beam quality is determined by the kilovoltage used and filtration levels. Increases in either kilovoltage or filtration will harden the x-ray beam, making it more penetrating and lowering differential absorption. This will produce an image with long scale or low contrast. Screen speed and milliampere-seconds primarily influence beam quantity, thus affecting density. To solve this problem for the combination that produces the *lowest* radiographic contrast, find the highest kilovoltage, highest filtration, and lowest grid ratio.

415. The answer is B. *(Bushong, 5/e, pp 317–318. Carroll, 5/e, pp 332, 340.)* Automatic exposure control devices (AEC) terminate the exposure when a predetermined level of radiation has been sensed. A properly calibrated AEC will compensate for changes in patient thickness and pathology by increasing or decreasing the exposure (mAs) as required. To utilize the AEC to its fullest advantage, the radiographer should select the optimum kilovoltage for the part being irradiated to ensure proper penetration and contrast. The positioning and centering of the part within the beam must be accurate to place the anatomy of interest over the sensing chamber for proper exposure. Additionally, collimation of the beam to the part is necessary to reduce scattered radiation, which may cause the AEC to terminate earlier than it should.

416. The answer is D (1, 2, 3). *(Bushong, 5/e, pp 317–318. Carroll, 5/e, pp 332, 340.)* The AEC will select the proper amount of exposure (mAs) to sufficiently expose the part of interest. This is achieved by selection of sensing chambers, which sample the exit beam and terminate the exposure when a predetermined level is received. The radiographer should select the optimum kilovoltage for the part irradiated, utilize good collimation to minimize the influence of scattered radiation on the AEC, and correctly position and center the part of interest within the beam. While the AEC can compensate for changes in patient thickness, pathology, and, to some extent, incorrect kilovoltage, it cannot adjust for variations in image receptor speed or improper processing of the image.

417. The answer is B. *(Bushong, 5/e, p 320. Carroll, 5/e, p 339.)* The typical AEC device employs three sensing chambers. These components are arranged with one center chamber corresponding with the central ray and two side chambers, one to each side of the center chamber. When selected, these sensors receive the exit beam and cause the exposure to terminate when a predetermined level has been achieved. These chambers may be used singly or in various combinations. When more than one is activated, the radiation received by each chamber is averaged until the predetermined level has been received. When performing the usual PA view of the chest, one or two side chambers are generally selected in order to provide proper exposure of the lungs. Use of the center chamber, located under the mediastinum, would result in higher exposure to demonstrate the mediastinum and overexposure of the lungs.

418. The answer is C. *(Bushong, 5/e, p 270. Curry, 4/e, p 149. Selman, 8/e, p 331.)* The expression for optical density is the ratio of the *light intensity incident* (I_o) on the radiograph to the *light intensity transmitted* (I_t) through the radiograph, using the $\log_{10}$ number system. The exposed and processed radiograph will demonstrate an accumulation of black metallic silver that will absorb some of the light from the view box, reducing its transmission in proportion to the varying amounts of black metallic silver. The reduction in light transmission will be indicated by an increase in the numerical value for density. Use of the logarithmic number system allows for a more manageable method of expressing a large range of numbers. To make it easier to understand this system, the reader should know specific equivalent values between the decimal and logarithmic number systems. These include the following:

Decimal Value	Log Equivalent
2	0.3
10	1.0
100	2.0
1000	3.0

Using these equivalents, one can see that as light transmission is reduced by a factor of 2.0, the density value will be expressed as an increase by a log value of 0.3. For example:

100% transmission = 0.0 density

50% transmission = 0.3 density

25% transmission = 0.6 density

12% transmission = 0.9 density.

The other mathematical expressions offered as answers represent *film speed, average gradient,* and *magnification factor.*

419. The answer is B (2, 3).   *(Bushong, 5/e, pp 269–271, 273–277. Carroll, 5/e, pp 504–506.)*   The H&D chart shown in the question is used to graphically demonstrate the response of radiographic film to exposure and processing. The characteristics of film speed, contrast, latitude, and base plus fog are illustrated. Changes in film response will be evidenced by changes in the position and shape of the curve on the H&D chart. More specifically, quantified data may be obtained by calculating the differences in film speed and contrast as portrayed by these curves.

420. The answer is B.   *(Bushong, 5/e, p 277.)*   Film contrast is associated with latitude in an inversely proportional relationship. This means that a high-contrast film has less (or narrower) latitude and low-contrast film has more (or wider) latitude. Latitude refers to the ability of a film to record densities at the toe-body and body-shoulder transition points. A film with wide latitude is more "forgiving" of exposure errors than is narrow-latitude film. However, wide latitude may not bring out the density differences as well. A proper matching of the film's characteristics with the imaging requirements of the human anatomy must be made in order to obtain the best possible results. Mottle, speed, and grain size are all factors of radiographic film, but are independent of film contrast.

421. The answer is B.   *(Bushong, 5/e, pp 270–272, 276–278. Carroll, 5/e, pp 506–507.)*   The shape of the H&D curve provides a relative indication of inherent film contrast. Film contrast may be significantly influenced by processing conditions, specifically development. If development time, temperature, or chemical strength is increased or decreased from the optimum conditions set, both density and contrast will be altered. Overdevelopment will increase density and vice versa, but contrast will decrease whether over- or underdevelopment occurs. Screen and film speed contribute to the density response of the film only. Mottle is speed-related and contributes to a loss of image quality due to the presence of noise.

422. The answer is B.   *(Bushong, 5/e, p 299. Carroll, 5/e, pp 68–69.)*   Milliampere-seconds (mAs) are the product of milliamperage and exposure time. Exposure time may be stated in terms of fractions, decimals, or milliseconds (1/1000 of a second). In order to calculate milliampere-seconds, one must be familiar with multiplying by fractions and decimals. When time is expressed in milliseconds, it must be converted to seconds before being multiplied. For this problem the solution is

$$400 \times \frac{1}{60} = \frac{400}{60} = 6.66 \approx 7 \text{mAs}$$

The decimal form for 1/60 may be found by dividing the numerator (top number) by the denominator (bottom number), which equals $0.01666 \approx 0.017$. The equivalent of this value in milliseconds is 17 ms (move decimal point three places to the right).

423. The answer is C.   *(Bushong, 5/e, pp 231–233, 444. Carroll, 5/e, pp 212, 482–483. Selman, 8/e, pp 285–288. Sweeney, p 10.)*   Intensifying screens act to amplify the photographic effect of x-rays on film by converting their energy to numerous light photons to which film is more sensitive. Improper use or damage of the screens can result in images of poor quality and the appearance of artifacts. Examples of such problems include the presence of dust, dirt, or other debris in the cassette, which will obstruct the transmission of light to the film-producing areas of low (white) density. Equally important is the need for complete physical contact between the film and screen, which is maintained by the design of the cassette. Areas of poor contact will cause localized blur and loss of recorded detail (sharpness). Crescent marks are caused by mishandling of the film. Regularly repeating artifacts are the result of a problem with the roller transport system of the processor.

424. The answer is A.   *(Selman, 8/e, pp 287–288. Sweeney, pp 50, 362.)*   Of the actions listed as answer options, only routine screen cleaning will minimize or prevent the formation of artifacts on the radiographic image. This action will remove dirt, dust, and other debris from the screen surface that would decrease the transmission of light from the phosphors to the film. Focal-spot size has no effect on artifact formation. The proper method for storing unopened boxes of film is to stand them on end. Laying them flat, on top of each other, will induce pressure artifacts. In general, pillows should not be used to position or support the anatomic structure of interest, unless they have been radiographed to ensure their contents are radiolucent. The fill of most bed pillows is not radiolucent and will cause a low-density, mottled appearance on the image.

425. The answer is C (1, 3). *(Bushong, 5/e, pp 211–213. Carroll, 5/e, p 475. Cullinan, 2/e, pp 110–111. Selman, 8/e, p 312.)* The transport system of the automatic processor serves to move the film through each phase of processing. This action is achieved through a system of various types of roller assemblies connected to a drive motor via gears and pulleys. The drive motor turns the gear system, which then turns the rollers to pull the film along their path. The rate at which the rollers turn must be accurately adjusted and monitored in order to maintain correct processing time. The speed at which the rollers turn will determine the length of time the film is in each solution tank. The turning action also contributes to the agitation process of the chemicals. The designs of the crossover and squeegee roller sets further act to remove excess chemicals from the film as it leaves each tank.

426. The answer is D. *(Bushong, 5/e, p 214. Carroll, 5/e, p 456.)* Optimum processing results rely on three development variables: *time, temperature,* and *chemical strength.* These variables must be monitored for changes that would degrade radiographic image quality. Exposure factors are based on the assumption that the processor variables are appropriately set. The radiographer must be able to determine the correct source of poor image quality, whether it is related to exposure or the processor. The use of *extended* processing in some areas of radiography has altered the usual relationship between these variables to warrant a change in exposure factors. Generally, this system of processing is restricted to a specialized imaging area for which the exposure factors have been sufficiently altered. Extended processing increases the immersion time for the film in the developer. Longer development times allow more thorough development of the silver crystals, particularly those close to the film base, and essentially increases film speed. An increase in film speed is accompanied by a decrease in exposure (mAs). The end results are sufficient density, better contrast, and less patient dose. Extended processing is generally limited to mammography.

427. The answer is B. *(Bushong, 5/e, p 211. Selman, 8/e, p 311.)* The transport system controls the overall processing time. The speed at which the rollers turn determines how long the film is in each tank. In the typical 90-s processor, the film spends approximately 20 s each in the developer, fixer, and washer, and about 30 s in the dryer. Roller speed is set and maintained by a drive system consisting of a motor and an arrangement of belts, chains, pulleys, and gears. When the transport system is operating properly, all rollers turn at the same rate.

428. The answer is B. *(Bushong, 5/e, p 212. Carroll, 5/e, p 477. McKinney, p 96. NCRP No. 99, p 54.)* The temperature of the developer is the most critical of the three processing solutions. Automatic processors contain a temperature control system that includes a thermostat and heater to continually monitor and maintain developer temperature. Generally, developer temperature will be between 92 and 95° F. Fixer and wash water temperatures are lower than that of the developer (usually about 5° F. lower). Fixer temperature is controlled by either a heat exchange system from the developer or by convection through the walls of the tanks. The wash water temperature is controlled by a mixing valve (combining hot and cold water), heat from the dryer, or a heat exchanger from the developer.

429. The answer is B. *(Bushong, 5/e, pp 442, 444. Carroll, 5/e, p 481. McKinney, pp 131–132.)* Cleaning of the transport rollers is necessary to remove debris from the roller surface. This is especially important for the rollers that sit outside the solution, such as the crossover racks. Being exposed to the air provides an increased opportunity for debris to dry and harden on the roller. During development the emulsion is softened to allow the chemicals to reach the exposed silver halide crystals. Insufficient hardener in the developer or fixer may cause pieces of the emulsion to lift off the film base and stick to the roller. This debris may cause wet pressure sensitization on the film or pi lines/marks. The rollers must be cleaned carefully to avoid damage to their surface. All rollers turn at the same rate, which is controlled by a drive system. A change in the speed of the rollers will have an adverse effect on image quality if other processing variables are not also altered to maintain the required balance. Oxidation of the chemicals is influenced by the presence of air within the chemicals and by overheating.

430. The answer is C. *(Bushong, 5/e, p 196. Carroll, 5/e, p 205. Curry, 4/e, p 161.)* In order to achieve optimum image quality with the least exposure to the patient, the spectral sensitivity of radiographic film must be matched with the primary spectral emission of the intensifying screens. Standard silver halide film is naturally sensitive to light emissions in the blue/UV range, which is produced by calcium tungstate phosphors. The newer rare-earth phosphors, particularly gadolinium, emit light well into the green range. Orthochromatic film is manufactured to absorb the predominant photon energies associated with green light emissions as well as blue emissions. The use of improperly matched film and screens results in a loss of imaging system speed and an increase in patient dose.

431. The answer is B. *(Bushong, 5/e, pp 293, 295. Carroll, 5/e, pp 194–195.)* Assuming the single emulsion film and screen are manufactured to be the same speed as the double film and screen, the single film and screen system will be half the speed of the double system. A change in imaging system speed should be compensated for by an inverse change in exposure (mAs). For this situation, the milliampere-second would need to be increased. The use of a double screen will result in two screens to be stimulated by the x-rays, increasing the quantity of light produced. Each film emulsion is then exposed and their combined densities yield the proper level of blackening. Single screen systems require more exposure to stimulate sufficient light emissions to blacken the single emulsion appropriately.

432. The answer is B (2 only). *(Bushong, 5/e, p 196. Carroll, 5/e, p 205. Curry, 4/e, p 161.)* Orthochromatic film is manufactured to be used with intensifying screens that predominantly emit light in the green range. Standard silver halide film is most sensitive to light emissions in the blue/UV range. In order to sensitize film to absorb the green emissions, a light absorbing dye (magenta in color) is added to the emulsion. This is the only physical difference between the two films. The dye causes the green emissions to be absorbed, thus depositing energy in the silver halide crystals and initiating latent image formation.

433. The answer is B. *(Bushong, 5/e, p 287. Carroll, 5/e, pp 248–249. Selman, 8/e, pp 320–321.)* OID influences radiographic density, magnification, and recorded detail; however, the effect is not always direct. An increase in OID will cause an increase (direct effect) in magnification and a decrease (indirect effect) in density and recorded detail. Magnification is affected by the change in SID/SOD ratio caused by changes in OID. Recorded detail is lost because of the increased geometric blur caused by an increased OID. The air-gap effect of OID will lower density because of the reduction of scattered photons reaching the image receptor. Shape distortion occurs when there is unequal OID. Optimum image quality relies on as little OID as possible.

434. The answer is C. *(Bushong, 5/e, pp 287–288. Carroll, 5/e, p 254.)* On occasion, the set-up for a radiographic exam may be limited by the condition of the patient or equipment. As a result, an unavoidable OID may exist, which may be compensated for by an increase in SID, if conditions allow. This is explained by the law of similar triangles, which indicates that geometric integrity can be sustained by maintaining the same SID/SOD ratio. An example of this situation is demonstrated by the air-gap technique for reducing the amount of scatter reaching an image receptor. This technique employs an OID of about 8 inches and SID of about 9 feet (108 inches). This results in a magnification factor (SID/SOD) of 1.08. With the usual imaging conditions of a SID of 40 inches and an OID of 3 inches (for bucky work), the same magnification factor is achieved (1.08).

435. The answer is B. *(Carroll, 5/e, pp 195–196, 243.)* Screen speed has an indirect effect and SID has a direct effect on radiographic density. Therefore, a change in these two factors will require a change in milliampere-seconds in order to maintain image density. The milliampere-seconds compensation may be initiated with either factor. The original 48 mAs will be reduced to 12 mAs in compensation for changing to a screen four times faster (50 speed to 200). Then, using the milliampere-second/distance ratio, the new 12 mAs will be increased to 20 mAs to compensate for the increase in SID (40 to 52 inches).

436. The answer is C. *(Carroll, 5/e, pp 102–106, 181–182.)*   Kilovoltage has a direct effect, while grid ratio has an indirect effect on radiographic density. Therefore, changes in both these factors must be accompanied with changes in milliampere-seconds in order to maintain image density. The 15 percent rule is applied in the process of adjusting milliampere-seconds for the kilovoltage change. The difference between 80 and 106 kV is equal to two steps of 15 percent; therefore, milliampere-seconds must be halved twice: 24 to 6 mAs. Next the milliampere-seconds must be increased to compensate for the increased grid ratio. The grid ratio change factors for the 5:1 and 12:1 grids are 2 and 5, respectively. The final result is 15 mAs.

437. The answer is D. *(Bushong, 5/e, pp 283–286. Carroll, 5/e, p 259. Curry, 4/e, pp 221–222.)*   Angling of the x-ray beam, while maintaining a parallel relationship between the object and the image receptor, will most noticeably affect the radiographic quality factor of *shape,* or *true distortion.* While shape distortion is generally an undesirable effect, angling of the x-ray beam is commonly used to improve visualization of structures of interest by distorting superimposed structures (e.g., AP axial projection of the skull). The difference between size (magnification) and shape distortion is whether the magnification of the object on the image is universal or varies across the object. Shape distortion is defined as *unequal magnification of the portions of the object,* while size distortion is recognized as *uniform or equal magnification of the entire object.* It is possible that angulation of the x-ray beam will have an effect on density and contrast. However, this effect is more due to the increased thickness of tissue through which the beam will pass.

438. The answer is B. *(Bushong, 5/e, p 282. Carroll, 5/e, p 47. Curry, 4/e, p 221.)*   The stated definition best describes *shape,* or *true, distortion.* The control of shape distortion is through the proper alignment of the x-ray beam, the part, and the image receptor. This alignment should place the part parallel to the plane of the image receptor and the central ray perpendicular to the part. This relationship will image the true shape of the object. Magnification is controlled by the relationship of the SID/SOD and results in all aspects of the object being equally enlarged. Absorption and geometric blur refer to object characteristics and distance factors between the tube, part, and image receptor that determine the quality of recorded detail (sharpness of structures imaged).

439. The answer is B. *(Carroll, 5/e, p 261. Curry, 4/e, p 222.)*   The proper alignment of the beam, part, and image receptor is necessary to accurately record the shape of an object. When one factor is incorrectly aligned, it will appear as either foreshortened or elongated. The situation in the question placed the object at an angle in reference to the image receptor, yet maintained proper alignment between the central ray and image receptor. The resulting image will show foreshortening of the part (see figure A below). If the central ray were to be directed perpendicular to the part, rather than the image receptor, the result would still be substandard, but the part would be elongated (see figure B below). When the part cannot be properly aligned to the image receptor, every attempt should be made to align the image receptor parallel to the part with the central ray directed to both. Another option is to employ Ceszynski's law of isometry, which directs the central ray at an angle one-half the degree of angle formed between the part and image receptor.

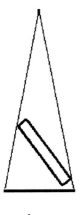

A.

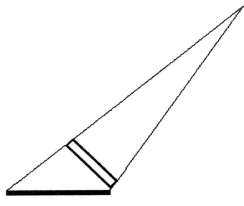

B.

440. The answer is C. *(Bushong, 5/e, p 294. Carroll, 5/e, pp 138–139.)* Collimation is the final change to the primary beam between the x-ray tube and the patient. Its function is to eliminate the peripheral photons of the beam, thereby restricting the area covered by the beam. This action reduces the quantity of photons in the beam. However, there is no effect on the beam quality because the collimator does not alter average beam energy. The fact that image contrast is altered by collimation is due to the decreased number of Compton interactions, which contribute to scattered radiation within the exit beam. Milliampere-seconds may need to be increased in order to compensate for the reduction in photon quantity.

441. The answer is A. *(Bushong, 5/e, pp 295, 298. Carroll, 5/e, p 285.)* There are many sources of patient motion that must be considered in order to provide optimum image quality. These include involuntary motion of the heart, respiration, peristalsis, tremors, and voluntary muscular movement. Such motion during the exposure will result in image blur and reduced recorded detail (sharpness). Of the answers offered, decreasing exposure time will reduce or eliminate motion blur recorded on the image. However, this technique must also be accompanied by other motion reduction techniques. These include using immobilization devices, having the patient suspend respiration, and effectively communicating with the patient to allay fears and gain cooperation.

442. The answer is D. *(Bushong, 5/e, pp 295, 298. Carroll, 5/e, pp 285, 379–380.)* When motion blur is a factor on a suboptimum image, using a shorter exposure time is the only successful technical adjustment of those mentioned. Each of the answer options will produce the same density as the original technique; however, other factors of image quality will also be affected. The factors in answers A and C will lower exposure time and increase kilovoltage to maintain density, which will increase penetration of the part and lower image contrast. Answer B will reduce SID to compensate for the reduced milliampere-seconds. The low SID will increase patient entrance dose and cause magnification and geometric blur of the image. The factors in answer D increase milliamperes and lower exposure time to maintain the original milliampere-seconds. These factors will reduce motion blur without altering contrast or geometric sharpness.

443. The answer is A. *(Bushong, 5/e, pp 317–320. Carlton, p 506. Carroll, 5/e, p 333.)* The combination of technical factors stated in the question provide satisfactory results for the majority of patients. AEC is commonly used for chest radiography. However, the AEC must be correctly used in accordance with the asymmetric structures of the thorax and the varying conditions of the patient. For PA projection, it is commonly recommended to use either one or both side chambers in order to measure the proper exposure levels to image the lung fields. A very small, emaciated patient must make the radiographer consider whether minimum reaction time will be a problem. The size of the patient would call for an exposure time shorter than the radiographic unit can provide, causing the image to be overexposed. Minimum reaction time is a limiting factor for all AECs. The best method for correcting this problem is to lower the milliamperage, which would increase the exposure time required (milliamperage and time are inversely proportional). A lower kilovoltage would also call for a longer exposure time and would alter the desired level of image contrast. A longer SID would also increase the time needed, but is generally not possible due to room limitations. Selection of the center sensing chamber would cause the exposure time to increase and further overexpose the image because of the increased density and thickness of the mediastinal structures.

444. The answer is B. *(Carlton, pp 505–507. Carroll, 5/e, pp 333–334.)* The proper use of an AEC requires the radiographer to manually select an appropriate kilovoltage station to stay within the limits of safe operation of the unit and provide optimum penetration of the part. The exposure time is determined by the unit's minimum response time and the selection of one or more sensing chambers, density level, and backup time. The use of a lower milliamperage station will cause the exposure time to be longer, while a higher milliamperage station may initiate the unit's overload protection circuit (no exposure) or the minimum response time (overexposure of the image). The use of all three sensing chambers is a common practice for the imaging of the abdomen; the radiation from the chambers is averaged for optimum exposure. If the beam is collimated tighter than usual, causing a portion of the side chamber(s) to be cut off, the AEC would respond by lengthening the exposure time to acquire sufficient radiation exposure (overexposed image). The density control is usually set at the "normal" position to produce the predetermined density level. This control option allows for the occasional increase (+1 or +2) or decrease (−1 or −2) in optimum density level to compensate for an anatomic structure that is difficult to accurately align with the sensing chamber. The backup time must always be set as a safety feature in the event the unit malfunctions or is improperly set. If the backup time is set too low, it will terminate the exposure early, causing an underexposed image. Of the answer options, only the factor related to insufficient backup time would cause an *underexposed* image.

445. The answer is C. *(Carlton, pp 505–506. Carroll, 5/e, p 335.)* The proper use of the AEC relies on the accurate centering of the structure of interest over the appropriately selected sensing chamber(s) and the selection of the correct kilovoltage. Furthermore, the beam must be adequately collimated to alleviate the effect of scattered radiation, which can undercut the part and terminate the exposure too early, causing a light (underexposed) image. Increasing kilovoltage or milliamperage will produce a shorter exposure time, but result in the same level of total exposure. The selection of the side chamber will not correlate with the proper location of the central ray (which is associated with the center chamber) as it is located lateral to the area of interest. If the selected chamber is not covered by a structure, but is exposed to raw radiation, a light image will be produced. Conversely, if the dense structure of the thoracic spine overlies the chamber, a dark image will result.

446. The answer is D. *(Bushong, 5/e, pp 280–281. Carroll, 5/e, pp 256–257. Selman, 8/e, pp 347–350.)* The presence of magnification on a radiographic image is controlled by the relationship between the SID and SOD. Changes in OID will indirectly alter the SOD. For the majority of radiographic procedures, magnification should be kept to a minimum. This is because as magnification of the imaged object increases, any blur present on the image will also be magnified, thus reducing recorded detail (sharpness). When macro-radiography is to be performed, a fractional focal spot (0.3 mm or less) must be available to reduce the geometric blur in order for the magnified image to be useful. Focal-spot size plays no direct role in creating or decreasing magnification; it only influences the amount of geometric blur on the image.

447. The answer is B. *(Carlton, pp 505. Carroll, 5/e, pp 334–336.)* The quantity of barium in the stomach will vary with each patient. The usual positioning of the stomach will result in some barium-filled and some unfilled areas over the sensing chamber, producing an averaged exposure. However, if only the barium-filled area is over the sensing chamber, the exposure time will be increased to compensate for the radiopaque nature of the barium and the result will be an overall dark image.

448. The answer is A. *(Carlton, p 504. Carroll, 5/e, pp 334, 339.)* The density controls associated with the AEC are designed to provide incremental increases or decreases in exposures (densities) under certain limited circumstances. The properly operating AEC will routinely have the control set at "normal" density, which was determined when the device was calibrated. The AEC should be capable of producing repeatable image densities of the same body part, regardless of the thickness of the part. The density control may be used to provide for exposure compensation on a temporary basis, while one waits for service to be performed on the AEC unit. The density control should *not* be used to correct for difficulties in accurate positioning of structures over the chamber; perhaps a more appropriate chamber should be selected or a manual technique used. Nor should it be used when the object is smaller than the chamber and a portion of the chamber thus receives direct radiation exposure; again manual technique may be more appropriate.

449. The answer is D. *(Carlton, pp 506. Carroll, 5/e, p 333. Thompson, p 389.)* Running into the minimum response time of the AEC will result in an overexposed (dark) image. The factors likely to cause this problem include having the milliamperage or kilovoltage set too high or imaging a very small patient who requires a small exposure level. Selecting a lower milliamperage will usually compensate for each of these factors. Using very tight collimation with the AEC may cause a portion of the activated sensing chamber to be cut off, resulting in a *longer* than necessary exposure time and also an overexposed image.

450. The answer is D. *(Carroll, 5/e, pp 334–336. Thompson, p 383.)* The lumbar spine should be located in the center of the image receptor, regardless of which projection is used. For this reason the center sensing chamber should be used for all projections of the LS spine. However, in order for the image to be properly exposed when using the AEC, extremely accurate centering of bony structures over the chamber is required to prevent early termination of the exposure. If proper centering for this projection is a common problem, manual selection of technique may be more appropriate.

451. The answer is C. *(Bushong, 5/e, pp 293, 299–300. Carroll, 5/e, pp 277–281. Thompson, pp 382, 389, 390.)* The use of a faster speed imaging system than indicated for a particular exam will result in an under-exposed image. High-speed systems are able to produce more light per exposure, thereby requiring less exposure to provide the desired results. When a particular exam calls for the use of a detail imaging system, more exposure (mAs) will be required to provide sufficient density than is needed for a 200 speed system. It is important to be sure one has the correct type of image receptor in order to avoid unnecessary repeats.

452. The answer is B. *(Bushong, 5/e, p 210. Carroll, 5/e, p 449. Selman, 8/e, p 308. Thompson, p 250.)* Although development and fixing of the radiographic image are most responsible for the quality and longevity of the image, proper washing is also extremely important. This is particularly important in ensuring proper archival quality (maintenance of optimum image quality over time). Proper washing requires a continuous flow of clean water to thoroughly remove all chemicals from the film. Failure to do so may cause fixer retention and a fading of the image during storage. Image density and contrast are determined by the development phase of processing. Sources of image fog related to processing include excessive development or inappropriate safelight conditions. Emulsion softening may result from insufficient hardener in the fixer or very high wash water temperatures.

453. The answer is B. *(McKinney, pp 134, 138.)* The developer, fixer, and wash tanks of an automatic processor should be emptied and cleaned on a monthly basis. Following the cleaning of their surfaces, the tanks should be repeatedly filled with and emptied of water, which is then allowed to circulate, before being refilled with fresh chemicals. At this same time period, all the deep racks of rollers should be thoroughly cleaned. When adding chemicals, the fixer tank should be filled before the developer tank to minimize the possibility of developer contamination.

454. The answer is C. *(McKinney, p 139. NCRP No. 99, p 45.)* The proper storage of processing chemicals requires a cool, dry environment similar to that for the storage of film. The temperature should not be greater than 70° F and the humidity should be around 60 percent. These conditions will provide sufficient shelf life for the chemicals. Proper rotation of stored products should be monitored to ensure timely use.

455. The answer is B. *(McKinney, pp 131–135.)* The processor plays an important role in the final outcome of the radiographic image and for this reason it needs to be attended to on a daily basis. In addition to running a daily sensitometric strip, the feed tray and crossover rollers (developer/fixer; fixer/wash) should be cleaned to prevent artifact formation. Also the developer temperature should be checked. The schedule for cleaning of the deep racks varies with recommendations of the manufacturers and use of the unit. It is generally recommended that the developer deep rack be cleaned weekly and all others be cleaned at least monthly.

456. The answer is B. *(Carroll, 5/e, p 459. McKinney, pp 61, 62.)* Exhausted or diluted developer may result in a number of effects due to low activity levels. Insufficient action by the developing agents causes low density and contrast on the final image. Insufficient hardener (glutaraldehyde) may allow the emulsion to swell too much, causing transport problems and film jams between the rollers. The lack of hardener will also make it difficult for the fixer hardener to sufficiently shrink and harden the emulsion, resulting in tacky films as they exit the processor. A lack of restrainer may cause chemical fog due to the development of some unexposed silver halide crystals. Proper replenishment rates must be set and maintained, and the chemicals for replenishment must be properly mixed.

457. The answer is D. *(Carroll, 5/e, p 460. McKinney, pp 70, 114–115.)* The proper concentration of fixer is required to provide optimum archival quality to the final image. As the image is stored, it should not deteriorate over time. Insufficient replenishment of fixer or overdilution of fixer during mixing may cause the following effects. *Poor clearing action*, due to low concentration of thiosulfate, will cause the image to appear milky or slightly opaque, detracting from the detail visibility of the image. *Insufficient hardener* in the fixer will cause the emulsion to remain soft and tacky on exiting the processor. The *reduction in activator* (low acetic acid) will cause a higher pH level than desired and insufficient neutralization of the developer action. The retained developer will continue to act on the uncleared silver halide crystals, causing the image to darken over time. A *brittle* film may result from *overfixation* (increased concentration or fixer temperature), whereby too much hardening occurs and the film may crack.

458. The answer is A. *(Carroll, 5/e, p 509. McKinney, p 45.)* The contamination of various processing solutions is very possible because of their close proximity. However, some cross mixing is more serious than others. The order of processing requires the film to move through the developer, into the fixer, then the wash water, and finally the dryer. With each move into the next tank (except entrance of dry film into developer), a small amount of solution is carried forward. The replenishment action and chemical nature of the fixer will usually counter any effect of developer carried into fixer. Fixer content in the wash water is overcome by the continuous overflow of dirty water and the addition of fresh clean water. The most serious problem would arise if some fixer solution spilled into the developer, even a small amount. This contamination would be sufficient to require draining the developer tank, cleaning it, and refilling it with fresh chemicals. Any action that may risk spilling solutions should be performed away from the developer tank.

459. The answer is B. *(Bushong, 5/e, p 208. Carroll, 5/e, p 451. McKinney, p 60.)* The developing agents work most effectively in an *alkali* solution (pH 10 to 11.5). For this reason, sodium carbonate or sodium hydroxide is included as the activator to maintain the alkali pH level. The activator also works to soften the emulsion. A low pH level may cause the image to be underdeveloped. The pH level of the fixer is acidic and acts to neutralize the developer action.

460. The answer is D. *(Carroll, 5/e, pp 160–161.)* The destructive nature of osteoporosis is evident in the image presented in the figure. Due to the loss of bone tissue and resulting low atomic number, fewer photoelectric interactions are taking place. This decrease in photoelectric/Compton (PE/C) ratio causes lower image contrast. This situation can be improved by using a lower kilovoltage and maintaining density by increasing milliampere-seconds according to the 15 percent rule. The effect will be to increase the PE/C ratio and subsequently the image contrast. Changes in milliampere-seconds will not affect the PE/C ratio; therefore, there will be no effect on image contrast.

461. The answer is D. *(Bushong, 5/e, pp 444–445. Carroll, 5/e, pp 492–493. McKinney, p 6.)* The artifact seen on the image represents a static mark, which results from friction between two surfaces that produces a small spark of light. This type of artifact is more likely to occur when storage or processing conditions are very dry (low humidity). Care must be taken when removing films from the bin or cassette, sliding a film into a cassette, or feeding film into the processor. Antistatic solution should be used when cleaning screens or processor feed trays. In some cases, a humidifier may be needed during very cold, dry times. Other types of plus density marks are caused by sensitization of the film emulsion from pressure, wet spots, or creases in the film as from fingernails. Guide shoe marks are white or minus densities due to scratching of the emulsion from the film base.

462. The answer is C. *(Bushong, 5/e, pp 444–445. Carroll, 5/e, pp 492–493. McKinney, p 6.)* The artifact type seen on the image is caused by static discharge in the darkroom. This is most likely to occur when the darkroom is cold and dry and there is friction between film and screen, or feed tray, or another film surface. A humid, hot darkroom is most likely to cause increased base-plus-fog density or tacky emulsion, which will cause the films to stick together. Other types of artifacts may result from the rollers of the processor transport system. A damaged roller may cause emulsion pickoff or smudge spots. A misaligned roller assembly may cause guide shoe scratches or film jams.

463. The answer is D. *(Bushong, 5/e, pp 443–445. Carroll, 5/e, pp 482–484. Cullinan, 2/e, p 94.)* Minus density artifacts will appear as white or clear areas on the radiograph. This is due to handling or processing problems that resulted in the emulsion's being scratched from the film base. No density will be present where there is no emulsion. Improperly seated guide shoes and emulsion pickoff due to dirty rollers coming in contact with the softened emulsion are the most common causes of this type of artifact. However, rough handling of the film before the emulsion has been sufficiently hardened will also cause emulsion removal. A less common cause of minus density areas would be fixer splashes on a film prior to processing. This would cause the silver halide crystals to be dissolved, leaving only the film base in these areas. Wet pressure or creasing or bending the film will sensitize the film, causing dark, or plus density, artifacts. Static discharges create a flash of light that exposes the film, causing plus density artifacts.

464–466. The answers are 464-B, 465-A, 466-C. *(Bushong, 5/e, pp 306–308. Carroll, 5/e, pp 378–381.)* To solve for the greatest density, each variable may be converted to the same value along with a change in milliampere-seconds for compensation. By making each variable (except mAs) the same, these variables no longer need to be considered. The highest mAs will provide greatest density. Refer to the list of conversion formulas at the beginning of this book to work through these problems. These problems may be solved as follows:

464.

Find mAs	Convert kV/mAs		Convert SID/mAs	
(A) 10	(A) 10	75	(A) 10	40″
(B) 20	(B) 40	75	(B) 30	40″
(C) 10	(C) 10	75	(C) 10	40″
(D) 10	(D) 10	75	(D) 10	40″

The answer is (B) 30 mAs, 75 kV, 40″ SID.

465.

Convert kV/mAs		Convert SID/mAs		Convert grid/mAs	
(A) 32	74	(A) 32	40″	(A) 32	10:1
(B) 5	74	(B) 5	40″	(B) 25	10:1
(C) 18	74	(C) 18	40″	(C) 22	10:1
(D) 48	74	(D) 15	40″	(D) 15	10:1

The answer is (A) 32 mAs, 74 kV, 40″ SID, 10:1 grid.

466.

Convert kV/mAs		Convert SID/mAs		Convert screen speed/mAs	
(A) 10	70	(A) 10	40″	(A) 20	200
(B) 10	70	(B) 10	40″	(B) 30	200
(C) 60	70	(C) 42	40″	(C) 42	200
(D) 40	70	(D) 28	40″	(D) 28	200

The answer is (C) 42 mAs, 70 kV, 40″ SID, 200 speed screen.

467–469.   The answers are 467-B, 468-B, 469-A.   *(Bushong, 5/e, pp 306–308. Carroll, 5/e, pp 378–381.)* To solve for the least density, each variable may be converted to the same value along with a change in milliampere-seconds for compensation. By making each variable (except mAs) the same, these variables no longer need to be considered. The least density is achieved with the lowest mAs. Refer to the list of conversion formulas at the beginning of this book to work through these problems. These problems may be solved as follows:

467.

Find mAs		Convert kV/mAs			Convert grid/mAs*		
(A)	10	(A)	10	72	(A)	10	10:1
(B)	4	(B)	4	72	(B)	4	10:1
(C)	3	(C)	6	72	(C)	6	10:1
(D)	4	(D)	8	72	(D)	8	10:1

The answer is (B) 4 mAs, 72 kV, 10:1 grid. *12:1 and 10:1 have the same conversion factors.

468.

Convert kV/mAs		Convert SID/mAs			Convert grid/mAs	
(A)	11	70	(A)	17	40″	(A)	42	12:1
(B)	18	70	(B)	18	40″	(B)	23	12:1
(C)	36	70	(C)	36	40″	(C)	36	12:1
(D)	48	70	(D)	33	40″	(D)	28	12:1

The answer is (B) 23 mAs, 70 kV, 40″ SID, 12:1 grid.

469.

Convert kV/mAs		Convert SID/mAs		Convert grid/mAs		Convert screen/mAs	
(A)	16	80	(A)	16	100 cm	(A)	16	10:1	(A)	4	400
(B)	24	80	(B)	24	100 cm	(B)	24	10:1	(B)	12	400
(C)	36	80	(C)	11	100 cm	(C)	9	10:1	(C)	9	400
(D)	48	80	(D)	15	100 cm	(D)	12	10:1	(D)	18	400

The answer is (A) 4 mAs, 80 kV, 100 cm SID, 10:1 grid, 400 speed screen.

470–473.   The answers are 470-C, 471-D, 472-C, 473-B.   *(Bushong, 5/e, pp 273–277.)*   The H&D curve—also known as a characteristic, or sensitometric, curve—provides a picture of the characteristics of a film in terms of how it responds to exposure and processing. This method allows various types of films to be compared graphically. The specific characteristics that can be evaluated are base plus fog, speed, contrast, and latitude. The numbered items on the charts represent the following: (1) base-plus-fog density; (2) toe—low density range; (3) body—useful density range; (4) shoulder—high density range; (5) speed point—1.0 above base plus fog; and (6) contrast value based on the average gradient of the useful density range. All radiographic film has some level of inherent density, which is referred to as base plus fog. For this reason, the H&D curve will never start at 0.0 density. The mathematical value for film contrast is obtained by calculating the average gradient of the curve between the densities of 0.25 and 2.0. The higher the average gradient value, the higher the film contrast. Most medical x-ray film has an average gradient between 2.5 and 3.5.

474–475.   The answers are 474-B, 475-D.   *(Bushong, 5/e, p 288. Curry, 4/e, p 224. Selman, 8/e, p 321.)* The quality of recorded detail on a radiographic image is influenced by numerous factors, including sources of geometric blur, motion blur, screen blur, and absorption blur. Of the factors stated in these problems, geometric and screen blur must be considered. It is assumed that motion and absorption blur are constant. To solve for the best recorded detail, one may use a check method of ticking off the factors most favorable for recorded detail. The option with the most checks is the best choice. In the first item, answer B has the longest SID, shorted OID, smallest focal spot, and slowest speed image receptor. The answer in the second item is a little closer with both A and D being possibilities. Closer evaluation can be made using the mathematical equation for geometric blur (OID/SOD × focal-spot size). The numerical value for geometric blur for A and D is found as follows:

(A) $\dfrac{10}{70} \times 1.2 = 0.14 \times 1.2 = 0.17$ (D) $\dfrac{20}{100} \times 0.3 = 0.2 \times 0.3 = 0.06$

Although the screen speed is slower (offering better recorded detail), geometric blur is more of an influencing factor. Also the conditions in option D result in one-third the geometric blur of option A, making the former the best answer.

476–477.   The answers are 476-A, 477-B.   *(Bushong, 5/e, p 288. Curry, 4/e, p 224. Selman, 8/e, p 321.)* Recorded detail is the quality factor that refers to the structural sharpness of the object imaged on the radiograph. Of the technical factors included in the answer options, milliampere-seconds and kilovoltage may be ignored as they are electrical factors that influence the quantity and quality of the x-ray beam, but have no influence on the geometric integrity of the imaging chain. However, SID, OID, and focal-spot size have a major impact on recorded detail in the area of geometric blur. Assuming motion blur is not a problem, the geometric factors will weigh more heavily than screen speed in determining the level of recorded detail. To solve for which combination will produce the worse recorded detail as evidenced by the most geometric blur, use the check off method of identifying the factors most likely to cause blur: *long OID, short SID,* and *large focal-spot size*. In the first question, answer A has the most blur, even though it has a slower screen speed. Using the mathematical equation for blur, the numerical values for blur in each of the options is (A) 0.2; (B) 0.05; (C) 0.04; and (D) 0.07.

The same method may be applied to the second question. The numerical values for blur for these answer options are (A) 0.06; (B) 0.17; (C) 0.10; (D) 0.13.

478–479.   The answers are 478-B, 479-A.   *(Bushong, 5/e, pp 273–277.)*   The characteristics of a film may be visualized by the location and shape of the H&D curve. The diagram presents two curves. The curve *located* closer to the vertical axis generally indicates a faster film type. More specific determination is made by comparing the points on the curve associated at the density value of 1.0, which is the speed reference point. For these curves, *A* is faster. Film contrast may be estimated by the *shape* of the curve. Low-contrast film will produce a more horizontal curve (*B*), while high-contrast film will appear as a vertical curve (*A*). Finally, film latitude is indicated by the shift in the curve at the transition points of toe-to-body and body-to-shoulder. The gradual shift, as in curve *B*, indicates that the film was wide latitude, which is associated with low contrast film. Curve *A* represents narrow latitude.

480–484.   The answers are 480-A, 481-A, 482-B, 483-B, 484-C.   *(Bushong, 5/e, pp 301–308, Carlton, pp 368–375. Carroll, 5/e, pp 136–138, 176–177, 192–196, 221, 456–458.)*   Radiographic density is the amount of blackening on the film as a result of exposure and processing. As the quantity of radiation reaching the film increases, density will increase. However, without chemical processing, the level of density is not visible. Optimum exposure delivered to the film can be destroyed by improper processing. Numerous technical factors influence the level of exposure reaching the film. These factors include grid ratio, imaging system speed, beam restriction, and processing. Focal-spot size has no effect on radiation quantity or quality, thus no effect on density.

Grid ratio indicates the ability of a grid device to remove scattered radiation from the exit beam. As grid ratio increases, scatter absorption increases and contrast improves. However, since scattered radiation contributes to radiographic density in the form of fog, its removal will cause a reduction in density on the image. Therefore, when employing high-ratio grids, an appropriate increase in exposure must be made to maintain the desired level of radiographic density.

Imaging systems are available in a variety of relative speeds for the purpose of obtaining the best possible image with the least amount of radiation exposure for various parts of the body and exam requirements. As system speeds increase, less exposure is needed to produce the desired radiographic density; therefore, faster speed imaging systems require less radiation. However, as system speeds increase there is a loss of recorded detail due to screen blur. This makes it necessary for the radiographer to select the imaging system best suited to the needs of an exam and to vary the amount of exposure as required. If no compensation is made to the exposure factors, radiographic density will increase when higher speed imaging systems are used in place of slower speed systems.

Beam restriction determines the amount of tissue that will be exposed. The advantages of collimation (reducing the field size) include decreased patient dose, less scattered radiation produced, and increased contrast. Since collimation reduces the quantity of primary and scattered photons, there will be fewer photons in the exit beam. This will reduce the amount of exposure to the recording medium and result in less radiographic density.

Processing influences the radiographic density in a variety of ways. Optimum processing requires a careful balance of developing temperature, time, and chemical activity. An increase in any of these variables will cause overdevelopment and an increase in density.

485–487.   The answers are 485-A, 486-C, 487-D. *(Bushong, 5/e, pp 311–312. Carlton, pp 400–401, 412–425. Carroll, 5/e, pp 233–234, 248, 284–286. Curry, 4/e, pp 221–222.)* Optimum radiographic quality relies on the ability to recognize the radiographed structures for what they are, as well as adequate density and contrast. The factors that determine this aspect of radiographic quality are *recorded detail* and *distortion* (size and shape). This question diagrams the effects of the relationship between the tube, object, and image receptor on how well the image resembles the object. Size distortion, or magnification, is controlled by the SID/SOD ratio and is explained by the law of similar triangles. In this example, the SID/SOD ratio between the four objects varies because each has a different OID. Object A has the greatest OID and therefore will be the most magnified.

Shape distortion is controlled by the alignment of the central ray, the part of interest, and the image receptor. Ideal alignment exists when the part is parallel to the image receptor and the central ray perpendicular to both part and image receptor. Variations in this ideal alignment include not positioning the part within the central ray; not directing the central ray to the middle of the part or the image receptor; and angling the central ray, or the part, or the image receptor without also aligning the other factors accordingly. Objects B and C are positioned in the periphery of the beam and will be imaged with the more divergent photons of the beam, causing elongation of both objects. However, object B has more OID and thus will be projected more laterally than object C and demonstrate more elongation on the radiograph.

Recorded detail refers to the sharpness of structures on the image; i.e., how well their edges can be visualized. The geometric factors that control sharpness are focal-spot size (smaller is better), SID (longer is better), and OID (shorter is better). This diagram portrays a situation in which the focal-spot size and SID are constant, but the OID varies for each part. Object D has the least OID and is aligned closely to the central ray; therefore, it will have the best recorded detail.

488–491.   The answers are 488-D, 489-B, 490-A, 491-C. *(Bushong, 5/e, pp 206–209. Carlton, p 293. Carroll, 5/e, pp 450–454.)* Specific chemical agents are mixed together in the developer and fixer tanks to perform the many activities involved in the processing of an image.

Glutaraldehyde acts as a hardener in the developer solution to control the amount of swelling of the emulsion. Due to the specific spacing of the rollers of the transport system, excessive emulsion swelling would cause films to jam. Exhausted developer, with associated low levels of hardener, may be a cause of such transport problems.

Hydroquinone is one of the two reducing or developing agents responsible for converting the exposed silver halide crystals to black metallic silver (latent to manifest image formation). The second is phenidone. Each reducing agent has its own role in the developing process. Hydroquinone acts to gradually develop the black tones of the image. Phenidone builds the gray shades very quickly. Together these agents produce the optimum level of image contrast.

Potassium bromide is a restrainer agent in the developer. Its primary action is to limit the action of the reducing agents to only *exposed* silver halide crystals. This action is important in minimizing the occurrence of chemical fog, which would cause a loss of image contrast. The bromine content of the restrainer is the active component and is of primary importance in the mixing of fresh chemicals. Since the reduction process of the silver halide crystals results in the liberation of bromine atoms, a sufficient supply is generally produced as films are processed.

Ammonium thiosulfate is the clearing agent in the fixer solution. In order to achieve an archival quality for the radiographic image, all unexposed, undeveloped silver halide crystals must be removed (cleared) from the film. Exhausted fixer will result in improper clearing, producing an image with a milky appearance that will darken over time. Equally important is the proper level of washing of the film to remove excess fixer, which, if retained, will lead to the occurrence of a brown stain and degradation of image quality over time.

Sodium sulfite is common to both the developer and fixer and serves as a preservative. In the developer, the specific action of the sodium sulfite is that of minimizing the oxidation of the reducing agents and thereby extending the life of the developer. In the fixer, sodium sulfite assists in the action of the ammonium thiosulfate as a clearing agent; it also continues to minimize the oxidation of developer carried over to the fixer and reduces the occurrence of discoloration of the fixer.

492–496. The answers are 492-C, 493-E, 494-B, 495-A, 496-D. *(Bushong, 5/e, pp 206–209. Carlton, p 293. Carroll, 5/e, pp 450–454.)*   Sodium carbonate is referred to as the *activator* of the developer. Its primary action is to maintain the required alkaline nature (pH 10 to 11.5) of the developer for maximum efficiency of the reducing agents. It also contributes to processing by assisting in the softening of the emulsion to allow the reducing agents to reach as many exposed crystals as possible and improve total development.

Phenidone and hydroquinone are the two *reducing agents* in the developer solution. Each has its own specific action in the development of the exposed radiograph. Phenidone acts to build the gray scale of the image very quickly. Hydroquinone gradually develops the darkest shades (the black tones) of the image. Together they provide the optimum contrast level.

Acetic acid is the *activator* of the fixer and is responsible for maintaining its acidic nature (pH about 4 to 4.5). This will act to neutralize the developer solution carried by the film as it enters the fixer tank. In addition, an acidic environment enables the fixer hardener to be more efficient.

Potassium alum is the *hardener* used in the fixer and thus performs the second major function of the fixing cycle of processing, that of shrinking and hardening the emulsion following clearing of the unexposed silver. Proper hardening of the emulsion is important in achieving the desired archival quality of the image and in allowing handling of the radiograph without damaging the image.

Sodium sulfite is included in both the developer and the fixer as a *preservative* component. This agent is included to reduce air oxidation of the reducing agents in the developer solution itself and continues such action on the developer carried over to the fixer. The preservative also assists the clearing agent in the fixer. The net result of the preservative is the extension of the life of chemical activity for a reasonable amount of time.

497–499. The answers are 497-B, 498-B, 499-B. *(Bushong, 5/e, pp 180–181, 310. Carlton, pp 379, 381. Carroll, 5/e, pp 37–40.)*   The images in the figure are of an aluminum penetrometer, also known as a *step wedge.* As the x-ray beam exposes this device, the varying thickness of the aluminum will attenuate the beam differently, producing an image of various densities. When exposure factors are altered to maintain density while varying kilovoltage, different scales of contrast will be demonstrated. Image A was produced using 100 kV, and 2 mAs; image B was produced using 60 kV and 30 mAs. Low kilovoltage is less penetrating and more likely to be absorbed by the penetrometer. Image B, therefore, yields fewer shades of gray between black and white, and when measured with a densitometer, the difference between adjacent steps is great. In comparison, image A demonstrates more shades of gray between black and white, and the measured density differences are smaller than on image B. This demonstrates that low kilovoltage results in high differential absorption, producing high contrast with a short scale of density differences. Conversely, high kilovoltage produces low differential absorption, creating low contrast with a long scale of density variations.

500–503.   The answers are 500-B, 501-A, 502-B, 503-B. *(Bushong, 5/e, pp 314–315. Carlton, pp 460–461. Carroll, 5/e, pp 300–307.)* Technique charts are employed to provide the radiographer with appropriate combinations of technical factors for imaging various aspects of human anatomy. Since not all patients are exactly the same, some adjustment must be made to the exposure factors to maintain acceptable results, regardless of part size. Technique charts most commonly exist in one of two forms: *fixed* or *variable* kilovoltage peak types. The fixed kilovoltage peak is based on the optimum kilovoltage to best penetrate a particular anatomic structure. Variations in the size of the part are then compensated for by changes in milliampere-seconds. The part sizes are grouped into small, medium, and large categories. The fixed kilovoltage peak chart tends to use higher kilovoltage than variable kilovoltage peak charts, thus producing images of longer scale with less patient dose.

Variable kilovoltage peak charts are based on an acceptable level of exposure (mAs) for a specific part, which is held constant while kilovoltage is altered to accommodate changes in thickness. This type of chart lists a range of measurements in centimeters corresponding to the possible sizes of the part. An initial kilovoltage level is determined based on the measurement of an average knee (phantom) and then increased or decreased by 2 kV for every increase or decrease in thickness of 1 cm. The variable kilovoltage peak chart tends to use lower kilovoltage, resulting in higher contrast and short-scale images at a higher dose to the patient.

504–509.   The answers are 504-D, 505-A, 506-C, 507-C, 508-C, 509-A. *(Bushong, 5/e, pp 295, 313. Carlton, pp 376, 395–396.)* Radiographic density and contrast are influenced by factors that affect the quantity or quality of the x-ray beam. Quantity factors increase or decrease the number of photons in the exit beam, thus determining the amount of radiation to expose the film. Quality factors alter average energy of the beam, making it more or less penetrating and again determining the availability of photons to expose the film. Factors related to the geometric relationship between the x-ray tube, body part, and image receptor primarily influence the sharpness (recorded detail) and distortion of the image. The controlling factor of density is milliampere-seconds, while the influencing factors include kilovoltage, SID, processing, image receptor speed, grid ratio, beam restriction, filtration, generator type, and patient factors. The controlling factor of contrast is kilovoltage, while the influencing factors include grid ratio, beam restriction, filtration, processing, patient factors, and milliampere-seconds (in extremes). The obvious overlapping of effects these factors can have makes it essential to adjust technical factors with great care.

510–514.   The answers are 510-D, 511-A, 512-B, 513-A, 514-B. *(Bushong, 5/e, pp 182–185, 187, 307. Carlton, pp 243, 247.)* In order to choose the best method of correcting a suboptimum image or a change in imaging conditions, one must determine whether there is sufficient density and contrast to effectively demonstrate the structures of interest. The density should be such as to provide sufficient blackening to adequately visualize the structures recorded. It is controlled by the amount of exposure the image receptor receives and by proper chemical processing. Contrast provides the ability to differentiate between the various structures recorded. It is controlled by the penetrability of the beam and the presence or absence of scattered radiation. If the part is underpenetrated, not all information will be recorded. Overpenetration will cause adjacent structures to blend together, making differentiation difficult. If the problem or imaging condition leads to under- or overexposure, an increase or decrease in milliampere-seconds is required. Increases or decreases in kilovoltage should be applied to compensate for under- or overpenetration. Since milliampere-seconds directly controls beam quantity only, it will not correct for inadequate image contrast. However, kilovoltage will influence both beam quality and quantity; it could be used to correct for density problems, but will also alter the contrast. If contrast is adequate, milliampere-seconds should be the variable selected to regulate density. For the situations stated in these questions, changes in grid ratio, SID, and patient thickness affect beam quantity and radiographic density, which should be corrected for by changing milliampere-seconds. Changes in atomic number or molecular density of the part require a change in beam quality, which is controlled by kilovoltage peak selection. With the use of the contrast medium barium sulfate, the kilovoltage must be increased to adequately penetrate the medium and milliampere-seconds must be decreased to maintain density.

515–520.   The answers are 515-D, 516-B, 517-C, 518-E, 519-A, 520-A.   *(Bushong, 5/e, pp 291–293. Carroll, 5/e, pp 202, 469, 482, 488. Selman, 8/e, pp 328–329. Sweeney, pp 27, 45, 50, 106–107, 266.)*   Radiographic artifacts arise from numerous sources, including darkroom safelights, radiographic equipment (tube, table, collimator) and grids as well as those listed as answer options.

Radiographic film is sensitive not only to light and x-rays, but to pressure, chemicals, and environmental conditions (e.g., heat, humidity). Proper storage conditions for radiographic film include room temperature of 70°F or less and humidity in the 40 to 60 percent range. Improper conditions could lead to fogging of the film and ultimately increased base-plus density, which would lower overall radiographic contrast. Boxes of film should be placed on end rather than flat when stored prior to being loaded into a film bin. Laying boxes of film flat is one method of causing pressure artifacts that may appear as either high- to low-density marks in a linear or circular shape.

Another source of pressure artifacts caused by improper film handling is creasing or folding the film prior to exposure or processing. The film should be handled by the edges and be placed directly into a film holder upon removal from the film bin.

Processing of the imaging offers many sources from which artifacts may appear. The roller transport system of the automatic processor will generally exhibit a regularly repeating mark due to damage or buildup of debris on the rollers. As the roller turns and the film moves through the processor, the defect repeatedly comes into contact with the film, causing the artifact. Such an example is the improperly positioned crossover rack that causes the guide shoes to scratch the film, leaving white lines along the film surface parallel with the direction of film movement through the processor. Other examples include pi lines and emulsion pickoff. Improperly mixed or exhausted chemicals will cause stains to appear on the film and decrease the archival quality of the radiographic image. Proper mixing and replenishment rates must be monitored to prevent this problem.

Dirty or damaged screens or cassettes may also contribute to artifact formation. Dust specks within the cassette will cause a random pattern of small, white specks on the image due to interference with light from the phosphors of the dirt particles. Larger pieces of debris may also get trapped within the cassette, which emphasizes the need to keep the darkroom and work areas clean. Routine cleaning of the fronts of cassettes will prevent artifacts formed by spilled contrast media or other contaminants.

Motion artifacts can arise from the patient or radiographic equipment. Prevention of these problems includes carefully instructing patients on remaining still and holding their breath, using short exposure times and proper immobilization techniques, and locking the tube and cassette into their positions.

521–526.   The answers are 521-A, 522-B, 523-B, 524-B, 525-A, 526-A.   *(Carroll, 5/e, pp 161–163. Laudicina, pp 30, 74–75, 92, 138–141. Selman, 8/e, p 340.)*   Understanding the classification of various disease processes is necessary in order to properly select exposure factors to ensure an optimum radiographic image. Generally, pathologic conditions may be assigned to one of two types: *additive* conditions (characterized by an increase in absorption factors) or *destructive* conditions (characterized by a decrease in absorption factors).

The additive conditions in this question group are ascites, cirrhosis, and hydropneumothorax. *Ascites* and *hydropneumothorax* are characterized by an accumulation of fluid in the abdomen and pleural cavity, respectively. In the case of hydropneumothorax, the fluid collection is associated with a collapse of the lung. *Cirrhosis* of the liver is characterized by the abnormal presence of fibrotic tissue, which is very dense. Each of these conditions would require an increase in exposure (mAs) to compensate for the increased thickness of the part from the normal status.

The remainder of the stated conditions are of the destructive type. Both *emphysema* and *bowel obstruction* are characterized by trapped air within the organ (lungs and intestine, respectively). This air results in a lower molecular density of the part, which makes it more radiolucent. A decrease in either milliampere-seconds or kilovoltage may be made to adjust for this change. *Osteoporosis* is characterized by demineralization of bony structures. This effectively lowers the atomic number of bone and requires a lower kilovoltage to optimize differential absorption.

527–531.   The answers are 527-C, 528-C, 529-D, 530-B, 531-A. *(Carroll, 5/e, pp 160–163. Laudicina, pp 5–6, 31–33, 156–157, 187.)*   Various changes that occur to parts of the human body due to aging, trauma, and disease processes alter the usual absorption characteristics of the body. Understanding these changes is necessary for the selection of proper exposure factors. Changes in the *thickness of a part* can usually be best compensated for by a direct change in milliampere-seconds (increased thickness; increased mAs). A change in the overall *average atomic number* will require a direct change in kilovoltage (increased Z; increased kV). However, the change in *molecular density* may be compensated for by a direct change in either milliampere-seconds or kilovoltage, depending on the part being imaged and the initial set of exposure factors.

Paget's disease and the formation of *callus* around a fracture site result in an increase in bone tissue and an increase in the average atomic number. This should be addressed by increasing beam penetration (kV). Conversely, *soft tissue* imaging is not necessarily a change in the condition of the part, but in the radiographic perspective. Instead of proper penetration of bony structures, the emphasis is optimum visualization of the soft tissue. This requires a less penetrating beam for more differential absorption, thus a decrease in kilovoltage. (This is the basis for imaging of the breast.)

Atrophy of any part of the body may occur for a variety of reasons. The result is a decrease in the size of the part, requiring a reduction in milliampere-seconds.

Pneumonia is an inflammatory process marked by the accumulation of fluid within the lung tissues or bronchial tree. This condition alters the usual gaseous molecular density of the lungs to fluid density. The commonly recommended change in exposure is an increase in milliampere-seconds rather than kilovoltage, since high kilovoltage is generally already employed for chest imaging.

532–536.   The answers are 532-D, 533-C, 534-A, 535-D, 536-E. *(Bushong, 5/e, pp 279–288. Carroll, 5/e, pp 284–286, 292–293. Selman, 8/e, pp 319–322, 347–355.)*   The factors that influence the geometric integrity of the radiographic image ultimately determine how well the image resembles or represents the object irradiated. These factors include recorded detail (sharpness of structures), magnification (size distortion), and shape (true) distortion. *Recorded detail* is influenced by increasing or decreasing the amount of blur of the anatomic details of the image. *Magnification* is the misrepresentation of the object's size. *Shape*, or *true, distortion* is the misrepresentation of the object's shape.

The sources of poor recorded detail are geometric blur, motion blur, screen blur, and absorption blur. Of these, geometric blur (the factors of beam geometry relative to the object and image receptor) may also influence distortion (size or shape). Optimum geometric integrity is achieved by using the most vertical x-ray photons located in the central core of the beam, as opposed to using the more divergent rays of the peripheral beam. This is made possible by using a long SID and further improved upon by keeping OID to a minimum. These two conditions will increase recorded detail and decrease magnification. Focal-spot size will also influence the beam's geometry, but it only has an effect on the recorded detail of the image. Shape distortion is controlled by the alignment of the central ray to the anatomic part and image receptor. Any changes in this alignment will influence shape distortion only, as long as SID, OID, and focal-spot size remain unchanged.

For the conditions set in these items, a *change in SID* will have a direct effect on recorded detail, an indirect effect on magnification, and no effect on shape distortion. *Changing the central ray angle* will affect shape distortion only.. *Changing focal–spot size* will alter recorded detail only. *Increasing OID* to 20 inches and decreasing focal-spot size to 0.3 mm or less is the recommended procedure for magnification imaging. The OID will have a direct effect on magnification while the use of a fractional focal spot will reduce the blur created and improve recorded detail.

537–541.   The answers are 537-E, 538-C, 539-A, 540-B, 541-E. *(Bushong, 5/e, pp 632–633. Carlton, pp 153–155. Carroll, 5/e, p 16.)*   The nomenclature of the x-ray beam encompasses many terms. The origin of the x-ray beam is the focal spot of the target. The design of the target bevel is such as to direct the majority of the newly created photons toward the window of the x-ray tube (toward the patient). Those photons that do manage to exit the tube at this point make up the *primary beam* to which the patient is exposed. These photons will have the highest energy level of the beam. The photons that project away from the tube window may exit the tube through the housing, which is designed to minimize the amount of this *leakage radiation.* As the primary beam encounters objects in its path, various interactions occur, changing the characteristics of the primary photons. Compton interactions cause a primary photon to lose energy and have its direction altered as it becomes a *scattered photon.* This photon has sufficient energy to penetrate the object and ultimately expose the film (fog) and radiology personnel (occupational exposure). Another interaction is photoelectric effect, which results in the total absorption of the primary photon and the ejection of an inner shell electron from an atom of the object irradiated. The vacancy in the orbit is filled by the movement of an outer shell electron inward and an associated energy emission in the form of a secondary photon termed *characteristic radiation.* The energy level of these photons is very low, as is their penetrability, resulting in these photons being absorbed locally. Those primary and scattered photons that successfully penetrate the object compose the *exit (remnant) beam* and are the source of exposure to the image receptor.

542–544.   The answers are 542-B, 543-C, 544-A.   *(Bushong, 5/e, p 214. Carroll, 5/e, pp 461, 509–510. Thompson, pp 385, 389, 391.)*   The developer is chiefly responsible for the visibility of details on the image, that is, density and contrast levels. Optimum development is based on the appropriate balance of developer time, temperature, and chemical activity level. Automatic processing maintains developer time by the precise speed at which the rollers of the transport system turn to move the film through each section of the processor. The reduced processing time, made possible by automatic processing, is further achieved by using a higher developer temperature and more concentrated chemicals to produce the optimum density level in this reduced time frame (average of 90 s). Careful monitoring of the transport, replenishment, and temperature control systems is required to ensure optimum operation of the processor and proper density and contrast levels on the images. This monitoring is most commonly achieved through daily sensitometric evaluation and then plotting the results on a control chart in order to watch for trends or gradual changes. An increase in the developer replenishment rate will increase the activity of the developer and lead to overdevelopment of the image, causing an increase in density and decrease in contrast (loss of low densities). The opposite condition, whereby developer activity is less than desired (either overdiluted or exhausted), will produce an image with a decrease in both density and contrast (loss of high densities). These effects will also be noted if developer time or temperature is less than optimum. A variation of rapid processing is the use of *extended processing,* which provides for longer development times, still at high temperatures and using more standard chemicals (less highly concentrated). This action allows for more thorough development of the exposed silver. The effect is increased film speed (density) and image contrast, allowing the use of less exposure. The positive results of longer developer time are due to the balance of the developer chemicals. Any increase in developer time must be carefully monitored as there is a point beyond which further increases in time will cause contrast to be lowered (due to chemical fog).

545–550.   The answers are 545-A, 546-C, 547-C, 548-A, 549-C, 550-D.   *(McKinney, pp 131–135. NCRP No. 99, pp 191–193.)*   The actual frequency for cleaning and general maintenance of the processor depends on its use. The recommendations for *daily* activities include checking the developer temperature and replenishment rates, cleaning of the crossover racks (developer/fixer, fixer/wash) as well as any rollers that sit above the solution level, and running a sensitometric test strip. On a *weekly* basis, the deep rack of the developer should be cleaned. *Monthly,* all tanks should be drained and cleaned, then filled with water that is allowed to circulate before the tank is refilled with chemicals. All deep racks should also be cleaned at this time. *Quarterly* maintenance would include emptying and cleaning the replenishment tanks. These actions are only a portion of the maintenance procedures that should be performed.

Radiographic Procedures

Radiographic View:
> Describes the body part as seen by an x-ray film or other recording media, such as a fluoroscopic screen. Restricted to the discussion of a *radiograph* or *image*.

Radiographic Position:
> Refers to a specific body position, such as supine, prone, recumbent, erect, or Trendelenburg. Restricted to the discussion of the patient's *physical position*.

Radiographic Projection:
> Restricted to the discussion of the *path of the central ray*.

POSITIONING TERMINOLOGY:

A. Lying Down:
  1. *Supine* — lying on the back
  2. *Prone* — lying face downward
  3. *Decubitus* — lying down with a horizontal x-ray beam
  4. *Recumbent* — lying down in any position

B. Erect or upright:
  1. *Anterior position* — facing the film
  2. *Posterior position* — facing the radiographic tube
  3. *Oblique positions* — (erect or lying down)
      a. Anterior — facing the film
          i. *Left anterior oblique* — body rotated with the left anterior portion closest to the film
          ii. *Right anterior oblique* — body rotated with the right anterior portion closest to the film
      b. Posterior — facing the radiographic tube
          i. *Left posterior oblique* — body rotated with the left posterior portion closest to the film
          ii. *Right posterior oblique* — body rotated with the right posterior portion closest to the film

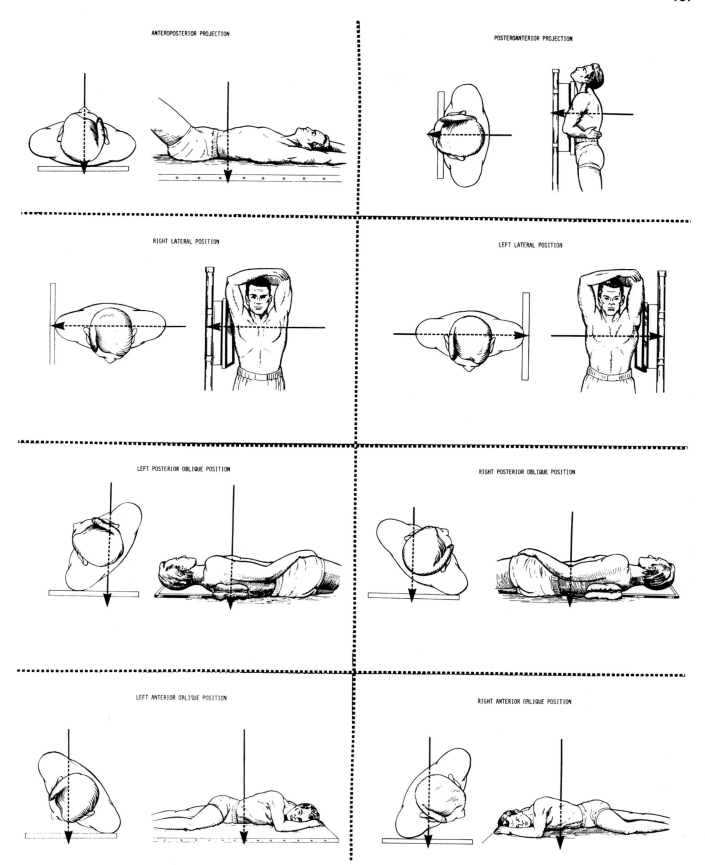

ANTEROPOSTERIOR PROJECTION

POSTEROANTERIOR PROJECTION

RIGHT LATERAL POSITION

LEFT LATERAL POSITION

LEFT POSTERIOR OBLIQUE POSITION

RIGHT POSTERIOR OBLIQUE POSITION

LEFT ANTERIOR OBLIQUE POSITION

RIGHT ANTERIOR OBLIQUE POSITION

DIRECTIONS: Each numbered question or incomplete statement below contains lettered responses. Select the **one best** response.

551. A radiograph of the finger should include the distal

(A) through proximal phalanges
(B) and middle phalanges only
(C) phalanx through distal end of metacarpal
(D) phalanx through proximal end of metacarpal

552. Positioning instructions for a lateral projection of the fourth finger would include:
1. Lateral surface of finger closest to image receptor
2. Medial surface of finger closest to image receptor
3. Distal phalanx in contact with image receptor
4. Entire finger parallel to image receptor

(A) 1 & 3
(B) 1 & 4
(C) 2 & 3
(D) 2 & 4

553. For what purpose are patients required to fold their fingers into a loose fist when positioning the wrist for the PA projection?

(A) To make patients more comfortable
(B) To better separate the two rows of carpal bones
(C) To improve magnification of the carpal bones
(D) To bring the wrist closer to the image receptor

554. The anatomic structures demonstrated by the basic projections of the hand should include the

(A) distal phalanges through the proximal ends of the metacarpals
(B) distal phalanges through the proximal row of carpals
(C) distal phalanges through the distal end of the radius and ulna
(D) metacarpals only

555. Members of the proximal row of carpal bones include:
1. Trapezium
2. Pisiform
3. Lunate

(A) 1 only
(B) 2 & 3
(C) 3 only
(D) 1, 2, & 3

556. The positions used for radiography of the thumb include the

(A) anteroposterior (AP), lateral, oblique
(B) posteroanterior (PA), lateral, oblique
(C) AP and lateral
(D) PA and oblique

557. Proper positioning of the forearm for the AP projection requires the hand to be

(A) pronated
(B) supinated
(C) lateral
(D) flexed

558. Positioning instructions for the lateral projection of the forearm include:
1. Shoulder joint to be level with the elbow
2. Hand to be pronated
3. Humerus and forearm to form a 45° angle

(A) 1 only
(B) 2 & 3
(C) 3 only
(D) 1, 2, & 3

559. Which of the following projections will best demonstrate the radial head completely free of superimposition?

(A) AP projection of the wrist
(B) Lateral projection of the elbow
(C) Medial oblique projection of the wrist
(D) Lateral oblique projection of the elbow

560. When radiographing the elbow in the acute flexion position, how should the central ray be directed to demonstrate the proximal forearm?

(A) Perpendicular to the humerus
(B) Perpendicular to the forearm
(C) At a 25° angle to the forearm
(D) At a 45° angle to the humerus

561. Proper positioning for a true AP projection of the humerus requires the

(A) humeral epicondyles to be parallel to the image receptor
(B) humeral epicondyles to be perpendicular to the image receptor
(C) hand to be pronated
(D) hand and forearm to be externally rotated 45°

562. A breathing technique may be beneficial when performing which radiographic procedure?

(A) Inferosuperior axial projection of the shoulder
(B) Transthoracic lateral projection of the humerus
(C) Oblique scapular Y position
(D) AP position of the sternoclavicular joints

563. The patient is recumbent in the supine position with the arm of the affected shoulder abducted to form a 90° angle with the body. The hand is externally rotated. The image receptor is placed vertically above the shoulder and as close to the patient's neck as possible. The central ray is directed horizontally, through the glenohumeral joint at an angle between 15 and 30° (depending on the amount of abduction of the arm). What radiographic position of the shoulder is being described?

(A) Transthoracic lateral projection of the humerus
(B) Scapular Y position
(C) Inferosuperior axial position
(D) Grashey method for glenoid cavity

564. The shoulder joint is formed through articulation between the

(A) glenoid cavity of the scapula and greater tuberosity of the humerus
(B) glenoid cavity of the scapula and head of the humerus
(C) sternal end of the clavicle and manubrium of the sternum
(D) acromial process of the scapula and acromial end of the clavicle

565. Which of the following positions would be safe for a patient with a suspected fracture of the proximal humerus?

(A) Transthoracic lateral position
(B) Inferosuperior axial position
(C) AP projection of acromioclavicular joints with weights
(D) Axial position of the shoulder

566. The projection that best demonstrates the clavicle free from superimposition by the ribs is the

(A) PA position; central ray (CR) directed 30° cephalad
(B) PA position; CR directed 30° caudal
(C) AP position; CR directed 30° caudal
(D) AP position; CR directed perpendicular to clavicle

567. Proper positioning of the scapula for the AP projection requires the

(A) patient to be erect
(B) affected arm to be rotated medially so that the hand is pronated
(C) body to be rotated toward the side of interest and the affected arm abducted to 90° with the body
(D) body to be in true AP position (no rotation) and the affected arm abducted to 90° with the body

568. In order to best demonstrate the interphalangeal joints of the foot in the dorsoplantar projection, the central ray should be directed

(A) 5° toward the toes
(B) 15° toward the toes
(C) 5° toward the heel
(D) 15° toward the heel

569. The average number of metatarsal bones in the foot is

(A) 5
(B) 7
(C) 8
(D) 14

570. The largest bone in the foot is the

(A) navicular
(B) cuboid
(C) first cuneiform
(D) os calcis

571. The ankle joint is formed by which bones?

(A) Os calcis, radius, ulna
(B) Talus, radius, ulna
(C) Os calcis, tibia, fibula
(D) Talus, tibia, fibula

572. The projection that best demonstrates the sesamoid bones of the foot is the

(A) dorsoplantar
(B) plantodorsal
(C) medial oblique
(D) tangential

573. The position that best demonstrates the base of the fifth metatarsal is the

(A) anteroposterior
(B) posteroanterior
(C) lateral oblique
(D) medial oblique

574. The criteria for producing an optimum radiograph of the foot in the lateral position includes:
    1. Superimposition of metatarsals
    2. Inclusion of distal tibia and fibula
    3. Superimposition of the tibia and fibula

(A) 1 & 2
(B) 2 & 3
(C) 1 & 3
(D) 1, 2, & 3

575. Which projection is performed to evaluate the longitudinal arch of the foot?

(A) Recumbent lateromedial
(B) Recumbent dorsoplantar
(C) Standing lateromedial
(D) Standing dorsoplantar

576. The axial projection of the os calcis requires the central ray to be directed

(A) perpendicular to the image receptor
(B) 30° cephalad entering the dorsum of the foot
(C) 40° cephalad entering the plantar surface of the foot
(D) 50° caudad entering the dorsum of the foot

577. The medial oblique position of the ankle to demonstrate the mortise joint requires the leg to be rotated

(A) 15° internally
(B) 30° internally
(C) 15° externally
(D) 30° externally

578. In order to properly demonstrate the knee joint in the anteroposterior position, the central ray should be directed

(A) perpendicular to the image receptor
(B) 5° cephalad
(C) 8° caudad
(D) 10° medially

579. A correctly positioned AP radiograph of the knee should demonstrate the patella overlapping the

(A) proximal end of the tibia
(B) proximal end of the fibula
(C) medial aspect of the femur
(D) distal end of the femur

580. A correctly positioned lateral position of the knee should demonstrate:
1. A lateral profile of patella
2. Superimposition of femoral condyles
3. An open space between femur and patella

(A) 1 & 2
(B) 2 & 3
(C) 1 & 3
(D) 1, 2, & 3

581. The radiographic projection of the knee below is the

(A) AP
(B) PA
(C) medial oblique
(D) lateral oblique

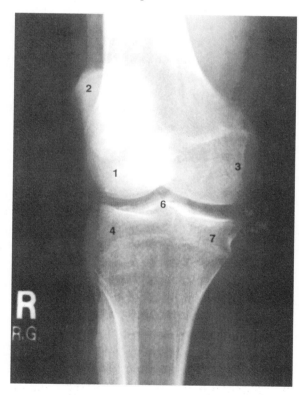

582. The Homblad method for obtaining a postero-anterior axial projection of the knee joint requires the relationship between the femur and image receptor to be

(A) perpendicular
(B) 70°
(C) 45°
(D) 20°

583. The Camp-Coventry method for imaging the posteroanterior axial position of the knee requires the central ray to be directed

(A) 90° to the image receptor
(B) 5 to 10° caudad
(C) 20 to 30° caudad
(D) 40 to 50° caudad

584. A properly positioned tangential projection of the knee will demonstrate the

(A) intercondyloid fossa
(B) tibia spines
(C) patellofemoral articulation
(D) tibiofibular articulation

585. The image of the knee is this figure represents the

(A) lateral oblique projection
(B) tangential (axial) projection
(C) oblique axial position
(D) PA axial position

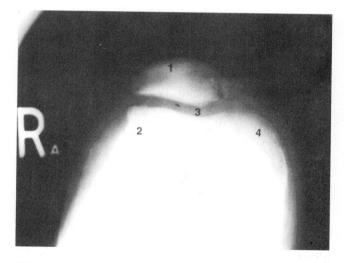

586. The hip bone is composed of the

(A) ilium, ischium, sacrum
(B) ileum, ischium, pubis
(C) ischium, sacrum, coccyx
(D) ilium, ischium, pubis

587. The AP projection of the pelvis requires the patient's legs to be

(A) extended with feet everted
(B) extended with feet inverted
(C) flexed with feet flat on table
(D) abducted with plantar surfaces of feet against each other

588. The long axis of the femoral neck is located by forming an imaginary line

 (A)   perpendicular to a line between the anterior superior iliac spine (ASIS) and symphysis pubis
 (B)   parallel to a line between the ASIS and symphysis pubis
 (C)   perpendicular to a line between the sacral promontory and symphysis pubis
 (D)   parallel to a line between the sacral promontory and the ASIS

589. A correctly positioned AP projection of the pelvis demonstrates:
  1. The greater trochanters in profile
  2. Symmetric opening of the obturator foramen
  3. Inclusion of the proximal half of the femoral shafts

 (A)   1 & 2
 (B)   2 & 3
 (C)   1 & 3
 (D)   1, 2, & 3

590. Radiography of a suspected hip fracture should include an AP

 (A)   and axial lateral of the affected hip
 (B)   and horizontal beam lateral of the affected hip
 (C)   pelvis only
 (D)   pelvis and axial lateral pelvis

591. The patient is supine with legs flexed and abducted about 40°. The central ray is perpendicular and enters about 1 inch above the symphysis pubis. What anatomic projection will be best demonstrated by this position?

 (A)   AP pelvis
 (B)   Horizontal beam lateral hip
 (C)   Oblique projection of femoral necks
 (D)   AP axial projection of femoral necks

592. The patient is supine with the right leg extended. The left leg is flexed, raised off the table, and supported in this elevated position. The image receptor is placed vertically, parallel to the x-ray tube. A horizontal x-ray beam is used with the central ray directed perpendicular to the midpoint of a line bisecting the patient's right ASIS and symphysis pubis. What anatomic projection will be best demonstrated by the position described?

 (A)   AP of right hip
 (B)   AP of left hip
 (C)   Axiolateral of right hip
 (D)   Axiolateral of left hip

593. An optimum image of an AP projection of the hip should

 (A)   include the entire sacrum and coccyx
 (B)   include the entire fixation device, if present
 (C)   include the distal two-thirds of the femur
 (D)   demonstrate the lesser trochanter in profile

594. How many vertebral bones are found in the average human body?

 (A)   22
 (B)   24
 (C)   33
 (D)   38

595. Which segments of the spine have a lordotic curvature?
  1. Lumbar
  2. Thoracic
  3. Cervical

 (A)   1 & 2
 (B)   2 & 3
 (C)   1 & 3
 (D)   1, 2, & 3

596. Which structure is not considered part of a "typical" vertebra?

(A) Body
(B) Spinous process
(C) Transverse foramen
(D) Superior articular facet

597. At what level does the spinal cord generally terminate?

(A) T8
(B) T12
(C) L2
(D) S1

598. The articulations of the vertebral column are primarily of which type?

(A) Gliding
(B) Hinge
(C) Saddle
(D) Cartilaginous

599. Which statement best describes the articulation between the atlas and axis vertebral bones?

(A) Anterior aspect of the dens articulates with the posterior aspect of the anterior arch
(B) Posterior aspect of the dens articulates with anterior aspect of the posterior arch
(C) Anterior aspect of the dens articulates with posterior aspect of the posterior arch
(D) Posterior aspect of the dens articulates with anterior aspect of the anterior arch

600. The costotransverse joint is formed by the articulation between the

(A) costal cartilage and the sternum
(B) head of a rib and costal cartilage
(C) head of a rib and a thoracic transverse process
(D) tubercle of a rib and a thoracic transverse process

601. What relationship is formed between the intervertebral foramen of the lumbar spine and the midsagittal plane of the body?

(A) 30°
(B) 45°
(C) 60°
(D) 90°

602. The central ray for the AP projection of the cervical spine should be directed

(A) 5 to 10° caudad
(B) 5 to 10° cephalad
(C) 15 to 20° caudad
(D) 15 to 20° cephalad

603. Which line should be placed perpendicular to the image receptor when positioning for the AP (open mouth) projection of C1–2?

(A) Orbitomeatal line
(B) Infraorbitomeatal line
(C) Line extending from lower edge of upper incisors to mastoid tip
(D) Line extending from upper edge of lower incisors to mastoid tip

604. For the AP (open mouth) projection of C1–2, the central ray should be directed

(A) perpendicular to the image receptor
(B) 5 to 10° cephalad
(C) 5 to 10° caudad
(D) 15 to 20° cephalad

605. The AP projection of the cervical spine will demonstrate

(A) C1–7
(B) C1–4
(C) C2–5
(D) C3–T1

606. Positioning instructions for the lateral projection of the cervical spine include:
1. Patient may be erect or recumbent in the lateral position
2. Shoulders should be depressed as much as possible
3. The central ray is angled 15° caudad to C4
4. Long SID of 72 inches or more is used

    (A)   1, 2, & 3
    (B)   1, 2, & 4
    (C)   1, 3, & 4
    (D)   2, 3, & 4

607. The right anterior oblique position of the cervical spine will best demonstrate the

    (A)   spinous processes
    (B)   intervertebral foramina of the right side
    (C)   intervertebral foramina of the left side
    (D)   vertebral foramen

608. In order to visualize the left intervertebral foramina of the cervical spine, which position should be used?

    (A)   Right posterior oblique (RPO)
    (B)   Right anterior oblique (RAO)
    (C)   Left posterior oblique (LPO)
    (D)   Left lateral

609. The intervertebral foramina of the lumbar spine are best demonstrated by the

    (A)   AP position
    (B)   lateral position
    (C)   45° oblique position
    (D)   70° oblique position

610. The oblique position of the lumbar spine will best demonstrate the

    (A)   spinous processes
    (B)   intervertebral foramina
    (C)   vertebral foramen
    (D)   zygapophyseal joints

611. The position that will best demonstrate the zygapophyseal joints of the thoracic spine is the

    (A)   AP
    (B)   lateral
    (C)   swimmer's lateral
    (D)   oblique

612. The position that will best demonstrate the intervertebral foramina of the thoracic spine is the

    (A)   AP
    (B)   lateral
    (C)   prone oblique
    (D)   supine oblique

613. For which position would a breathing technique be advantageous?

    (A)   AP lumbar
    (B)   Lateral lumbar
    (C)   Oblique thoracic
    (D)   Lateral thoracic

614. The composition of the intervertebral disk includes

    (A)   a cartilaginous center surrounded by a soft, gelatinous exterior
    (B)   a soft, highly elastic center surrounded by a fibrocartilaginous exterior
    (C)   alternating layers of fibrocartilaginous rings and soft, highly elastic interspace material
    (D)   a solid structure of hyaline cartilage

615. The annulus fibrosus is the

    (A)   external portion of the vertebral body
    (B)   internal portion of the vertebral body
    (C)   external portion of the intervertebral disk
    (D)   internal portion of the intervertebral disk

616. The positioning instructions for the AP projection of the sacrum includes:

1. Patient supine with midsagittal plane centered to middle of image receptor
2. Central ray directed at an angle of 15 to 20° caudad
3. Central ray entering at a point midway between the symphysis pubis and the ASIS

(A) 1 & 2
(B) 2 & 3
(C) 1 & 3
(D) 1, 2, & 3

617. The soft, highly elastic core of the intervertebral disk is referred to as

(A) cancellous bone
(B) fibrocartilage
(C) annulus fibrosus
(D) nucleus pulposus

618. How should the central ray be directed for the AP projection of the coccyx?

(A) 15° caudad
(B) 15° cephalad
(C) 10° caudad
(D) 10° cephalad

619. Which of the following structures are demonstrated on an AP projection of the lumbar spine?

(A) Intervertebral joint spaces, spinous processes, intervertebral foramina
(B) Spinous processes, vertebral bodies, zygapophyseal joints, vertebral foramen
(C) Transverse processes, intervertebral joint spaces, vertebral foramen
(D) Spinous and transverse processes, vertebral bodies, intervertebral joint spaces

620. For which reason would the PA projection of the lumbar spine be more advantageous than the AP projection?

(A) Improved recorded detail of structures
(B) Less magnification of the part
(C) Easier centering of the patient
(D) Lower gonadal dose

621. The union of the vertebral column with the pelvis occurs at the

(A) lumbosacral joint
(B) ileocecal junction
(C) sacroiliac joint
(D) zygapophyseal joints

622. If the patient is rotated 25 to 30° toward the left from the supine position and the central ray is perpendicular and enters one inch medial to the right ASIS, what anatomic structures will be best demonstrated?

(A) Right lumbar zygapophyseal joints
(B) Left lumbar zygapophyseal joints
(C) Right sacroiliac joints
(D) Left sacroiliac joints

623. How should a 14 by 17 inch image receptor be aligned when performing a scoliosis survey?

(A) Crosswise with bottom at level of iliac crest
(B) Crosswise with top at level of xiphoid
(C) Lengthwise with top at suprasternal notch
(D) Lengthwise with bottom 1 inch below iliac crest

624. Which of the following are recommendations for reducing patient dose when performing scoliosis studies?

1. Use of low kilovoltage (60 to 70)
2. PA projection rather than AP
3. Use of specific area shields

(A) 1 & 2
(B) 2 & 3
(C) 1 & 3
(D) 1, 2, & 3

625. The bony structure for which ASIS serves as a landmark is

(A) L3
(B) L4–5
(C) S1–2
(D) S5

626. The number of true ribs (those which attach to the sternum) that make up the bony thorax is

(A) 5
(B) 7
(C) 10
(D) 14

627. The makeup of the bony thorax includes:
1. Ribs
2. Sternum
3. Clavicles
4. Thoracic vertebrae

(A) 1, 2, & 3
(B) 2, 3, & 4
(C) 1, 3, & 4
(D) 1, 2, & 4

628. How many ribs attach directly to the sternum?

(A) 7
(B) 14
(C) 18
(D) 24

629. The most superior portion of the sternum is termed the

(A) gladiolus
(B) body
(C) manubrium
(D) xiphoid

630. The following statements referring to radiography of the ribs are all true EXCEPT

(A) the upper anterior ribs should be imaged on full expiration
(B) the upper anterior ribs should be imaged in the prone position
(C) the upper posterior ribs should be imaged on full inspiration
(D) the lower posterior ribs should be imaged in the supine position

631. The patient is rotated 45° toward the left from the supine position with the left arm abducted from the body. The central ray is directed perpendicular to a point midway between the sternum and left lateral aspect of the body at the level of the seventh thoracic vertebra. The patient is instructed to stop breathing on full inspiration. This position will best demonstrate the axillary aspect of the

(A) first through tenth ribs on left side
(B) eighth through twelfth ribs on left side
(C) first through tenth ribs on right side
(D) eighth through tenth ribs on right side

632. When imaging the right anterior ribs, what oblique position should be used?

(A) Left posterior oblique (LPO)
(B) Left anterior oblique (LAO)
(C) Right posterior oblique (RPO)
(D) Right anterior oblique (RAO)

633. What positions are commonly used for imaging the sternum?
1. AP or PA
2. Left lateral
3. Oblique

(A) 1 & 2
(B) 2 & 3
(C) 1 & 3
(D) 1, 2, & 3

634. What breathing instructions should be given to the patient when you are radiographing the sternum in the lateral position?

(A) Suspend respiration at full inspiration
(B) Suspend respiration at full expiration
(C) Suspend respiration whenever patient is comfortable
(D) Continue shallow breathing during exposure

635. Which of the following statements is true regarding the visceral anatomy of the thorax?

  (A) The right lung has two lobes
  (B) The left lung has two lobes
  (C) The hilum is the cavity that accommodates the heart
  (D) The most inferior portion of the lung is termed the *apex*

636. What is the correct descending (largest to smallest) order of the following bronchial structures?
      1. Alveoli
      2. Main stem bronchus
      3. Trachea
      4. Bronchioles

  (A) 2, 3, 1, 4
  (B) 3, 4, 2, 1
  (C) 1, 4, 2, 3
  (D) 3, 2, 4, 1

637. All the following are criteria for obtaining an optimum PA chest radiograph EXCEPT

  (A) rotation of scapulae away from lung fields
  (B) elevation of clavicles above apex of lungs
  (C) maximum depression of diaphragm by full inspiration
  (D) adequate penetration of lower lungs on patients with large breasts

638. Chest radiography requires the central ray to enter the patient at the level of

  (A) T5
  (B) T7
  (C) T9
  (D) the xiphoid process

639. For the patient who is unable to stand for chest radiography, what position should be used to demonstrate air-fluid levels?

  (A) Supine AP
  (B) Dorsal decubitus with vertical x-ray beam
  (C) Lateral decubitus with horizontal x-ray beam
  (D) Semierect AP and lateral

640. A patient is recumbent in the left lateral position. The image receptor is placed vertically along the anterior aspect of the patient with its midpoint aligned with T7. The x-ray beam is directed horizontally to the midpoint of the film. The patient is instructed to stop breathing on full inspiration. This describes which patient position?

  (A) Dorsal decubitus
  (B) Left lateral decubitus
  (C) Right lateral decubitus
  (D) Ventral decubitus

641. Which statement is true regarding routine oblique positions for chest radiography?

  (A) The LAO best demonstrates the left lung
  (B) Chest obliques require body rotation of 60°
  (C) The RAO best demonstrates the left lung
  (D) Respiration should be suspended on the first full expiration

642. A patient is in the erect anteroposterior position and is instructed to step forward slightly from the image receptor and then lean back, so that the shoulders rest against the image receptor. This places the clavicles parallel with the floor. The central ray is directed perpendicularly and enters at the midpoint of the sternum. This position will best demonstrate the

  (A) sternoclavicular joints
  (B) costophrenic angles
  (C) clavicles
  (D) apices of the lungs

643. Radiography of a foreign body made of glass or wood requires the use of

  (A) high kilovoltage
  (B) low kilovoltage
  (C) compression to immobilize the patient
  (D) a direct exposure imaging system

644. All the following are cranial bones that contribute to the structure of the orbit EXCEPT the

  (A) sphenoid
  (B) temporal
  (C) ethmoid
  (D) frontal

645. Each of the following facial bones is paired EXCEPT the

(A) mandible
(B) maxilla
(C) palatine
(D) inferior nasal concha

646. All the following paranasal sinuses are contained within cranial bones EXCEPT the

(A) frontal
(B) sphenoid
(C) ethmoid
(D) maxillary

647. The correct method for positioning and centering of the skull for a lateral projection includes all the following instructions EXCEPT

(A) midsagittal plane is parallel to the image receptor
(B) interpupillary line is perpendicular to the image receptor
(C) infraorbitomeatal line is parallel with the transverse plane of the image receptor
(D) perpendicular central ray enters the skull 2 inches posterior to the external auditory meatus (EAM)

648. The radiographic base line that should be placed perpendicular to the image receptor for the PA projection of the skull is the

(A) glabellomeatal line
(B) orbitomeatal line
(C) infraorbitomeatal line
(D) acanthiomeatal line

649. The skull projection that will demonstrate the dorsum sella projected through the foramen magnum is the

(A) submentovertical (full basal)
(B) verticosubmental (full basal)
(C) AP axial
(D) PA with 25° caudal tube angle

650. If the orbitomeatal base line cannot be adjusted as required for the AP axial projection of the skull, the recommended alternative base line is the

(A) glabellomeatal line
(B) infraorbitomeatal line
(C) acanthiomeatal line
(D) interpupillary line

651. The skull projection that requires the IOML to be parallel and the midsagittal plane to be perpendicular to the image receptor is the

(A) PA projection
(B) lateral projection
(C) AP axial projection
(D) submentovertical projection

652. A patient is placed in the anteroposterior (erect or recumbent) position with the midsagittal plane and OML perpendicular to the image receptor. The central ray is directed caudally at an angle of 30° and exits at the foramen magnum to best demonstrate the

(A) occipital bone
(B) zygomatic arches
(C) parietal bones
(D) mandibular rami

653. The use of the submentovertical position of the skull to demonstrate the zygomatic arches requires all the following positioning instructions EXCEPT

(A) alignment of IOML parallel to the image receptor
(B) a central ray that enters midway between the mandibular angles along a coronal plane just posterior to the outer canthus
(C) a central ray angle of 10° cephalad
(D) a decrease in exposure factors

654. A patient is positioned erect and facing the image receptor. The head is adjusted to place the midsagittal plane and mentomeatal line perpendicular to the image receptor. The central ray is also perpendicular to the image receptor and exits at the acanthion. This position will best demonstrate the

   (A) petrous portion of temporal bone
   (B) maxillary sinuses
   (C) sphenoid sinuses
   (D) temporomandibular joints

655. If the petrous ridges are seen within the lower portion of the maxillary sinuses on a parieto-acanthial projection, the positioning must be corrected by adjusting the head to place the

   (A) acanthiomeatal line perpendicular to the image receptor
   (B) acanthiomeatal line angled 37° to the image receptor
   (C) orbitomeatal line perpendicular to the image receptor
   (D) orbitomeatal line angled 37° to the image receptor

656. When performing the acanthioparietal projection of the facial bones on a patient with cervical spine trauma, what modification to the routine positioning instructions would be necessary?

   (A) Gently extend the head as much as the patient can tolerate and align the central ray parallel to the mentomeatal line
   (B) Without adjusting the extension of the patient's head at all, align the central ray parallel to the mentomeatal line
   (C) Without adjusting the extension of the patient's head, direct the central ray 30° caudad, entering at the nasion
   (D) Position the head with the acanthiomeatal line perpendicular and direct the central ray perpendicular to the image receptor

657. Positioning for the superoinferior tangential projection of the nasal bones requires alignment of the

   (A) orbitomeatal line perpendicular to the image receptor
   (B) glabellomeatal line parallel to the image receptor
   (C) mentomeatal line parallel to the image receptor
   (D) glabelloalveolar line perpendicular to the image receptor

658. The tangential projection of a depressed or flat zygomatic arch is achieved by rotating the patient's head

   (A) 30° from the supine position, away from the side of interest
   (B) 15° from the supine position, toward the side of interest
   (C) 30° from the prone position, away from the side of interest
   (D) 15° from the prone position, toward the side of interest

659. Which projection will best demonstrate both mandibular rami on the same image?

   (A) Neck extended, chin resting on image receptor, central ray angled 40 to 45° toward chin
   (B) Chin and nose rest on image receptor, central ray perpendicular and exiting at lips
   (C) Chin and nose rest on image receptor, central ray angled 30° cephalad
   (D) Head positioned as for a true lateral projection, central ray angled 25° cephalad

660. The axiolateral projection places the patient's head in the lateral position and the central ray is directed 25° cephalad, entering just behind the mandibular angle furthest from the image receptor. This will best demonstrate the

   (A) ramus of side closest to image receptor
   (B) ramus of side furthest from image receptor
   (C) symphysis
   (D) body

661. The positions that will demonstrate the TMJs include:

1. Axiolateral position with central ray 25° caudad
2. AP axial position with central ray 35° caudad
3. Axiolateral oblique position with central ray 15° caudad

(A) 1 & 2
(B) 2 & 3
(C) 1 & 3
(D) 1, 2, & 3

662. In the lateral position, the sphenoid sinuses are located directly

(A) inferior to the frontal sinuses
(B) posterior to the ethmoid sinuses
(C) anterior to the ethmoid sinuses
(D) posterior to the maxillary sinuses

663. All the following statements pertaining to the paranasal sinuses are true EXCEPT

(A) paranasal sinuses are fully developed at birth
(B) maxillary sinuses are generally the largest set
(C) sphenoid sinuses are located in the body of the sphenoid bone
(D) frontal sinuses may be single, paired, or completely absent

664. Radiography of the paranasal sinuses in the lateral position requires the central ray to enter

(A) 2 inches superior to the EAM
(B) at the EAM
(C) 3/4 inch anterior and 3/4 inch superior to the EAM
(D) midway between the outer canthus and EAM

665. Demonstration of air-fluid levels within the paranasal sinuses requires:

1. Horizontal x-ray beam
2. Patient erect
3. Vertical image receptor

(A) 1 & 2
(B) 2 & 3
(C) 1 & 3
(D) 1, 2, & 3

666. Positioning for the PA axial projection of the paranasal sinuses requires the

(A) infraorbitomeatal line perpendicular and central ray angled 20° caudad
(B) infraorbitomeatal line perpendicular and central ray angled 15° caudad
(C) orbitomeatal line perpendicular and central ray angled 20° caudad
(D) orbitomeatal line perpendicular and central ray angled 15° caudad

667. The parietoacanthial projection will demonstrate the sphenoid sinuses if the positioning is modified by

(A) a 15° cephalad central ray angle
(B) a 15° caudad central ray angle
(C) opening the patient's mouth
(D) having the central ray exit at the nasion

668. The eustachian tube is located between

(A) laryngopharynx and stomach
(B) middle ear and nasopharynx
(C) laryngopharynx and right and left main stem bronchi
(D) orifice of the external acoustic meatus and the tympanic membrane

669. All the following are considered parts of the organs of hearing EXCEPT the

(A) semicircular canals
(B) cochlea
(C) ossicles
(D) tympanic membrane

670. The organs of hearing are located within the

(A) mastoid process of the temporal bone
(B) petrous portion of the temporal bone
(C) body of the sphenoid bone
(D) greater wings of the sphenoid bone

671. The axiolateral oblique projection of the mastoid process may be performed with a central ray angle of 15° caudad and the head rotated from the lateral position

(A) 45° toward the table
(B) 15° toward the table
(C) 45° away from the table
(D) 15° away from the table

672. A patient is placed in an erect or recumbent position facing the image receptor. The head is rotated toward the side of interest, placing the midsagittal plane at a 45° angle with the image receptor. The head is further adjusted to place the IOML perpendicular to the image receptor. The central ray is directed 12° cephalad and exits 1 inch anterior to the EAM closest to the image receptor. This position will best demonstrate the

(A)   posterior profile of the petrous portion (Stenver method)
(B)   anterior profile of the petrous portion (Arcelin method)
(C)   axioposterior oblique of the mastoid portion (Mayer method)
(D)   axiolateral oblique of the mastoid portion (Law method)

673. Proper radiographic imaging of the mastoids requires

(A)   removal of the patient's dentures
(B)   use of a large focal spot
(C)   taping of the auricles in a forward position
(D)   use of high kilovoltage (>100)

674. When performing an AP tangential projection of the mastoid process, the head should be rotated

(A)   15° toward the side of interest
(B)   15° away from the side of interest
(C)   55° toward the side of interest
(D)   55° away from the side of interest

675. The projections that will demonstrate both petrous ridges on the same image include:
   1. Submentovertex projection
   2. AP axial projection
   3. Posterior profile (anterior oblique)

(A)   1 & 2
(B)   2 & 3
(C)   1 & 3
(D)   1, 2, & 3

676. A correctly positioned parieto-orbital oblique projection should demonstrate the optic canal in the

(A)   upper outer quadrant of the orbit
(B)   upper inner quadrant of the orbit
(C)   lower outer quadrant of the orbit
(D)   lower inner quadrant of the orbit

677. The positioning instructions for the parieto-orbital oblique projection of the optic canal requires the

(A)   IOML to be perpendicular to the image receptor
(B)   central ray to be angled 12° cephalad
(C)   side of interest to be furthest from the image receptor
(D)   midsagittal plane to form a 53° angle with the image receptor

678. High-quality radiographs of the fine anatomic structures of the cranium or facial bones require
   1. Close collimation
   2. Small focal spot
   3. 80 to 90 kV

(A)   1 & 2
(B)   2 & 3
(C)   1 & 3
(D)   1, 2, & 3

679. The PA projection of the cranium may be modified to demonstrate the floor of the orbits by directing the central ray

(A)   perpendicularly to exit at the nasion
(B)   10° caudad
(C)   20° caudad
(D)   30° caudad

680. Radiographic exams of the orbit for foreign body localization requires:

> 1. Cleaning of screens prior to exam
> 2. Immobilization of skull position
> 3. Instruction that patients should not move their eyeballs during the exposure

(A)   1 & 2
(B)   2 & 3
(C)   1 & 3
(D)   1, 2, & 3

681. All the following radiographic procedures for the cranium would be useful for foreign body localization of the eye EXCEPT

(A)   PA axial projection
(B)   lateral position
(C)   submentovertex projection
(D)   parietoacanthial projection

682. Imaging the soft tissue of the neck in the lateral position requires all the following EXCEPT

(A)   use of low kilovoltage
(B)   depression of shoulders
(C)   entrance of central ray anterior to C3
(D)   slight elevation of chin

683. *Cholecystography* is the radiographic examination of the

(A)   gallbladder
(B)   bile ducts
(C)   gallbladder and bile ducts
(D)   blood vessels of the liver

684. The methods by which contrast media can be introduced into the biliary system include:

> 1. Oral
> 2. Intravenous injection
> 3. Direct injection

(A)   1 & 2
(B)   2 & 3
(C)   1 & 3
(D)   1, 2, & 3

685. Where is the gallbladder most likely to be located within a patient with an *asthenic* body type?

(A)   Horizontal position, high in abdomen, lateral to midline
(B)   Semivertical position midway between most lateral aspect of abdomen on right side and midline
(C)   Semivertical position midway between most lateral aspect of abdomen on left side and midline
(D)   Vertical position, low in abdomen, close to midline

686. The technique that directly introduces contrast media into the biliary ducts via the ampulla of Vater is the

(A)   transhepatic cholangiogram
(B)   oral cholecystogram
(C)   hypertonic duodenogram
(D)   endoscopic retrograde cholangiopancreatography (ERCP)

687. In what position should the patient be placed in order to demonstrate layering of calcifications within the gallbladder?

(A)   RAO
(B)   LAO
(C)   Right lateral decubitus
(D)   Left lateral decubitus

688. Routine preliminary radiography of the gallbladder would include which projections?

> 1. PA
> 2. AP
> 3. RAO
> 4. LAO

(A)   1 & 3
(B)   1 & 4
(C)   2 & 3
(D)   2 & 4

689. The C loop of the duodenum and retrogastric area will best be demonstrated by which projection of the stomach?

(A) RAO
(B) LPO
(C) Upright left lateral
(D) Recumbent right lateral

690. A coned-down (10 by 12) PA image of the stomach will require the central ray to enter at

(A) T10
(B) L2
(C) L4
(D) S2

691. A patient is rotated approximately 45° toward the left from the recumbent supine position. The central ray is directed in a perpendicular manner along the sagittal plane, which is midway between the vertebral column and left lateral border of the body at the level of L1. This projection is the

(A) LPO of the stomach
(B) LAO of the gallbladder
(C) RPO of the colon
(D) RAO of the esophagus

692. Placing a patient in the AP Trendelenburg position during a UGI series may be useful to

(A) improve filling of the pylorus
(B) demonstrate the pyloric stenosis
(C) demonstrate a hiatal hernia
(D) open the duodenal loop

693. All the following statements regarding a double contrast GI series versus a single contrast UGI series are true EXCEPT

(A) it is easier for the patient to tolerate
(B) it offers better visualization of the mucosa
(C) it provides better visualization of small lesions on the mucosa
(D) it employs thick barium

694. The fluoroscopic imaging of the terminal ileum is generally included as part of the

(A) UGI series
(B) small bowel series
(C) esophagram
(D) barium enema

695. A poorly prepared colon may cause retained fecal material to resemble

(A) diverticulosis
(B) ulceration
(C) polyposis
(D) inflammation

696. A patient is placed in the prone, recumbent position. The central ray is directed at a caudal angle of about 35°, entering the midsagittal plane at the level of the ASIS. This position will best demonstrate the

(A) hepatic flexure
(B) splenic flexure
(C) cecum
(D) rectosigmoid

697. All the following projections are part of both the double contrast and single contrast barium enema routines EXCEPT the

(A) PA axial of the rectosigmoid colon
(B) right and left lateral decubitus of the abdomen
(C) right and left posterior oblique of the abdomen
(D) lateral rectum

698. The correct centering points for the lateral rectum projection are the

(A) iliac crest and midsagittal plane
(B) ASIS and midaxillary plane
(C) symphysis pubis and midsagittal plane
(D) iliac crest and midaxillary plane

699. For radiography of the colon on a patient with a colostomy, how is the barium administered?

(A) Rectally, as usual
(B) Orally, allowing time for the barium to reach the colon
(C) Through the stoma
(D) Barium cannot be administered in these patients

700. The aspect of the kidney on which the renal *hilum* is located is the

(A) superior border
(B) inferior border
(C) lateral border
(D) medial border

701. Which of the following statements is true regarding the position of the kidney within the abdomen?

(A) Upper pole of kidney is anterior to lower pole
(B) Lower pole of kidney is anterior to upper pole
(C) Medial border of kidney is anterior to lateral border
(D) Lateral border of kidney is anterior to medial border

702. What is the correct sequence of macroscopic structures of the kidney through which the filtered material flows to reach the ureter?

(A) Pelvis, major calyces, minor calyces, pyramids
(B) Pelvis, pyramids, major calyces, minor calyces
(C) Major calyces, minor calyces, pyramids, pelvis
(D) Pyramids, minor calyces, major calyces, pelvis

703. The congenital condition in which the lower poles of the two kidneys are fused together is:

(A) agenesis
(B) horseshoe kidneys
(C) ectopic kidneys
(D) polycystic kidneys

704. A common reason for the appearance of a large filling defect in the bladder of men over 50 years old is

(A) acute urinary tract infection (UTI)
(B) benign prostatic hypertrophy (BPH)
(C) bifid collecting systems
(D) renal failure

705. All the following statements are true pertaining to the scout radiograph for an intravenous urography (IVU) procedure EXCEPT

(A) the prone abdomen radiograph, centered at the ASIS, is most commonly requested
(B) patients should first be instructed to empty their bladder
(C) the image demonstrates from the kidneys to the bladder
(D) patients should be instructed to suspend breathing on expiration

706. Methods to enhance filling of the renal pelvis and proximal ureter include:
  1. Compression band over lower abdomen
  2. Patient in prone position
  3. Exam table in Trendelenburg position

(A) 1 & 2
(B) 2 & 3
(C) 1 & 3
(D) 1, 2, & 3

707. Positioning the abdomen for an AP oblique projection as part of an IVU exam generally requires the body to be rotated

(A) 15°
(B) 30°
(C) 45°
(D) 60°

708. A patient is rotated 60° toward the right, with the left leg remaining in an extended position. The perpendicular central ray enters at a point 2 inches above the symphysis pubis and 2 inches medial to the left ASIS. This position will best demonstrate the

(A) left ureterovesical junction
(B) right ureterovesical junction
(C) male urethra
(D) female urethra

709. An abdominal radiograph in the upright position may be requested as part of the IVU procedure to demonstrate

(A) motility of kidneys
(B) suprarenal glands
(C) vesicoureteral junction
(D) prevertebral space

710. When nephrotomograms are part of the IVU exam, they should be obtained

(A) prior to injection of contrast media
(B) within 1 to 5 min following injection of contrast media
(C) within 5 to 10 min following injection of contrast media
(D) at least 20 min following injection of contrast media

711. Which of the following are readily visible on the plain film abdominal radiograph?

(A) Kidneys, ureters, bladder
(B) Kidneys, gas within the stomach, full bladder
(C) Gas within colon, bladder, uterus
(D) Bladder, urethra, psoas muscles

712. An AP nephrogram or nephrotomogram is achieved by centering

(A) at the xiphoid process
(B) midway between the iliac crest and xiphoid process
(C) midway between the iliac crest and symphysis pubis
(D) at the level of the iliac crest, along the midsagittal plane

713. What radiographic image will best demonstrate *nephroptosis?*

(A) Posterior oblique of kidney region
(B) AP Trendelenburg of kidney region
(C) Prone KUB
(D) AP upright KUB

714. Which of the following statements is true regarding the hysterosalpingogram?

(A) It is a retrograde procedure
(B) The contrast media is injected into the vagina
(C) Iodized oil-based contrast media is used
(D) An AP projection of the collimated pelvis, centered at the midpoint of the symphysis pubis, is required as part of the exam

715. The type of contrast media used during hysterosalpingography is

(A) barium sulfate
(B) iodized oils
(C) water-soluble iodine compounds
(D) air

716. All the following statements are true regarding the correct method for imaging the abdomen in the supine AP position EXCEPT

(A) the image receptor is centered at the iliac crest
(B) the bottom of the image receptor is placed 2 inches below the symphysis pubis
(C) the patient's knees are slightly flexed
(D) two crosswise images may be needed for the hypersthenic patient

717. What variation from the recumbent AP projection must be made to image the abdomen in the erect AP projection?

(A) Center more to the left side of the midsagittal plane
(B) Center more to the right side of the midsagittal plane
(C) Center at the ASIS
(D) Center 2 to 3 inches above the iliac crest

718. If an AP nephrotomogram obtained at the 8 cm level best demonstrates the lower poles of the kidneys, what additional level should be used to demonstrate the upper poles of the kidneys?

(A) 4 cm
(B) 6 cm
(C) 10 cm
(D) 12 cm

719. Nephrotomography is generally performed at multiple fulcrum levels (cuts), which are usually separated by about

(A) 0.5 cm
(B) 1.0 cm
(C) 2.0 cm
(D) 3.0 cm

720. A tomographic image of the kidneys is obtained using the 5 cm fulcrum setting and a 10° linear amplitude. The image demonstrates the transverse processes of the vertebral column and poor visualization of the kidneys. The best correction would be to change to

(A) a 2 cm fulcrum setting
(B) an 8 cm fulcrum setting
(C) an amplitude of 5°
(D) an amplitude of 20°

721. A suspicious area is noted on a lateral chest radiograph at a point 10 cm posterior to the sternum. If the patient measures 26 cm in the AP diameter and 38 cm in the lateral diameter, at what level should the fulcrum be set for an AP tomogram of the area in question?

(A) 28 cm
(B) 20 cm
(C) 16 cm
(D) 10 cm

722. Tomographic imaging may be advantageous in which of the following?
    1. Evaluation of healing fractures
    2. Demonstration of subtle skull fractures
    3. Diagnosis of vascular disease

(A) 1 & 2
(B) 2 & 3
(C) 1 & 3
(D) 1, 2, & 3

723. Tomographic images are frequently a part of the radiographic exam of the biliary system referred to as

(A) an intravenous cholangiogram (IVC)
(B) an oral cholecystogram (OCG)
(C) a percutaneous transhepatic cholangiogram (PTC)
(D) an endoscopic retrograde cholangiopancreatogram (ERCP)

724. Tomographic images of the skull should be obtained at section intervals of

(A) 1 to 5 mm
(B) 5 to 10 mm
(C) 1 to 2 cm
(D) 2 to 3 cm

725. Structures of the brainstem include:
    1. Medulla oblongata
    2. Cerebellum
    3. Pons

(A) 1 & 2
(B) 2 & 3
(C) 1 & 3
(D) 1, 2, & 3

726. Which section of the brain is divided into two equal halves?

(A) Cerebrum
(B) Midbrain
(C) Medulla oblongata
(D) Pons

727. The section of the brain to which the spinal cord is directly attached is the

(A) cerebrum
(B) cerebellum
(C) medulla oblongata
(D) pons

728. Arrange the following structures in the order through which cerebrospinal fluid flows within the ventricular system:
    1. Lateral ventricle
    2. Third ventricle
    3. Fourth ventricle
    4. Cerebral aqueduct
    5. Interventricular aqueduct

(A) 2, 4, 3, 5, 1
(B) 1, 4, 3, 5, 2
(C) 3, 5, 2, 4, 1
(D) 1, 5, 2, 4, 3

729. The body system NOT demonstrated with contrast media on the image in the figure below is the

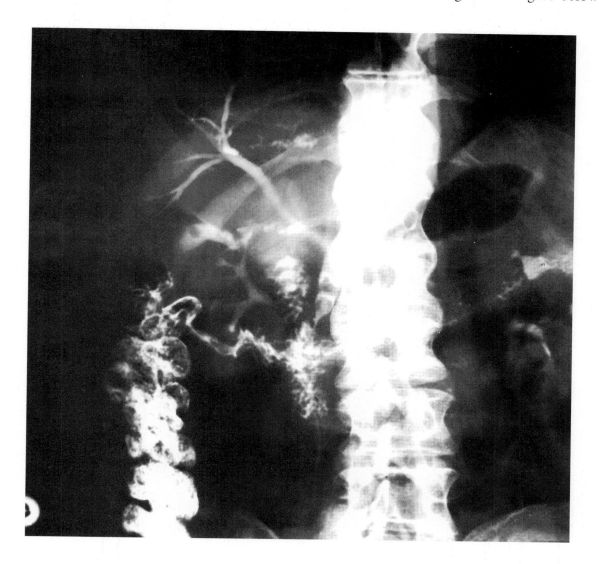

(A)   urinary system
(B)   gastrointestinal system
(C)   lymphatic system
(D)   biliary system

730. The structure marked number 2 on the image below is the

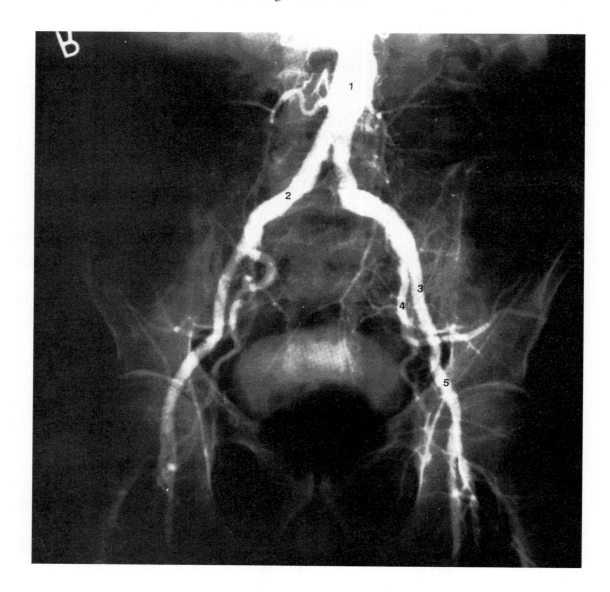

(A) aorta
(B) common iliac artery
(C) femoral artery
(D) external iliac artery

Questions 731–734

Refer to the radiographic images below to answer these questions.

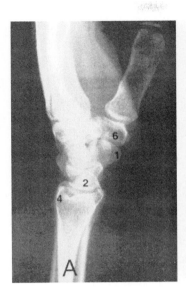 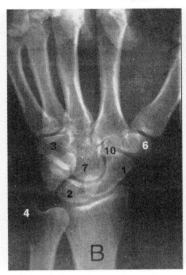 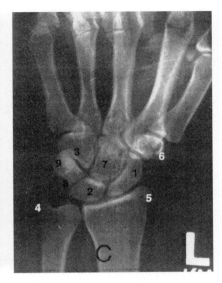

731. The radiographic position demonstrated in film B is the

(A) lateral wrist
(B) PA wrist
(C) oblique wrist
(D) PA wrist with radial deviation

732. What anatomic structure is indicated by the number 7?

(A) Scaphoid
(B) Capitate
(C) Hamate
(D) Lunate

733. On image C, the *lunate* is number

(A) 2
(B) 3
(C) 8
(D) 9

734. What structure is labeled number 6?

(A) Scaphoid
(B) Hamate
(C) Trapezoid
(D) Trapezium

Questions 735–737

Use the image below to identify the following structures.

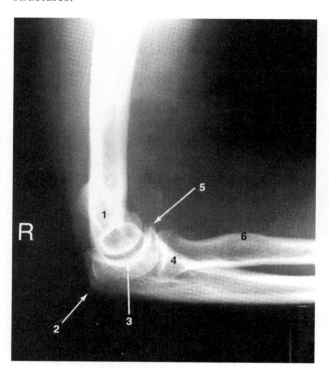

735.   The olecranon process is number

(A)   1
(B)   2
(C)   5
(D)   6

736.   Which of the following is the ulnar struc-
        ture that articulates with the trochlea of the
        humerus?

(A)   2
(B)   3
(C)   4
(D)   5

737.   The structure that articulates with the capitu-
        lum of the humerus is

(A)   2
(B)   3
(C)   4
(D)   5

Questions 738–739

Refer to the figure below to answer the following items.

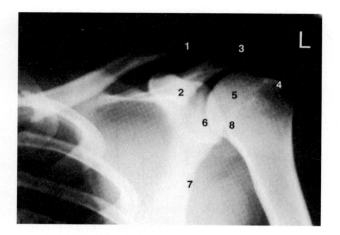

738.   The projection of the shoulder demonstrated in
        the figure is the

(A)   Grashey method
(B)   inferosuperior axial projection
(C)   PA oblique position
(D)   AP external rotation

739.   The acromion process of the scapula is labeled
        number

(A)   1
(B)   2
(C)   3
(D)   4

Questions 740–741

Refer to the diagram of the scapula in the figure below to answer these questions.

Questions 742–744

Use the radiographic image of the foot below to identify the following structures.

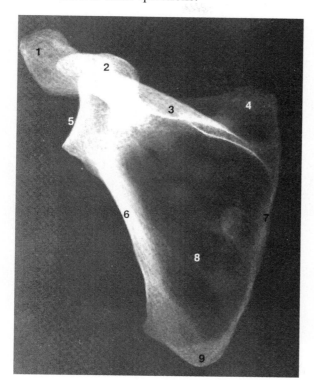

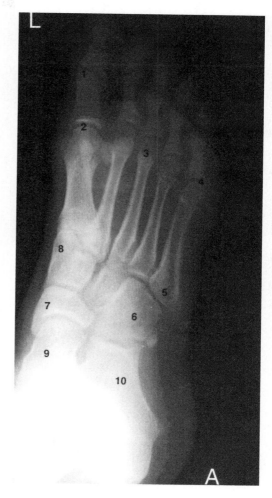

740. The structure labeled number 5 is the

   (A)   glenoid cavity
   (B)   acromion process
   (C)   coracoid process
   (D)   scapular notch

741. The structure labeled number 7 is the

   (A)   lateral (axillary) border
   (B)   medial (vertebral) border
   (C)   superior border
   (D)   inferior angle

742. The cuboid is the structure numbered

   (A)   6
   (B)   7
   (C)   8
   (D)   10

743. The head of the third metatarsal is number

   (A)   1
   (B)   2
   (C)   3
   (D)   4

744. The first interphalangeal joint is number

   (A)   1
   (B)   2
   (C)   3
   (D)   4

Questions 745–747

Refer to the radiographic image below to answer the following items.

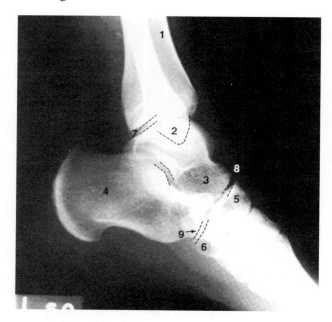

Questions 748–749

Refer to the figure below to locate the structures stated in each item.

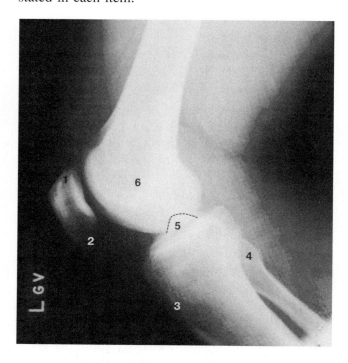

745. The joint space represented by number 7 is the

(A) talonavicular
(B) calcaneocuboid
(C) talocalcaneal
(D) tibiotalar

746. The talus bone is number

(A) 3
(B) 4
(C) 5
(D) 6

747. The navicular bone is number

(A) 3
(B) 4
(C) 5
(D) 6

748. The tibial tuberosity is labeled number

(A) 2
(B) 3
(C) 4
(D) 5

749. The base of the patella is number

(A) 1
(B) 2
(C) 3
(D) 5

Questions 750–752

Use the radiographic image below to identify the structures listed in these questions.

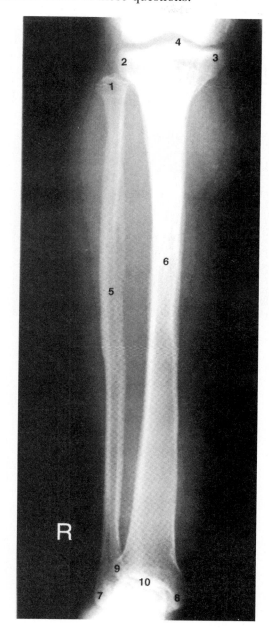

750. The lateral malleolus is the structure numbered

(A) 1
(B) 2
(C) 7
(D) 8

751. The head of the fibula is the structure numbered

(A) 1
(B) 3
(C) 5
(D) 7

752. The tibial spine is the structure numbered

(A) 2
(B) 4
(C) 6
(D) 8

Questions 753–756

Use the image of the hip bone below to identify the following anatomic structures.

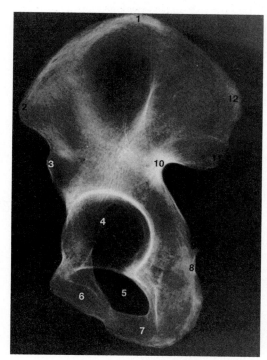

753. The greater sciatic notch is labeled

(A) 4
(B) 5
(C) 8
(D) 10

754. The acetabulum is labeled

(A) 4
(B) 5
(C) 8
(D) 10

755. The anterior superior iliac spine is labeled

(A) 2
(B) 3
(C) 9
(D) 11

756. The ischial ramus is labeled

(A) 4
(B) 6
(C) 7
(D) 10

Questions 757–758

Refer to the radiographic image below to answer the following items.

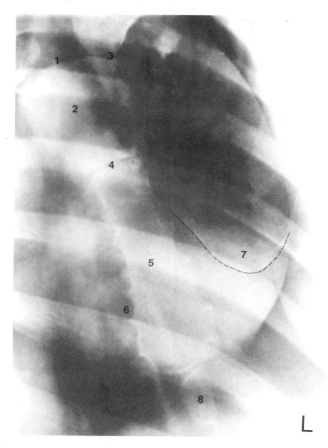

757. The special imaging technique for production of the image demonstrated in the figure was the use of

(A) the AEC with side chambers only
(B) linear tomography
(C) magnification via an air gap
(D) a breathing technique

758. The sternal angle is identified as number

(A) 1
(B) 4
(C) 6
(D) 7

Questions 759–761

Use the image below to identify the structures of a typical vertebra.

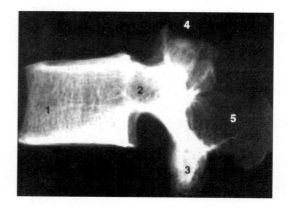

759. The pedicle is number

(A) 1
(B) 2
(C) 4
(D) 5

760. The spinous process is number

(A) 1
(B) 3
(C) 4
(D) 5

761. The superior articular facet is number

(A) 2
(B) 3
(C) 4
(D) 5

Questions 762–765

Refer to the radiographic image below to answer the following items.

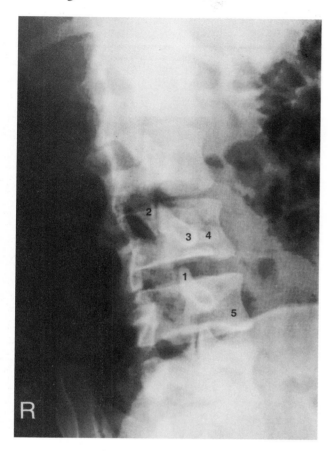

762. What position is demonstrated by the radiographic image?

(A) Left lateral
(B) AP
(C) Left posterior oblique
(D) Right posterior oblique

763. Which of the following joints is best demonstrated in the figure?

(A) Sacroiliac joints
(B) Intervertebral joints
(C) Zygapophyseal joints
(D) L5–S1 joint

764. The structure labeled number 2 represents

(A) an inferior articular facet
(B) a superior articular facet
(C) a pedicle
(D) a lamina

765. The pedicle is represented by the number

(A) 1
(B) 2
(C) 3
(D) 4

Questions 766-768

Use the radiographic image below to locate the following structures.

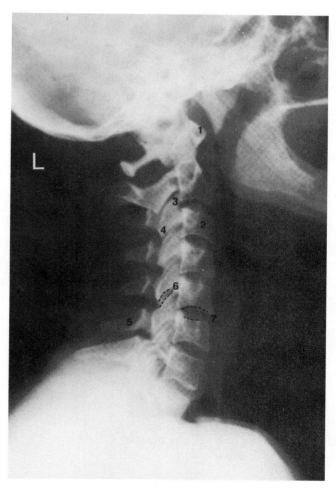

766. The structure numbered 3 is the

(A) spinous process of C3
(B) superior articular facet of C3
(C) inferior articular facet of C2
(D) transverse process of C2

767. The structure numbered 6 is the

    (A) zygapophyseal joint of C5–6
    (B) intervertebral joint of C5–6
    (C) intervertebral foramen of C5–6
    (D) zygapophyseal joint of C4–5

768. The structure numbered 1 is the

    (A) odontoid process
    (B) body of C1
    (C) lateral masses of C1
    (D) anterior arch

Questions 769–772

Use the radiographic image below to locate the structures indicated.

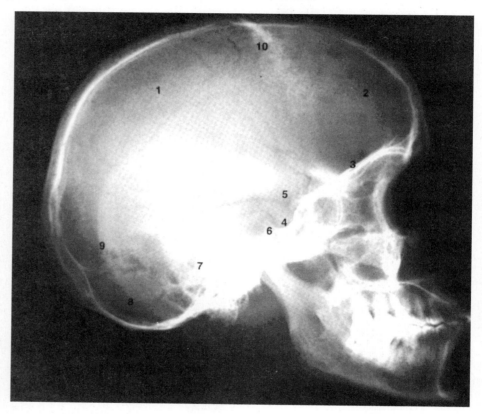

769. The mastoid portion of temporal bone is labeled

    (A) 3
    (B) 4
    (C) 7
    (D) 8

770. The dorsum sella is number

    (A) 3
    (B) 4
    (C) 5
    (D) 6

771. The lambdoidal suture is labeled

    (A) 3
    (B) 7
    (C) 9
    (D) 10

772. The greater wing of the sphenoid is number

    (A) 2
    (B) 3
    (C) 5
    (D) 7

Questions 773–776

Use the radiographic image below to identify the structures indicated in the following questions.

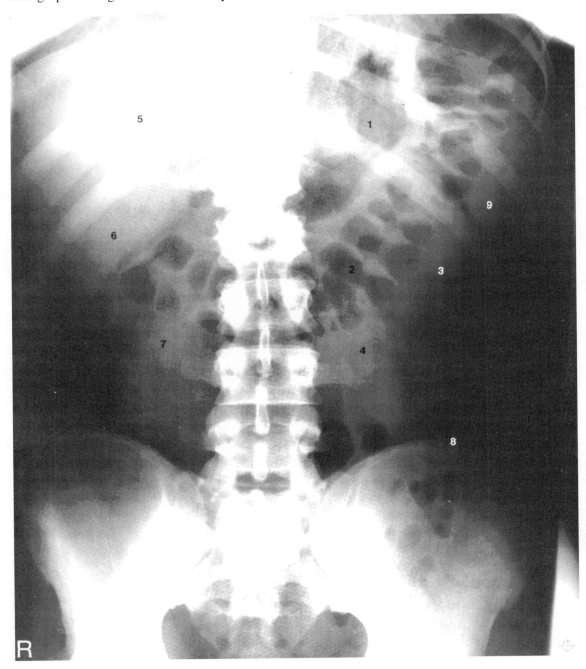

773. The liver is represented by number

    (A) 1
    (B) 2
    (C) 4
    (D) 5

774. The left kidney is represented by number

    (A) 2
    (B) 3
    (C) 5
    (D) 6

775. The right psoas muscle is represented by number

    (A) 3
    (B) 4
    (C) 6
    (D) 7

776. The transverse colon is represented by number

    (A) 2
    (B) 4
    (C) 7
    (D) 9

Questions 777–778

Use the radiographic image below to identify the structures in the following items.

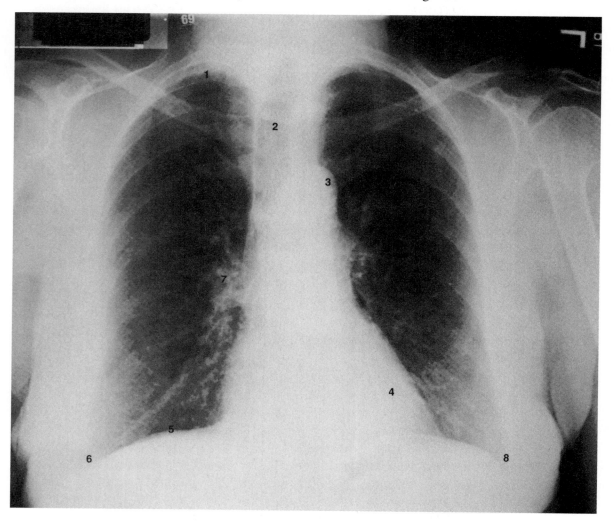

777. The right costophrenic angle is number

    (A) 1
    (B) 5
    (C) 6
    (D) 8

778. The aortic arch is marked number

    (A) 2
    (B) 3
    (C) 4
    (D) 5

Questions 779–781

Use the radiograph below to locate the anatomic structures indicated in each statement.

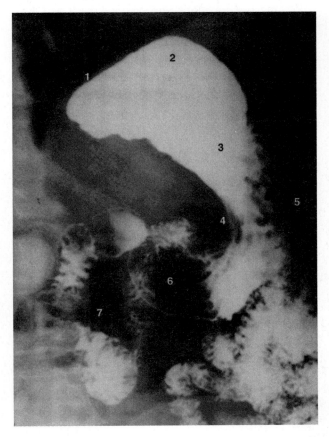

779. The pylorus is the structure numbered

    (A) 1
    (B) 2
    (C) 4
    (D) 6

780. The cardiac orifice is the structure numbered

    (A) 1
    (B) 2
    (C) 6
    (D) 7

781. The greater curvature of the stomach is number

    (A) 3
    (B) 4
    (C) 5
    (D) 7

Questions 782–785

Use the radiograph below to locate the anatomic structures indicated.

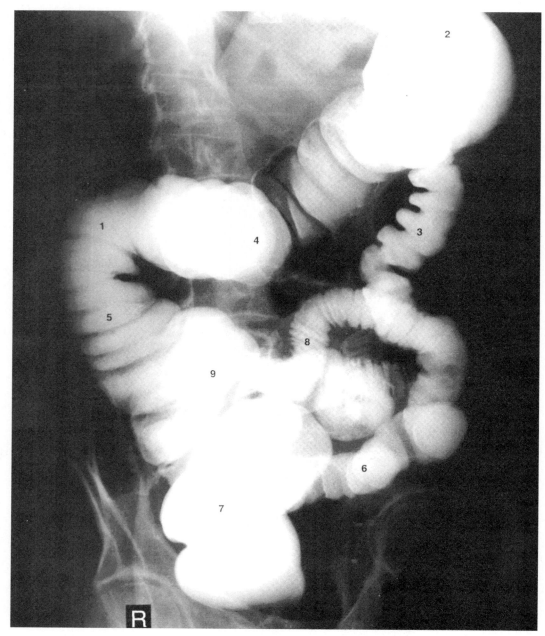

782. The splenic flexure is indicated by number

    (A) 1
    (B) 2
    (C) 5
    (D) 6

783. The cecum is indicated by number

    (A) 3
    (B) 6
    (C) 8
    (D) 9

784. The sigmoid colon is indicated by number

    (A) 3
    (B) 5
    (C) 6
    (D) 8

785. The ascending colon is indicated by number

    (A) 3
    (B) 4
    (C) 5
    (D) 7

Questions 786–787

Use the diagram of the cerebral ventricles below to answer the following questions.

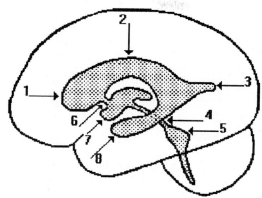

786. The third ventricle is represented by number

(A) 2
(B) 3
(C) 7
(D) 8

787. The inferior horn of the lateral ventricle is number

(A) 1
(B) 3
(C) 5
(D) 8

DIRECTIONS: Each group of questions below consists of lettered headings followed by a set of numbered items. For each numbered item select the **one** lettered heading with which it is **most** closely associated. Each lettered heading may be used **once, more than once, or not at all.**

Questions 788–791

Match each of the following descriptions with its correct vertebral component listed as answer options.

- (A) Spinous process
- (B) Transverse process
- (C) Vertebral foramen
- (D) Intervertebral foramen

788. Structure formed by the union of the posterior aspect of the body and anterior aspect of the vertebral arch

789. Structure most posterior on vertebral arch; most prominent on C7

790. Structure formed by the alignment of the vertebral notches in the formation of the zygapophyseal joints

791. Structure situated between a pedicle and lamina

Questions 792–799

For each skull structure, identify the cranial bone on which it is found.

- (A) Frontal bone
- (B) Occipital bone
- (C) Temporal bone
- (D) Sphenoid bone
- (E) Ethmoid bone

792. Cribriform plate

793. Supraorbital margin

794. Sella turcica

795. Inion

796. Mastoid process

797. Petrous portion

798. Greater wing

799. Perpendicular plate

Questions 800–804

Match each description to the correct structure.

- (A) Acanthion
- (B) Glabella
- (C) Outer canthus
- (D) Gonion
- (E) Nasion

800. The most superior midline landmark on the skull

801. Midline point marking the union of the nose and upper lip

802. Most lateral and inferior landmark on the skull

803. Site of the junction of nasal bones with the frontal bone

804. One of the reference points in forming the orbitomeatal line (OML)

Questions 805–809

Identify which facial bone is being described.

- (A) Vomer
- (B) Mandible
- (C) Maxilla
- (D) Zygoma

805. Contains the alveolar process on its inferior border

806. Articulates with the perpendicular plate of the ethmoid

807. Articulates with the temporal bone, forming a hinge type of joint

808. Contains a coronoid process

809. Contains a paranasal sinus

Questions 810–813

Identify which paranasal sinus is primarily demonstrated by each projection.

    (A)   Frontal
    (B)   Maxillary
    (C)   Sphenoid/ethmoid
    (D)   All sinuses

810.   Parietoacanthial projection

811.   PA axial projection

812.   Submentovertex projection

813.   Lateral position

Questions 814–817

Identify the *entrance* or *exit* points for the following skull projections.

    (A)   Nasion
    (B)   Acanthion
    (C)   Superior to EAM
    (D)   Foramen magnum

814.   Lateral projection of cranial bones

815.   AP axial projection of the sella turcica or dorsum sella

816.   Parietoacanthial projection of maxillary sinuses

817.   PA projection of the frontal paranasal sinuses

Questions 818–825

Identify the radiologic exam of the urinary system from the descriptions stated in the questions.

    (A)   Intravenous urography
    (B)   Retrograde urography
    (C)   Voiding cystourethrography
    (D)   Hypertensive intravenous urography
    (E)   Percutaneous antegrade urography

818.   Contrast media is injected through a retention catheter placed in the bladder

819.   Contrast media is injected directly into the renal pelves via catheters placed within the ureters

820.   This exam is also referred to as an *excretory urogram*

821.   Contrast media is directly injected into the renal pelvis via a nephrostomy tube for a patient with hydronephrosis

822.   This exam provides a functional study of the bladder and urethra

823.   This exam determines whether poor kidney function is a cause of a patient's high blood pressure

824.   This exam evaluates the presence and extent of ureteral reflux

825.   Several radiographs are obtained shortly after the bolus injection of contrast media

Questions 826–828

Identify the kidney structures labeled in the figure.

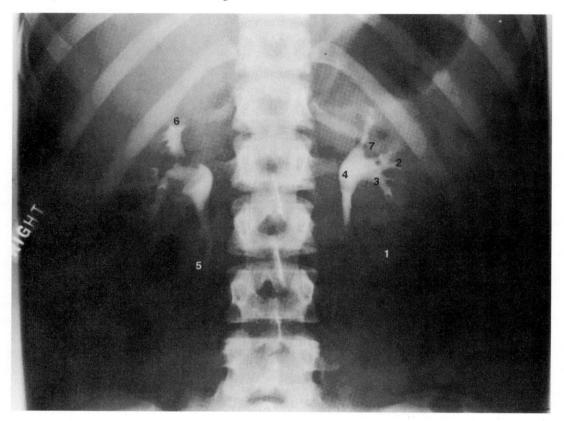

(A) Renal cortex
(B) Minor calyx
(C) Major calyx
(D) Renal pelvis
(E) Ureter

826.   Identify the structure labeled number 3

827.   Identify the structure labeled number 4

828.   Identify the structure labeled number 1

Questions 829–833

Identify the various pathological conditions of the urinary system from the descriptions stated in the questions.

    (A)   Hydronephrosis
    (B)   Cystitis
    (C)   Pyelonephritis
    (D)   Renal failure
    (E)   Ectopic kidney

829. Is commonly the result of an infection due to a vesicovaginal fistula

830. Results from a kidney that failed to ascend to the normal position

831. Involves infection of the kidney and renal pelvis

832. Is commonly due to a stricture or obstruction in a ureter

833. Results in dilatation of the renal pelvis, calyces, and, in extreme cases, the ureter

Questions 834–838

Identify which radiographic images will best demonstrate the areas or conditions described in each question.

    (A)   Upright AP bladder
    (B)   RPO abdomen
    (C)   Postvoid bladder
    (D)   AP Trendelenburg

834. Will provide enhanced filling of the renal pelvis and calyces

835. Will demonstrate the presence of an enlarged prostate gland

836. Will demonstrate prolapse of the bladder

837. Will demonstrate the distal ureters and vesicoureteral orifices

838. Will best demonstrate the entire left ureter and vesicoureteral junction

Questions 839–843

Identify which duct is being described in each question

    (A)   Stensen's duct
    (B)   Ampulla of Vater
    (C)   Common bile duct
    (D)   Wharton's duct
    (E)   Cystic duct

839. Its opening is guarded by the sphincter of Oddi

840. It extends from the gallbladder

841. It drains the parotid gland

842. It is formed by the union of the hepatic and cystic ducts

843. It is formed by the union of the common bile duct and the pancreatic duct

Questions 844–850

What radiologic procedure would most likely be performed on a patient with the symptoms or suspected condition stated in the following questions?

    (A)   Esophagram
    (B)   Oral cholecystogram
    (C)   Upper gastrointestinal series
    (D)   Lower gastrointestinal series
    (E)   Small bowel series

844. Diagnosis of cholelithiasis

845. Complaint of epigastric pain with dyspepsia

846. Complaint of heartburn or dysphagia

847. Follow-up exam for duodenal ulcer

848. Suspected diagnosis of regional enteritis (Crohn's disease)

849. Complaint of bloody diarrhea associated with significant weight loss

850. Diagnosis of diverticulosis

Radiographic Procedures

Answers

551. The answer is C. *(Ballinger, 7/e, vol 1, p 59. Bontrager, 3/e, pp 112–114.)* The request for a radiograph of any of the fingers requires the inclusion of the entire digit and the associated metacarpophalangeal joint. The inclusion of the distal end of the metacarpal (one of the five bones of the metacarpus) will ensure demonstration of the joint space. The proximal end of the metacarpal articulates with the carpal bones and is generally more inclusive than necessary.

552. The answer is D (2, 4). *(Ballinger, 7/e, vol 1, p 60. Bontrager, 3/e, p 114.)* Radiography of the fingers in the lateral position requires the digit to be positioned parallel to the image receptor to obtain the least amount of OID possible. The choice of whether to position the lateral or medial aspect of the digit on the image receptor is dictated by which digits are in question. The fourth and fifth digits should be positioned with their medial surface closest to the image receptor. The lateral projection of the first and second fingers is obtained with the lateral surface closest to the image receptor. (The third digit is imaged from either position.) To minimize distortion and open joint spaces, the distal phalanx of the fourth finger must be raised to maintain a parallel relationship between the long axis of the finger and the plane of the image receptor. This will necessitate some measure of OID at the distal phalanx.

553. The answer is D. *(Ballinger, 7/e, vol 1, p 75. Bontrager, 3/e, p 122.)* Extension of the hand when positioning for the PA projection results in a slight elevation of the wrist from the image receptor surface. This OID may contribute to a suboptimum quality image. In order to reduce this OID, the hand is arched slightly by folding the fingers and placing the wrist in contact with the image receptor surface. This position is also generally more comfortable for the patient, but this is not the primary reason for the positioning requirement.

554. The answer is C. *(Ballinger, 7/e, vol 1, pp 66–71. Bontrager, 3/e, pp 110, 118–121.)* Proper radiography of the hand should demonstrate all the phalanges, the metacarpals, the carpals, and the distal end of the radius and ulna. This requirement should be met for all the basic positions of the hand: PA, oblique, and lateral.

555. The answer is B (2, 3). *(Ballinger, 7/e, vol 1, p 74. Bontrager, 3/e, pp 102–103.)* The eight carpal (wrist) bones are separated into two rows. The proximal row, which articulates with the distal end of the radius and ulna, includes the scaphoid (navicular), lunate, triquetral, and pisiform (lateral to medial). The distal row, which articulates with the proximal ends of the five metacarpals, includes the trapezium (greater multangular), trapezoid (lesser multangular), capitate, and hamate (lateral to medial).

556. The answer is A. *(Ballinger, 7/e, vol 1, p 64. Bontrager, 3/e, p 115.)* The basic positions to be included when radiographing the thumb are the AP, lateral, and oblique. The AP position is desired over the PA position in order to include the entire digit and the distal end of the first metacarpal. Occasionally, the PA projection may be required instead of or in addition to the AP owing to patient limitations. The oblique and lateral positions are relatively easy for the patient to assume.

557. The answer is B. *(Ballinger, 7/e, vol 1, p 88. Bontrager, 3/e, p 130.)* The correct method for positioning of the forearm for the AP projection is to supinate the hand. This position will place the radius and ulna free of superimposition upon each other and maintain the humerus parallel to the image receptor. Pronation of the hand causes the radius and ulna to cross one another.

558. The answer is A (1 only). *(Ballinger, 7/e, vol 1, p 88. Bontrager, 3/e, p 130.)* In order to obtain an optimum radiograph of the forearm in the lateral position, the part must be positioned as follows: The forearm is flexed to form a 90° angle with the humerus; the humerus must be lowered to place the shoulder joint at the same level as the elbow joint; the hand must be extended with its lateral aspect in contact with the image receptor. These requirements are necessary to assure proper superimposition of the distal and proximal ends of the radius and ulna and demonstration of the shafts of the radius and ulna in the true lateral position.

559. The answer is D. *(Ballinger, 7/e, vol 1, p 95. Bontrager, 3/e, p 136.)* The radial head is located at the proximal end of the radius and forms part of the elbow joint. In order to demonstrate the radial head free of superimposition from the ulnar, the lateral oblique projection of the elbow should be used. This position requires the arm to be extended with the hand supinated. The entire extremity is then rotated laterally about 40°. The medial oblique position of the elbow causes the radial head to be completely superimposed by the ulna. The lateral position of the elbow demonstrates the radial head partially free of the ulna, but not completely.

560. The answer is B. *(Ballinger, 7/e, vol 1, pp 98–99. Bontrager, 3/e, p 138.)* The acute flexion position is used when trauma to the elbow prevents the patient from extending the arm for routine imaging of the elbow. Therefore, the elbow must be imaged in two segments in order to demonstrate the distal humerus and proximal forearm with minimal distortion. This is achieved through the following positioning steps: The humerus is placed on the image receptor with the humeral epicondyles parallel to the image receptor to avoid rotation; the central ray is then directed perpendicular to the forearm (in order to demonstrate the proximal forearm) or it is directed perpendicular to the humerus (in order to demonstrate the distal humerus). For either of these the central ray enters the part at about 2 inches superior to the olecranon process.

561. The answer is A. *(Ballinger, 7/e, vol 1, p 106. Bontrager, 3/e, p 143.)* Positioning a patient for the AP projection of the humerus may be performed in either the erect or recumbent position. The arm is slightly abducted from the body and the hand supinated to aid in placing the humeral epicondyles parallel to the image receptor. Pronation of the hand (or rotating the arm medially) will place the humeral epicondyles perpendicular to the image receptor as required for the lateral projection of the humerus. External rotation of the arm will generally place the humeral epicondyles at an angle with the image receptor, which will not produce the desired results.

562. The answer is B. *(Ballinger, 7/e, vol 1, p 108. Bontrager, 3/e, p 160.)* The use of a breathing technique is possible when performing the transthoracic lateral projection of the humerus. This projection is obtained on the trauma patient who is suspected of having a humeral fracture and is unable to move the arm for routine imaging. The patient is placed in the lateral position with the affected arm closest to the image receptor and the opposite arm raised overhead. The central ray is directed perpendicularly through the thorax at the level of the surgical neck of the affected arm. If suspended respiration is used, the humerus will be projected through the thorax with superimposition of the ribs and lung markings. Having the patient breathe normally and using a long exposure time with a low milliamperage will blur the rib and lung markings and improve visibility of the humerus. This technique may be used with various exams that require the object of interest to be imaged through the thorax, such as examination of the lateral dorsal spine. However, this does not include the other exams listed as answer options for this question. The scapular Y projection, the AP projection of the sternoclavicular joints, and the axial projection of the shoulder all should be obtained using suspended respiration.

563. The answer is C. *(Ballinger, 7/e, vol 1, pp 120–121. Bontrager, 3/e, p 157.)* The position described in the question is the inferosuperior axial position of the shoulder. This position provides demonstration of the glenohumeral joint, the acromioclavicular joint, and the coracoid process of the scapula. Due to the amount of abduction of the affected arm, this position is not routinely used and should only be attempted on a trauma patient when a physician is available to abduct the patient's arm.

564. The answer is B. *(Ballinger, 7/e, vol 1, p 115. Bontrager, 3/e, p 150.)* The shoulder or glenohumeral joint is one of three joints that make up the shoulder girdle. The shoulder joint is formed by the articulation between the glenoid cavity of the scapula and the head of the humerus. This diarthrotic joint allows free movement of the upper limb. The two other joints of the shoulder girdle are the acromioclavicular (articulation between the acromial process of the scapula and the acromial end of the clavicle) and the sternoclavicular joint (articulation between the sternal end of the clavicle and the manubrium of the sternum).

565. The answer is A. *(Ballinger, 7/e, vol 1, pp 118–119. Bontrager, 3/e, p 160.)* When radiographing a trauma patient with a suspected fracture of the humerus, the affected arm should not be moved for positioning unless a physician is available to do so. Therefore, exams of the shoulder in the axial or inferosuperior axial positions or a weight-bearing exam of the acromioclavicular (AC) joints should not be performed. The transthoracic lateral projection of the humerus is safe to perform as it does not require the affected arm to be moved. This position, along with the AP projection with the arm placed "as is," is the preferred method for demonstrating trauma to the proximal humerus.

566. The answer is B. *(Ballinger, 7/e, vol 1, pp 142–143. Bontrager, 3/e, p 163.)* Demonstration of the clavicle may be obtained with the patient either erect or recumbent (although erect is generally easier for the patient). The basic positions are the PA/AP and an axial projection. Generally the PA/AP position is obtained with the clavicle placed at the center of the image receptor and the central ray (CR) directed perpendicularly. The image will show some superimposition of the clavicle with the ribs. The axial projection may also be performed PA or AP, with the central ray angled to project the clavicle away from the ribs. When using the PA position, the CR should be angled 25 to 30° caudally, while the AP position requires a 25 to 30° cephalad angle.

567. The answer is D. *(Ballinger, 7/e, vol 1, pp 148–149. Bontrager, 3/e, p 166.)* Demonstration of the scapula in the AP projection requires the affected arm to be abducted to form a 90° angle with the body and the hand supinated. This position will draw the scapula away from the thorax, although not completely. Generally, the erect position is more comfortable for the patient; however, the recumbent supine position is also acceptable. A breathing technique with a long exposure and low milliamperage is desirable for blurring the ribs and providing a clearer view of the scapula.

568. The answer is D. *(Ballinger, 7/e, vol 1, pp 168–169. Bontrager, 3/e, p 187.)* The interphalangeal joints of the foot are demonstrated by the AP (dorsoplantar) projection of the toes. The natural wedge shape of the foot causes a nonparallel relationship between the phalanges and the image receptor when the foot is placed flat on the table. If the central ray is directed perpendicular to the image receptor with the foot in this position, the bones of the toes and forefoot would appear foreshortened. To minimize this distortion and open joint spaces, the forefoot should be raised on a 15° wedge (thin end toward heel), and a perpendicular central ray may then be used. If a wedge is not used, the central ray should be angled 15° toward the heel with the foot flat on the image receptor.

569. The answer is A. *(Ballinger, 7/e, vol 1, p 163. Bontrager, 3/e, p 170.)* The average foot is composed of fourteen phalanges, five metatarsals, and seven tarsal bones. The phalanges make up the five digits (toes): three in the second through fifth toes and two in the great toe. The distal ends of the metatarsals articulate with the five proximal phalanges. The proximal ends of the metatarsals articulate with four of the seven tarsal bones: the three cuneiform bones and the cuboid bone. The remaining tarsal bones articulate with the distal ends of the tibia and fibula to form the ankle joint.

570. The answer is D. *(Ballinger, 7/e, vol 1, p 163. Bontrager, 3/e, p 172.)* The os calcis (calcaneus), one of the seven tarsal bones, is the largest bone of the foot. It is located at the most posterior and inferior aspect of the foot.

571. The answer is D. *(Ballinger, 7/e, vol 1, p 167. Bontrager, 3/e, p 174.)* The bones of the ankle joint include the talus (tarsal bone) and the distal ends of the tibia and fibula. The talus, also known as the astragalus, is situated in the hind foot on top of the os calcis. The lateral malleolus of the fibula and the medial malleolus of the tibia articulate with the lateral and medial surfaces of the talus, respectively. Also included in the makeup of this distal joint is the tibiofibular articulation.

572. The answer is D. *(Ballinger, 7/e, vol 1, p 174.)* The tangential projection of the foot should be used to project the sesamoid bones of the foot free of overlying structures. These sesamoid bones are generally located at the distal end of the first metatarsal. The tangential projection is achieved by placing the patient prone and resting the foot on the toes in a flexed position. The plantar surface of the foot should be perpendicular to the image receptor. The central ray should also be perpendicular to the image receptor and tangential to the plantar surface of the foot.

573. The answer is D. *(Ballinger, 7/e, vol 1, pp 178–179. Bontrager, 3/e, p 192.)* The medial oblique position of the foot demonstrates the bases of the third through fifth metatarsals free of overlapping structures. The part is positioned by flexing the knee and placing the foot with the plantar surface on the image receptor. The leg and foot are then rotated medially so that the bottom of the foot forms a 30° angle with the image receptor. The central ray is directed perpendicular to the image receptor entering at the base of the third metatarsal. The lateral oblique is used to demonstrate the bases of the first and second metatarsals.

574. The answer is D (1, 2, 3). *(Ballinger, 7/e, vol 1, p 183. Bontrager, 3/e, p 193.)* The image of the foot in the lateral position should include the phalanges, metatarsals, tarsals, and the distal ends of the tibia and fibula. The metatarsal bones should be superimposed and the fibula overlapping the posterior aspect of the tibia. This is achieved by ensuring that the plantar surface of the foot is perpendicular to the image receptor. The medial lateral position may be used as an alternative method.

575. The answer is C. *(Ballinger, 7/e, vol 1, pp 186–187. Bontrager, 3/e, p 194.)* The standing or weight-bearing lateral projection of the foot is performed to demonstrate the longitudinal arch of the foot. With the patient standing, the image receptor is positioned vertically along the medial aspect of the foot to be examined. A horizontal x-ray beam is directed to the center of the image receptor at the level of the base of the fifth metatarsal. The patient should stand with weight balanced on both feet. Both feet should be examined in this manner for comparison purposes.

576. The answer is C. *(Ballinger, 7/e, vol 1, p 193. Bontrager, 3/e, p 195.)* Radiography of the os calcis commonly requires two images: the lateral and axial projections. To obtain the axial projection, the patient is supine with the leg extended and the heel placed on the lower half of the image receptor. The foot is held in a fully flexed position by wrapping a strap or length of tape, gauze, or other appropriate material around the foot and having the patient hold the material. This is necessary to minimize the chance of superimposition of the forefoot over the area of interest. The central ray is angled 40° cephalad and enters at the midpoint of the foot at the level of the base of the fifth metatarsal. This projection should demonstrate complete visualization of the os calcis to include its articulation with the talus bone.

577. The answer is A. *(Ballinger, 7/e, vol 1, p 207. Bontrager, 3/e, p 198.)* The correct amount of leg rotation for the oblique position of the ankle depends on which portion of the ankle is of interest. Visualization of the mortise joint requires the leg to be internally rotated between 15 and 20°. This position will usually place the malleoli parallel to the image receptor and sufficiently open the ankle joint space. A steeper oblique angle of 45° internal rotation may be used to open up spaces between the tarsal bones.

578. The answer is B. *(Ballinger, 7/e, vol 1, pp 214–215. Bontrager, 3/e, p 204.)* The anteroposterior position of the knee is obtained by placing the patient in the supine position with the affected leg extended and not rotated. The image receptor should be centered just below the apex of the patella. In order to visualize the joint space, the central ray is angled 5 to 7° cephalad and enters at the apex of the patella. If the radiographic procedure is to specifically demonstrate the distal femur or proximal tibia and fibula, rather than the joint space, the central ray should be perpendicular.

579. The answer is D. *(Ballinger, 7/e, vol 1, pp 214–215. Bontrager, 3/e, p 204.)* When the knee is correctly positioned for the anteroposterior projection (no rotation of the leg), the patella will be seen superimposed over the distal end of the femur. Rotation of the leg will cause the patella to be superimposed over either the lateral or medial aspects of the femur depending on the direction of the rotation. The posterior aspect of the patella articulates with the patellar surface of the femur. The most distal portion of the patella is the apex, which is located just above the joint space of the femur and tibia. No portion of the patella is superimposed over the tibia or fibula.

580. The answer is D (1, 2, 3). *(Ballinger, 7/e, vol 1, p 217. Bontrager, 3/e, p 206.)* The lateral position of the knee should demonstrate the knee in a flexed position with superimposition of the femoral condyles. The amount of flexion of the knee is generally about 20 to 30° except in the case of trauma to the patella, for which the knee should be flexed only slightly, about 10°. The central ray should be angled 5° cephalad in order to minimize the magnification of the medial condyle, which may obscure the joint space. The leg should be placed with the lateral surface closest to the image receptor and the patella perpendicular to the image receptor. This will provide a lateral profile of the patella and demonstrate the space between the patella and the femur.

581. The answer is D. *(Ballinger, 7/e, vol 1, pp 164–165, 214, 220. Bontrager, 3/e, pp 204–205. Weir, p 167.)* The figure demonstrates the lateral (external) oblique projection of the knee. This projection requires the leg to be rotated laterally 45° (foot is everted). As for the AP projection, the central ray is directed at a 5° cephalad angle to enter at the knee joint. This position will project the patella laterally and the proximal tibia superimposed over the proximal fibula. The labeled structures on the image are as follows: (*1*) lateral femoral condyle, (*2*) patella, (*3*) medial femoral condyle, (*4*) lateral tibial condyle, (*6*) tibial spine, and (*7*) medial tibial condyle.

582. The answer is B. *(Ballinger, 7/e, vol 1, pp 224–225. Bontrager, 3/e, p 207.)* The Homblad method of obtaining a posteroanterior axial position of the knee joint may be achieved with the patient upright or on the table on hands and knees. Either way, the patella is placed in contact with the image receptor. The knee is flexed to form a 70° angle between the femur and the image receptor. The central ray is directed through the joint space, perpendicular to the image receptor. This position demonstrates the tibial spine projected through the open intercondyloid fossa, as well as the joint space of the knee. See the diagram below.

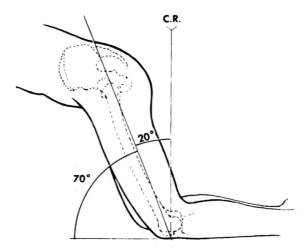

(Reprinted with permission from: Ballinger, PW: *Merrill's Atlas of Radiographic Positions and Radiologic Procedures*, ed 7, vol 1, St. Louis, Mosby–Year Book, p 224.)

583. The answer is D. *(Ballinger, 7/e, vol 1, pp 226. Bontrager, 3/e, p 207.)* The Camp-Coventry method for obtaining a PA axial position of the knee requires the patient to be prone with the lower leg flexed to form a 40 to 50° angle with the image receptor. This is achieved by bending the knee and resting the dorsum of the foot on a supportive surface, which will place the anterior aspect of the knee close to the image receptor. The central ray is then angled to match the angle formed by the lower leg and image receptor (40 to 50°). It is directed caudally and enters at the popliteal depression. See the diagram below.

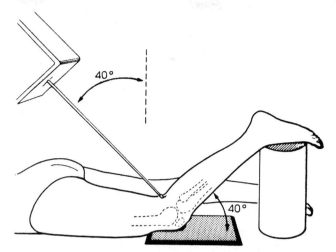

(Reprinted with permission from: Ballinger, PW: *Merrill's Atlas of Radiographic Positions and Radiologic Procedures*, ed 7, vol 1, St. Louis, Mosby–Year Book, p 226.)

584. The answer is C. *(Ballinger, 7/e, vol 1, pp 49, 231–235. Bontrager, 3/e, p 211.)* Many methods have been described for imaging of the knee in the tangential position. Each varies the recommended degree of flexion of the knee and the amount of central ray angle needed. The desired result of each method requires the central ray to be directed tangentially (central ray skims between two body parts) through the patellofemoral joint, thus demonstrating the relationship between the patella and the condyles of the femur. This position is useful in evaluating the patella for subluxation and fractures.

585. The answer is B. *(Ballinger, 7/e, vol 1, pp 165, 231–233. Bontrager, 3/e, pp 212, 213.)* The radiographic image in the figure represents the tangential (axial) projection for demonstration of the patellofemoral joint space, position of the patella, and possible transverse fracture of the patella. This perspective may be obtained with the patient in a variety of positions: recumbent in the prone, supine, or lateral positions or sitting up. For each, the knee is flexed and the image receptor is positioned extending beyond the distal femur. The central ray is directed tangentially through the patellofemoral space. The anatomic structures labeled on this image are as follows: (*1*) patella, (*2*) medial femoral condyle, (*3*) patellofemoral space, and (*4*) lateral femoral condyle.

586. The answer is D. *(Ballinger, 7/e, vol 1, p 242. Bontrager, 3/e, p 219. Pansky, 5/e, p 488.)* The hip bone (also known as the innominate, or os coxae) is composed of three bones: the ilium, ischium, and pubis. Two hip bones make up the pelvis. The pelvic girdle includes the two hip bones and the sacrum and coccyx bones. The pelvic girdle provides for the attachment of the lower limbs to the trunk. Note that the ilium bone of the hip is spelled with an "i" as opposed to the ileum of the small bowel, spelled with an "e."

587. The answer is B. *(Ballinger, 7/e, vol 1, p 246. Bontrager, 3/e, p 229.)* When positioning for the AP projection of the pelvis, the lower legs should be extended and the feet rotated medially (inverted) to overcome the anteversion of the femoral necks. This position will allow visualization of the greater trochanters in profile. Manipulation of the legs should only be performed on patients for whom a hip fracture or other condition that would be complicated by movement is not suspected. If desired, the patient's physician may manipulate the limbs themselves for this projection.

588. The answer is A. *(Ballinger, 7/e, vol 1, pp 244–245. Bontrager, 3/e, p 225.)* An imaginary line extending perpendicular to the midpoint of a line between the ASIS and superior aspect of the symphysis pubis may be used to locate both the femoral head and neck. The femoral head sits approximately 1.5 inches inferior to this intersection point, while the femoral neck is about 2.5 inches inferior. Alignment of the x-ray tube and image receptor to be parallel to this intersecting line will maintain proper perspective of the femoral neck and produce an image with little or no distortion of the hip in the axiolateral position.

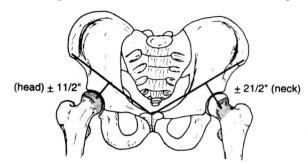

(head) ± 1 1/2"   ± 2 1/2" (neck)

(Reprinted with permission from: Bontrager, KL: *Textbook of Radiographic Positioning and Related Anatomy,* ed 3, St. Louis, Mosby–Year Book, p 225.)

589. The answer is A (1, 2). *(Ballinger, 7/e, vol 1, p 247. Bontrager, 3/e, p 229.)* A properly positioned radiograph of the pelvis should demonstrate the entire pelvis, including all the ilia, sacrum, coccyx and proximal one-fourth to one-third of the femoral shafts. To include such a large area, a 14 by 17 inch image receptor should be used crosswise. The optimum image will demonstrate a nonrotated pelvis as evidenced by symmetric shapes of both the alae of the ilia and opening of the obturator foramen. Proper centering will demonstrate equidistant location of the ilial alae and greater trochanters from the edges of the image, as well as the iliac crest located about 1 inch below the top of the image receptor. Correct inversion of the feet will place the greater trochanters in profile. The smaller patient may include more of the femoral shaft, but this is not necessary for the routine pelvic radiograph.

590. The answer is B. *(Ballinger, 7/e, vol 1, pp 256–261. Bontrager, 3/e, p 228.)* As with any trauma, two views at right angles to each other of the area of interest should be obtained. In the case of a trauma patient who is suspected of having a hip fracture or a patient with a healing hip fracture, the usual manipulation of the injured leg should not be performed by the radiographer. Images of the hip in the AP projection and using a horizontal beam for the lateral projection may be done (preferably on the stretcher) with the leg in its current position. A physician is the only person who should attempt to move a limb in this situation. A team approach should also be used to safely lift the patient for correct placement of the image receptor for the AP projection. Obtaining the horizontal beam lateral projection of the injured hip may also require careful lifting of the patient to build up the affected hip. Axial lateral projections of the hip or pelvis require flexing of the hip and, therefore, are not to be performed on trauma patients.

591. The answer is D. *(Ballinger, 7/e, vol 1, pp 252–255. Bontrager, 3/e, pp 231, 235.)* The position described is that of the modified Cleaves method for the AP axial projection of both femoral necks on the same image for comparison. This method can also be used for similar demonstration of a single hip joint. The original Cleaves method required the patient to be positioned as described, but employed a 40° cephalad tube angle for a more truly axial projection of the hips. The extensive manipulation of the legs for either method prohibits their use for patients with trauma or other restricted movement of the affected hip.

592. The answer is C. *(Ballinger, 7/e, vol 1, pp 260–261. Bontrager, 3/e, p 232.)* The position described in the question is the Danelius-Miller modification of the Lorenz method for axiolateral demonstration of the femoral neck. This is more commonly referred to as a "cross table" or "horizontal beam" lateral projection of the hip. The position should be used for trauma patients as it does not require movement of the affected hip. In this case, the left leg (unaffected) is moved out of the way by flexing and raising it. The long axis of the femoral neck is then identified by imaging a line perpendicular to the midpoint of a line between the ASIS and anterior portion of the symphysis pubis. The image receptor is placed parallel to the femoral neck in a vertical position. The x-ray tube is positioned horizontally and parallel to the femoral neck and image receptor with the central ray entering about 2 inches below the intersection point on the imaginary lines used for location of the femoral neck. The radiographic image should demonstrate the relationship between the femoral head and acetabulum, with the femoral neck superimposed over the greater trochanter and the proximal shaft of the femur.

593. The answer is B. *(Ballinger, 7/e, vol 1, pp 256–257. Bontrager, 3/e, p 230.)* A radiograph of the AP projection of the hip should include demonstration of the hip joint and the proximal third of the femur. If a fixation device or orthopedic appliance is in place, it should be completely included on the image. Portions of the hip bone should be included to adequately demonstrate the acetabulum and femoral head. The correct amount of leg inversion should demonstrate the greater trochanter in profile. The lesser trochanter will be minimally visible.

594. The answer is C. *(Ballinger, 7/e, vol 1, p 280. Bontrager, 3/e, p 244. Gray, 15/e, p 34.)* The human vertebral column is divided into five segments: the cervical, thoracic, lumbar, sacrum, and coccyx. On average, the number of bones in each segment are 7, 12, 5, 5, and 4, respectively. The bones of the cervical, thoracic, and lumbar regions are truly separate bones and form the most movable part of the spine; thus, these regions are referred to as the *true spine*. The sacrum and coccyx segments do not function independently and generally fuse together to form one sacrum and one coccyx, in later life. For this reason, these last two sections are referred to as the *false spine*. Some anatomy references count the sacrum and coccyx as one vertebra each, making the total count 26 vertebrae.

595. The answer is C (1, 3). *(Ballinger, 7/e, vol 1, p 281. Bontrager, 3/e, p 245.)* There are two types of curvatures associated with the spinal column: the lordotic (convex anteriorly) and kyphotic (concave anteriorly) curves. The cervical and lumbar regions of the spine are normally lordotic and the thoracic and sacral/coccyx regions are kyphotic. The kyphotic curvature is also referred to as a primary curve since it develops in utero. However, the lordotic curve is formed as the spine accommodates the weight of the head (cervical) and the body (lumbar) as the child grows. Thus the lordotic curve is considered a secondary curve. A third type of curve, scoliosis, is a side-to-side displacement of the thoracic and lumbar segments. The degree of curvature may be very subtle to extremely accentuated. The latter may become a source of interference for thoracic or abdominal structures.

596. The answer is C. *(Ballinger, 7/e, vol 1, p 281. Bontrager, 3/e, p 246.)* The "typical" components of the vertebra refer to those structures that may be found on vertebra in any section of the spinal column (cervical, thoracic, and so on). In general, each vertebra may be divided into two sections, a *body* and a *vertebral arch*. The body, or anterior portion, is a mass of bone. The formation of the vertebral arch arises from the posterior aspect of the body (with the exception of C1, which has no body). The arch is formed by two pedicles (anteriorly) and two laminae (posteriorly). Also arising from the arch are two transverse processes, two superior and two inferior articular facets (all formed by the junction of the pedicle and lamina), and one spinous process (at the junction of the laminae). Structures specific to a segment of the vertebral column include the transverse foramen, found only on the cervical vertebrae, and the rib facets, found only on the thoracic vertebrae (T1–10).

597. The answer is C. *(Ballinger, 7/e, vol 3, p 98. Pansky, 5/e, p 216.)* The spinal cord begins at the brainstem and continues to the lower level of L1 or upper part of L2. From that point on, the individual nerve roots, referred to as the *cauda equina*, continue to their respective intervertebral or sacral foramen. The meningeal covering of the brain also continues with the spinal cord to include the cauda equina.

598. The answer is A. *(Ballinger, 7/e, vol 1, p 289. Bontrager, 3/e, p 252. Pansky, 5/e, p 564.)* The majority of the joints within the vertebral column are gliding joints of the *diarthrotic* type. These include the zygapophyseal joints of the vertebral arch, the atlantooccipital joint, the atlantoepistrophic joint, costovertebral joints, and costotransverse joints. The articulations between vertebral bodies and disks and the sacroiliac joints are of the cartilaginous *amphiarthrotic* type, which permit only slight movement. Hinge and saddle joints are also diarthrotic types of joints, but are not found in the vertebral column.

599. The answer is A. *(Ballinger, 7/e, vol 1, p 282. Pansky, 5/e, p 204.)* The atlantoepistrophic joint is formed between the first and second cervical vertebrae. Specifically, it is formed by the dens (odontoid) of the axis (C2) projecting superiorly through the ring of the atlas (C1). The actual point of articulation occurs between the anterior surface of the dens and the posterior surface of the anterior arch of C1. This union provides a pivot and allows for rotation of the head.

600. The answer is D. *(Ballinger, 7/e, vol 1, pp 364–366. Ballinger, 3/e, p 272.)* The *costotransverse* joint is one of two articulations between the rib and the vertebral column; the second is the *costovertebral* joint. The costotransverse joint is formed by the articulation between the tubercle and neck of the rib with the rib facet on the transverse process of the thoracic vertebra. The costovertebral joint is formed by the articulation between the head of the rib and the demifacet of two vertebral bodies. Demifacets are located on the inferior and superior aspects of the posterior vertebral bodies of T2 through T9. The first thoracic vertebra has a full-size superior facet for the first rib and an inferior demifacet that joins with the superior demifacet of T2 for the second rib. The tenth through twelfth vertebral bodies have full rib facets on the superior vertebral body and no inferior facets. Anteriorly, the ribs connect with the sternum via costochondral unions.

601. The answer is D. *(Ballinger, 7/e, vol 1, p 287. Bontrager, 3/e, p 250.)* The orientation of the lumbar intervertebral foramina forms a 90° plane with the midsagittal plane of the body. This alignment indicates that visualization of these structures will be achieved by imaging the lumbar spine with the patient in the lateral position. Since this relationship is the same for the thoracic intervertebral foramina, their presence will also be best demonstrated by the lateral position of the thoracic spine. On the other hand, the cervical intervertebral foramina are located at a 45° angle with the midsagittal plane and are also projected at a 15° inferior angle. Therefore, visualization of these structures requires an oblique position with a compensatory tube angle of 15° (caudal for prone positioning; cephalad for supine positioning).

602. The answer is D. *(Ballinger, 7/e, vol 1, p 300. Bontrager, 3/e, p 287.)* The AP projection of the cervical spine is performed with the patient in the erect (sitting or standing) or recumbent anteroposterior position. The midsagittal plane should be aligned with the middle of the table and the shoulders on the same plane to avoid rotation. The neck is extended to place an imaginary line between the occlusal plane and the mastoid tips perpendicular to the table. This will minimize the effect of the mandible's being superimposed over the upper cervical vertebrae. The central ray is directed at a 15 to 20° cephalad angle and enters at the lower point of the thyroid cartilage (about C5). This tube angle will open the disk spaces between the vertebrae and further project the mandible away from the area of interest. Optimum visualization of C3–T1 should be possible. The open mouth method of the AP projection is generally also performed to demonstrate C1–2.

603. The answer is C. *(Ballinger, 7/e, vol 1, p 292. Bontrager, 3/e, p 288.)* When positioning the patient for an open mouth AP projection of C1–2, the radiographer must attempt to avoid superimposition of the teeth or back of the head over the area of interest. The optimum amount of anatomy demonstrated will be achieved by aligning the lower edge of the upper incisors with the back of the skull as located by the mastoid tips. Once this plane has been placed perpendicular to the image receptor, patients are asked to open their mouth as wide as possible by moving only their lower jaw. The radiographer should immobilize the head to maintain the position desired. The central ray is directed perpendicularly through the middle of the open mouth. If patients are able to remove their upper teeth, the alignment between the maxillary alveolar process and the mastoid tip will provide even less obstruction of the area of interest.

604. The answer is A. *(Ballinger, 7/e, vol 1, p 292. Bontrager, 3/e, p 288.)* The AP projection of the cervical spine demonstrates C3–T1; therefore, the open mouth method is performed to demonstrate C1–2 in the AP projection. This position requires the plane between the lower edge of the upper incisors and the mastoid tips to be perpendicular to the image receptor. The patient opens the mouth by moving only the lower jaw to maintain proper positioning. The central ray is directed *perpendicularly* through the center of the open mouth.

605. The answer is D. *(Ballinger, 7/e, vol 1, p 300. Bontrager, 3/e, p 287.)* The AP projection of the cervical spine demonstrates the bodies of C3 through T1. The open mouth AP projection should be included to demonstrate C1–2 and thereby provide complete visualization of the cervical spine. The central ray is directed 15 to 20° cephalad, entering at the lower edge of the thyroid cartilage, for the AP projection.

606. The answer is B. *(Ballinger, 7/e, vol 1, pp 302–303. Bontrager, 3/e, p 289.)* The lateral projection of the cervical spine may be performed with the patient erect (standing or sitting) or recumbent. If the patient has a history of trauma, the recumbent supine position with a horizontal x-ray beam should be employed. Ideally, it is most effective if the patient is erect, as this will improve the ability to depress the shoulder. This is important in ensuring demonstration of the entire cervical region. If the recumbent lateral position is used, it may be necessary to include a lateral of the cervicothoracic region using the "swimmer's" method. However, even this position is better achieved with the patient erect or supine using a horizontal beam. Because of the OID created by the shoulders, a long SID should be used to compensate for the magnification effect and to improve recorded detail. A 72 inch SID is commonly used. The central ray is directed perpendicular to the image receptor and enters the cervical spine at the level of C4 (upper edge of thyroid cartilage).

607. The answer is B. *(Ballinger, 7/e, vol 1, pp 308–309. Bontrager, 3/e, p 290.)* The oblique projection of the cervical spine is used to demonstrate the intervertebral foramina. These foramina are formed by the vertebral notches located below and sometimes above the pedicles of each cervical vertebra. These openings allow the passage of nerves from the spinal cord. Each vertebra has two such openings, one on the right and one on the left. These intervertebral foramina are located on a plane that forms a 45° angle with the midsagittal plane, thus requiring the body to be rotated 45° for imaging of them. Both oblique projections must be performed to demonstrate the right and left foramina. The oblique position may be obtained in either the anterior or posterior position. The tube angle and side demonstrated will be determined by which position is used. For *anterior obliques* (RAO or LAO), the central ray is directed at a 15 to 20° angle caudad, and the *side closest* to the image receptor will be best demonstrated. For the *posterior obliques* (RPO or LPO), the central ray is directed 15 to 20° cephalad, and the intervertebral foramina *furthest* from the image receptor will be demonstrated. For this question, the right anterior oblique position will best demonstrate the right intervertebral foramina. The spinous process is demonstrated by the lateral cervical spine position. The vertebral foramen is not demonstrated by any means.

608. The answer is A. *(Ballinger, 7/e, vol 1, pp 308–309. Bontrager, 3/e, p 290.)* The oblique position is used to demonstrate the intervertebral foramina of the cervical spine. This position may be obtained with the patient either prone or supine (erect or recumbent); however, the position selected will determine the tube angle used and whether the left or right intervertebral foramina are demonstrated. Anterior obliques require the central ray to be directed 15 to 20° caudad and will demonstrate the side closest to the image receptor. Posterior obliques require a 15 to 20° cephalad tube angle and will demonstrate the intervertebral foramina furthest from the image receptor. For this question, either the RPO or LAO position may be used to demonstrate the left intervertebral foramina.

609. The answer is B. *(Ballinger, 7/e, vol 1, pp 336–337, 339. Bontrager, 3/e, pp 250, 263.)* The intervertebral foramina of the lumbar spine form a 90° angle with the midsagittal plane of the body. The lateral position will place these structures superimposed over each other and visible on the same radiograph. Commonly, the left lateral position is used unless there is specific complaint on the right side or other indication for a right lateral position. However, only the joints on L1–4 will be open and round. The Kovacs method for demonstration of the L5–S1 intervertebral foramina requires the body to be rotated 30° forward from lateral and the use of a 15 to 30° caudad tube angle with the patient in the prone oblique position.

610. The answer is D. *(Ballinger, 7/e. vol 1, pp 339, 340–343. Bontrager, 3/e, p 262.)* The oblique position of the lumbar spine will best demonstrate the zygapophyseal joints. The zygapophyseal joints form a 45° angle with the midsagittal plane of the body, thus requiring a 45° body rotation for their demonstration. Both sides must be radiographed in order to demonstrate these joints. The *anterior oblique position* of the lumbar spine will demonstrate the zygapophyseal joints *furthest* from the image receptor and the *posterior oblique position* will demonstrate the *side closest* to the image receptor. The lumbar spinous processes and intervertebral foramina are demonstrated by the lateral position. The vertebral foramen is not visible by any position.

611. The answer is D. *(Ballinger, 7/e, vol 1, pp 285, 327–329. Bontrager, 3/e, pp 273, 286.)* The zygapophyseal joints of the thoracic spine form a 70° angle with the midsagittal plane of the body. To demonstrate these joints, both oblique positions must be radiographed. The body is rotated to place the midsagittal plane at a 70° angle with the image receptor. Either the anterior or posterior oblique position may be used. The central ray is directed perpendicular to the image receptor and enters at the level of T7. The *posterior* *oblique position* (RPO or LPO) will demonstrate the zygapophyseal *joints furthest* from the image receptor, while the *anterior oblique position* (RAO or LAO) will demonstrate the *side closest* to the image receptor.

612. The answer is B.   *(Ballinger, 7/e, vol 1, pp 285, 324–326. Bontrager, 3/e, pp 273, 285.)*   The intervertebral foramina of the thoracic spine form a 90° angle with the midsagittal plane of the body. When placed in the lateral position, these foramina will lie superimposed over each other and appear open and round on the radiograph. This projection may be performed with the patient in the erect or recumbent lateral position. The central ray is directed perpendicularly and enters at the level of T7.

613. The answer is D.   *(Ballinger, 7/e, vol 1, p 325. Bontrager, 3/e, p 285.)*   A breathing technique may be applied when radiographing the thoracic spine in the lateral position. This is done by using a long exposure time at a reduced milliamperage and allowing the patient to breathe quietly during the exposure. The effect will be blurring of the lung markings and ribs for better visualization of the thoracic vertebrae.

614. The answer is B.   *(Ballinger, 7/e, vol 1, p 281. Bontrager, 3/e, p 247. Gray, 15/e, pp 224–225. Pansky, 5/e, p 206.)*   The intervertebral disks are found between the vertebral bodies from C2 to the sacrum. The disks join the vertebrae together and form slightly movable (amphiarthrodial) joints that assist in the overall flexibility of the spinal column. They also act to absorb shock received by the spinal column as a result of any vigorous activity of the body. The composition of the disks themselves is twofold. The outermost portion consists of concentric rings of fibrous cartilage and is referred to as the *annulus fibrosus*. The center of the disk contains a matrix of soft, semigelatinous, highly elastic material referred to as the *nucleus pulposus*. The semirigid nature of the disks allows them to flatten out and return to their natural shape with movement of the vertebral column. The disk composite adheres to the inferior and superior surfaces of two adjacent vertebral bodies whose surfaces are covered by hyaline cartilage.

615. The answer is C.   *(Ballinger, 7/e, vol 1, p 281. Bontrager, 3/e, p 247. Gray, 15/e, pp 224–225.)*   The annulus fibrosus forms the exterior portion of the intervertebral disks, providing some structure for the containment of the soft, pulpy material in the center of the disk. It exists in the form of concentric rings and is composed of fibrous tissue at its outermost layer and fibrocartilaginous tissue in its inner rings. The makeup of the vertebral bodies consists of dense, compact bone tissue on the exterior and less dense, cancellous bone tissue filled with marrow on the interior.

616. The answer is C.   *(Ballinger, 7/e, vol 1, pp 350–351. Bontrager, 3/e, p 259.)*   The AP projection of the sacrum requires the patient to be placed in the supine position with the midsagittal plane of the body centered to the midline of the image receptor. The transverse plane of the shoulders and pelvis should be parallel with the table top to avoid rotation of the part. A small support under the knees will alleviate strain on the lower back and help maintain position. The central ray must be angled cephalad to compensate for the curve of the sacrum. Typically, a tube angle of 15° is satisfactory; however, the more pronounced curve of the female pelvis may require an angle of 20°. The central ray enters midway between the symphysis pubis and the ASIS. The PA projection may be obtained with the patient prone and using a 15° caudad angle on the tube. This position is advantageous in reducing the gonadal dose for female patients, but will cause an increase in OID that will vary with the thickness of the patient's pelvis.

617. The answer is D.   *(Ballinger, 7/e, vol 1, p 281. Bontrager, 3/e. p 247. Gray, 15/e, pp 224–225. Pansky, 5/e, p 206.)*   The intervertebral disk is composed of two parts, the *annulus fibrosus* and the *nucleus pulposus*. The inner core of the disk is the nucleus pulposus, which is a matrix of soft, highly elastic material. As a whole, the disk is capable of flattening out and then returning to its natural shape as required by the various movements of the spinal column. Cancellous bone is found in the inner portion of the vertebral body.

618. The answer is C.   *(Ballinger, 7/e, vol 1, pp 350–351. Bontrager, 3/e, p 257.)*   The AP projection of the coccyx is obtained by placing the patient in the supine position with the midsagittal plane centered to the midline of the image receptor. Adjust the shoulders and hips to eliminate rotation of the pelvis. Some form of support placed under the patient's knees will help maintain the correct position. The central ray is directed caudad at an angle of 10°. It should enter 2 inches superior to the symphysis pubis. An increased tube angle may be needed for the pelvis with a more prominent curvature. As with the AP projection of the sacrum, this view may be obtained in the prone position for the reduced gonadal dose, but at the price of a larger OID.

619. The answer is D. *(Ballinger, 7/e, vol 1, p 333. Bontrager, 3/e, p 261.)* The AP projection of the lumbar spine is obtained by placing the patient in the supine position with the midsagittal plane centered to the middle of the image receptor. To reduce the lordotic curve and thereby open the intervertebral joint spaces, the patient's knees should be flexed and the feet placed flat on the table. The central ray should be directed perpendicularly, entering at about 1 inch superior to the iliac crest. The radiograph should demonstrate the vertebral bodies, intervertebral joint spaces, spinous and transverse processes, laminae, and sacroiliac joints. The lumbar intervertebral foramina are best demonstrated with the patient in the lateral position and an oblique (45°) position is required to visualize the zygapophyseal joints.

620. The answer is D. *(Ballinger, 7/e, vol 1, p 330. Bontrager, 3/e, p 261.)* The PA projection of the lumbar spine has some advantages over the AP projection. The primary advantage is the significant reduction in dose delivered to the gonads, particularly in the female patient. Gonadal shielding is easily achieved with the male patient for the exam; however, the location of the ovaries in the pelvis makes it difficult to adequately shield the female patient without obscuring important anatomic structures. Placing the patient in the prone position prevents the ovaries from receiving the entrance dose. Further, the prone position is commonly more comfortable for patients with injury to their back or who are severely emaciated. This position also places the vertebral bodies parallel with the central ray and opens up the intervertebral joint spaces. However, the prone position does create an OID that will vary with the size of the patient. The magnification may be compensated for by using a longer SID, if possible. Selection of AP or PA projection must be considered within the context of each department's procedural policies.

621. The answer is C. *(Ballinger, 7/e, vol 1, pp 244, 289. Bontrager, 3/e, p 249.)* The union of the vertebral column with the pelvis occurs at the two sacroiliac joints. The specific points of articulation are the articular surface of the sacrum, located on each side of the sacral body as part of the sacral ala (lateral masses), and the articular surface on the medial aspect of the ilial ala. These joints are classified as the diarthrodial (gliding) type; however, their position is such that only slight movement is possible, causing some to consider the sacroiliac joints to be amphiarthrodial. The joint itself exists on an oblique plane with the midsagittal plane of the body and thus requires the body to be rotated in order to visualize the open joint space. The lumbosacral joint is the union of the lumbar and sacral regions of the vertebral column via the L5–S1 intervertebral joint and the zygapophyseal joints between L5 and S1. The ileocecal junction is the union between the third segment of the small bowel (ileum) with the first segment of the large bowel (cecum).

622. The answer is C. *(Ballinger, 7/e, vol 1, pp 344–345. Bontrager, 3/e, pp 240–241.)* The position describes the posterior (supine) oblique position for demonstrating the sacroiliac (SI) joints. Specifically, the posterior oblique position will demonstrate the joint furthest from the image receptor, as indicated by the centering of the beam medial to the right ASIS with the patient in the LPO position. An axial projection of the SI joints may be obtained using the same position and angling the central ray about 20° cephalad, entering 1 inch medial and 1.5 inches distal to the right ASIS. The anterior (prone) oblique position may also be used, but will demonstrate the SI joint closest to the image receptor. If the PA axial projection is preferred, the tube angle must be directed caudad, entering 1 inch lateral to the last spinous process (L5); the central ray should exit at the ASIS.

623. The answer is D. *(Ballinger, 7/e, vol 1, pp 358–359. Bontrager, 3/e, p 266.)* The scoliosis survey is performed to determine or evaluate the existence of a lateral curvature to the thoracic or lumbar spine. The radiographic images most commonly obtained are the AP or PA projections, erect or recumbent, and the erect lateral projection. In order to include as much of the thoracic and lumbar spines as possible when using a 14 by 17 inch image receptor, the cassette should be placed lengthwise with its bottom about 1 inch below the iliac crest.

624. The answer is B (2, 3). *(Ballinger, 7/e, vol 1, pp 358–359. Bontrager, 3/e, p 266.)* Scoliosis studies are most frequently performed on young patients and require periodic followup exams. These issues have raised concern for added radiation protection measures during this exam. Recommended methods for reducing patient dose include the use of high kilovoltage (80 to 100), the PA rather than the AP position, shielding of specific areas, and compensating filters. The use of high kilovoltage lowers the required milliampere-seconds and has the further advantage of producing a longer gray scale for a more even density range over the thoracic and lumbar regions of the spine. The PA projection prevents radiosensitive structures such as the thyroid, breasts, and gonads from receiving the entrance dose. Since the PA projection will create an OID, departmental policy as to whether this is acceptable must be considered. Either contact or shadow shielding devices will reduce exposure to the breasts and gonads, as will compensating filters.

625. The answer is C. *(Ballinger, 7/e, vol 1, p 38. Bontrager, 3/e, p 253.)*   Bony landmarks are useful for localizing anatomic structures and for positioning of the average size and shape body. The ASIS is on the same level as the first to second sacral segments and is thus useful in positioning for the SI joints and other pelvic structures. The landmark for L3 is the lowest margin of the ribs. The iliac crest locates the region of L4–5 and the symphysis pubis is used to locate the coccyx.

626. The answer is D. *(Ballinger, 7/e, vol 1, pp 364–365. Bontrager, 3/e, p 299.)*   The bony thorax encases and protects the lungs, heart, and great vessels of the mediastinum. The ribs form a type of cage that encircles these organs, and extends from the thoracic spine posteriorly to the sternum anteriorly. In total, there are 12 pairs of ribs (24 in total). Of these, the first 7 pairs (14 ribs) are considered to be *true* ribs because they each attach to costal cartilage and then attach to the 7 facets on each side of the sternum. In comparison, the remaining 5 pairs of ribs (10 ribs) are termed *false* ribs because they do not attach to the sternum, but rather to the costal cartilage of the seventh rib. Two pairs of the false ribs, the eleventh and twelfth, do not attach to any structure anteriorly. For this reason, they are termed *floating* ribs.

627. The answer is D (1, 2, 4). *(Ballinger, 7/e, vol 1, p 365. Bontrager, 3/e, p 298.)*   The bony thorax is composed of the 12 pairs of ribs, the sternum, and the twelve thoracic vertebrae. The head and tubercle of the ribs attach posteriorly to the thoracic vertebrae via two joints, the costotransverse and the costovertebral joints. Both of these are the diarthrodial (gliding) type joints. The shafts of the ribs project anteriorly and inferiorly, forming the lateral aspects of the thorax. The anterior portion of the ribs, referred to as the *sternal end*, attaches to costal cartilage, which then attaches to the sternum, with the exception of the last two pairs of ribs, which do not attach to the costal cartilage. The clavicles are part of the upper extremity and the shoulder girdle, which, with the scapula, attach the upper extremity to the trunk of the body.

628. The answer is B. *(Ballinger, 7/e, vol 1, pp 364–365. Bontrager, 3/e, p 298.)*   Of the 24 ribs (12 pairs), the first 7 ribs on each side of the thorax (14 ribs) attach directly to the manubrium and body of the sternum via costal cartilage. Six of the remaining ribs (3 on each side) connect to the costal cartilage of the seventh rib. The last 2 pairs of ribs (floating ribs) do not have anterior connections with any structure.

629. The answer is C. *(Ballinger, 7/e, vol 1, pp 364–365. Bontrager, 3/e, p 298.)*   The sternum is a relatively small, thin, flat bone that lies in the center of the anterior bony thorax. It has three distinct parts. The uppermost part is the *manubrium*, the middle part is the *body* or *gladiolus*, and the distal portion is the *xiphoid process*. As a whole, the sternum functions as an attachment point for the two clavicles (the sternoclavicular joints) at the manubrium and the direct attachment point for 7 of the 12 pairs of ribs. The first rib attaches to the manubrium, the second rib to the junction of the manubrium and body, and the remaining 5 pairs to the body of the sternum. At its most superior point, there is a depression in the manubrium referred to as the *jugular* (or *suprasternal*) *notch*; it serves as a landmark for the disk space of T2–3.

630. The answer is A. *(Ballinger, 7/e, vol 1, pp 384–387. Bontrager, 3/e, pp 303–304.)*   The best procedure for imaging of the ribs depends on the specific ribs of interest. As with any radiographic exam, the side of interest should be placed closest to the image receptor. Therefore, anterior ribs should be imaged in the prone position and posterior ribs in the supine. The point at which the patient should suspend breathing is also of concern owing to the relationship of the diaphragm to the ribs. To best visualize the upper ribs (those above the diaphragm), the patient should be instructed to suspend respiration on full inspiration; to visualize the lower ribs (below the diaphragm), suspension should be on full expiration. These exams may also be performed with the patient in the recumbent or upright (if able) positions. It is specifically recommended that the patient be erect for imaging of the upper ribs to get the diaphragm as low as possible. The recumbent position will assist in elevating the diaphragm for imaging of the lower ribs.

631. The answer is A. *(Ballinger, 7/e, vol 1, pp 388–389. Bontrager, 3/e, pp 310–311.)* The oblique position is used to demonstrate the axillary portion of the ribs. One side at a time is imaged. If the supine position is used, the side closest to the image receptor will be demonstrated. This question described the LPO position; thus the axillary portion of the left ribs will be recorded. The centering point and breathing instructions are consistent with the requirements for imaging the upper ribs (first through tenth). In order to image the left side using the prone oblique position, the RAO position would be used, demonstrating the side furthest from the image receptor. In order to image the lower ribs in the oblique position, the central ray should enter at the level of the tenth thoracic vertebra and respiration should be suspended on full expiration.

632. The answer is B. *(Ballinger, 7/e, vol 1, pp 390–391. Bontrager, 3/e, pp 310–311.)* The routine positions most commonly performed for imaging the ribs are the AP or PA and oblique. The AP and posterior oblique positions are specific for the posterior ribs. The PA and anterior oblique positions should be used for the anterior ribs. The prone oblique position requires the side of interest to be furthest from the image receptor. Therefore, the best oblique position for the right anterior ribs would be the LAO.

633. The answer is B (2, 3). *(Ballinger, 7/e, vol 1, p 368. Bontrager, 3/e, p 302.)* The sternum is a midline structure overlying the mediastinum and thoracic vertebrae. For this reason, a true frontal view (AP or PA) is not useful. In its place, a prone oblique (RAO) with only 15 to 20° of body rotation is recommended, along with a left lateral. The slight rotation should be just enough to move the sternum off the spine. The RAO position is used to project the sternum into the shadow of the heart, thereby providing a more homogeneous background to image the sternum against. The left lateral position may be performed with the patient erect, recumbent on the left side, or supine with a horizontal x-ray beam.

634. The answer is A. *(Ballinger, 7/e, vol 1, p 372. Bontrager, 3/e, p 307.)* Radiography of the lateral sternum requires the patient to suspend respiration during the exposure. In order to improve image contrast, it is recommended that the patient stop breathing on full inspiration. The use of a breathing technique is acceptable for the RAO as it will blur lung markings. However, the sternum does not overlap the lungs when imaged in the lateral position.

635. The answer is B. *(Ballinger, 7/e, vol 1, p 398. Bontrager, 3/e, pp 56–57.)* The visceral structures of the thorax include the lungs and the mediastinum. The two lungs are located on either side of the mediastinum and are considered the organs of respiration. The right lung is divided into three lobes: upper, middle, and lower. The left lung is divided into two lobes: upper and lower. The most superior portion of the lungs is termed the *apex.* The base of the lungs is located at the most inferior point of the thorax, resting on the diaphragm. The mediastinum is the area between the lungs and contains the heart, great blood vessels, trachea, and esophagus. The hilum refers to the mediastinal aspect of the lungs that provides access for the bronchus, vasculature, and nerves to and from the lungs.

636. The answer is D (3, 2, 4, 1). *(Ballinger, 7/e, vol 1, pp 397–398. Bontrager, 3/e, p 54.)* The *bronchial* structures of the respiratory system provide a passageway for the exchange of gases by the body. These "air tubes" begin at the pharynx via the nose or mouth. Air is conveyed through the pharynx and larynx and into the trachea. The trachea terminates through its bifurcation into the right and left main stem bronchi. These bronchi enter the lungs at the thoracic hilum and further subdivide into bronchioles of decreasingly smaller sizes, which project to all aspects of the lungs. At the most distal end of the terminal bronchioles are the alveolar air sacs, which are the site of the exchange of gases.

637. The answer is B. *(Ballinger, 7/e, vol 1, pp 410–413. Bontrager, 3/e, pp 60–61.)*   The optimum PA chest radiograph should demonstrate the lungs and heart without rotation, with inclusion of all aspects of the lung fields. The technique selection should provide proper penetration and exposure of the part to produce the desired image contrast. The ideal chest image is obtained with the patient in the erect position. To minimize magnification of the heart shadow, a 72 inch SID is most commonly employed. The patient is positioned with hands on hips and the shoulders depressed and rotated forward to pull the scapulae away from the lungs. The clavicle should be demonstrated as slightly lower than the apex of the lungs. To visualize as much of the lungs as possible, the patient should be directed to stop breathing on the *second* full inspiration (breathe in, let it out, and breathe in again). A long scale of contrast is preferred for chest radiography and is obtained by use of high kilovoltage with an appropriate imaging system. Women with large breasts overhanging their lungs may need to be instructed to draw them to the sides in order to clearly demonstrate the lower lobes and costophrenic angles of the lungs.

638. The answer is B. *(Ballinger, 7/e, vol 1, pp 412, 415, 416. Bontrager, 3/e, p 63.)*   Routine imaging of the chest in the PA, lateral, and oblique positions requires the central ray to be directed perpendicular to the midpoint of the thorax at the level of the seventh thoracic vertebra. This method provides complete inclusion of the thoracic cavity from just above the apex of the lungs to just below the costophrenic angles on the average patient. Exact location of T7 is recommended by measuring 7 inches down from the vertebra prominens (spinous process of C7) on females and 8 inches down on males. The fifth thoracic vertebra is located just below the sternal angle, making it too high for chest radiography. The ninth thoracic vertebra is just above the xiphoid, both of which are too low as centering points.

639. The answer is C. *(Ballinger, 7/e, vol 1, pp 430–432. Bontrager, 3/e, pp 70–71. Carlton, pp 539–541.)*   In order to demonstrate air-fluid levels, a horizontal x-ray beam must be used. This will place the central ray parallel to the fluid level. If the beam is perpendicular or even at a 45° angle, fluid may be noted, but no specific level will be discernible. For those patients who cannot stand up, a decubitus position and a horizontal x-ray beam may be required. Air will rise and be found in the uppermost portion of the cavity, while fluid will settle in the lowermost portion. It is often requested of the radiographer to demonstrate the presence of an air-fluid level or even free air in the thorax. The lateral decubitus position, with the patient's dependent side built up, is commonly used for this reason. This procedure must include the side down to demonstrate fluid and the side up to demonstrate free air. The supine position will not demonstrate air-fluid levels or free air. The semierect position with the beam horizontal to the floor will demonstrate air-fluid level better than if the tube were positioned parallel to the image receptor.

640. The answer is B. *(Ballinger, 7/e, vol 1, pp 430–431. Bontrager, 3/e, p 71.)*   The term *decubitus* means "to lie down." More specific to radiography, this term further infers the use of a horizontal beam. The patient may be radiographed in a variety of decubitus positions that are further defined by terms used to indicate the dependent side (body surface patient is resting on). This question is describing the left lateral decubitus position. The right lateral decubitus position would have the patient lying on his or her right side. The ventral and dorsal decubitus positions are synonymous with supine and prone positions, respectively. Chest radiography with the patient in the decubitus position is often performed to demonstrate the presence of free air or air-fluid levels in the thorax.

641. The answer is C. *(Ballinger, 7/e, vol 1, pp 416–417. Bontrager, 3/e, p 73.)*   Chest radiography in the oblique position is best performed from the prone position (anterior obliques); however, posterior obliques may be used on the patient with limitations. For a routine study, the patient is rotated 45° from the PA position. The thorax is centered to the midpoint of the film at the level of T7. Anterior obliques will best demonstrate the side furthest from the image receptor. (RAO shows left lung; LAO shows right lung.) As with PA and lateral chest images, respiration should be suspended after the second full inspiration.

642. The answer is D. *(Ballinger, 7/e, vol 1, pp 422–423. Bontrager, 3/e, p 72.)*   The lordotic position was described in this question. It is performed to demonstrate the apices of the lungs free from superimposition of the clavicles, which are projected above the apices. For patients with limitations, this position may be modified by placing the patient in the supine position and angling the central ray 15 to 20° cephalad.

643. The answer is B. *(Ballinger, 7/e, vol 1, p 461. Carroll, 5/e, pp 162–163.)* Foreign bodies made of radiolucent materials, such as wood, glass, or plastic, require short-scale contrast imaging to enhance their presence against the soft tissues of the body. Low kilovoltage should be used to increase the differential absorption between such foreign bodies and the surrounding tissues. High kilovoltage would lengthen the gray scale, lowering contrast and the ability to visualize such structures. Compression is useful in reducing the thickness of tissue to be penetrated; however, when trying to localize a foreign body, it is important to image the area as is. Compression may displace the position of the foreign body, making it difficult to extract. A direct exposure system provides excellent detail resolution, but the amount of exposure required negates its use. A modern extremity imaging system will demonstrate the detail with an acceptably low dose. Direct exposure systems may be used to image excised tissue, such as biopsy specimens, as the dose to that material is not of consequence.

644. The answer is B. *(Ballinger, vol 1, p 256. Bontrager, 3/e, p 349. Pansky, 5/e, p 136.)* The orbit is made up of portions of seven bones—three cranial and four facial bones. The cranial bones include the *frontal* bone, which forms a major part of the orbital roof, and portions of the *sphenoid* and *ethmoid* bones, which contribute to the medial wall of the orbital cavity. Part of the sphenoid bone also forms the posterior, lateral wall of the orbit.

645. The answer is A. *(Ballinger, 7/e, vol 1, pp 214–216. Bontrager, 3/e, p 342.)* There are fourteen facial bones, of which only two are not paired. These are the *mandible* and *vomer*. The maxilla, palatine, and inferior nasal conchae are all midline structures. The maxillae are solidly united just below the nasal septum and form the anterior portion of the upper face and contribute to the makeup of the oral, nasal, and orbital cavities. The palatine are located behind the palatine process of the maxillae and form the hard palate. The inferior nasal conchae project from the lateral walls of the nasal cavity and with the superior and middle conchae from the ethmoid bone form divisions within the nasal cavity.

646. The answer is D. *(Ballinger, 7/e, vol 2, pp 364–365. Bontrager, 3/e, pp 390–391.)* The average human skull contains four sets of paranasal sinuses. These are named for the bones in which they are situated. Three sets are contained within cranial bones: the *frontal*, *sphenoid*, and *ethmoid*. The fourth set is contained within the maxillary facial bones.

647. The answer is D. *(Ballinger, 7/e, vol 2, pp 222–223. Bontrager, 3/e, p 329.)* The steps for correctly imaging the skull in the lateral position are as follows. The patient may be either erect or recumbent. By placing the patient's body in the anterior oblique position, the head can turn sufficiently to place the midsagittal plane parallel to and the side of interest closest to the image receptor (RAO position for the right side of the skull and LAO for the left side). The head is then adjusted to place the infraorbitomeatal line (IOML) parallel to the transverse plane of the image receptor (this also aligns the IOML perpendicular to the front edge of the image receptor) and the interpupillary line perpendicular to the image receptor. The central ray is directed perpendicular to the skull, entering 2 inches superior to the EAM. The image should demonstrate superimposition of the orbital roofs, temporomandibular joints, EAMs, mastoids, and mandibular rami. The sella turcica should be seen in profile.

648. The answer is B. *(Ballinger, 7/e, vol 2, pp 226–227. Bontrager, 3/e, p 330.)* The PA projection of the skull requires the *orbitomeatal line* to be placed at right angles to the image receptor. This position places the frontal bone closest to the image receptor. To avoid rotation, the midsagittal plane is also perpendicular to the image receptor. The central ray may be directed perpendicularly or at a caudad angle of 15 to 30°, depending on the anatomic structures of interest. For either method, the central ray exits at the nasion. When no tube angle is used, the image will demonstrate the petrous portion of the temporal bone superimposed over the orbits. As the caudad tube angle is applied and increased, the petrous bones will be projected into the lower portion of the orbits or below.

649. The answer is C. *(Ballinger, 7/e, vol 2, pp 230–232. Bontrager, 3/e, pp 328, 332.)*   The AP axial projection of the skull will demonstrate the dorsum sella within the foramen magnum of the occipital bone. The patient is positioned with the back of the skull closest to the image receptor. The head is adjusted to place the midsagittal plane and orbitomeatal line (OML) at right angles to the image receptor. The central ray is directed caudally at an angle of 30° to exit at the foramen magnum. If the infraorbitomeatal line (IOML) must be used instead of the OML, the tube angle must be increased to 37°. For some patients, the PA axial projection may need to be performed. This method requires the central ray to be angled 25° cephalad, exiting about 1.5 inches above the nasion. The full basal projection of the skull (either the submentovertical or verticosubmental projections) will demonstrate the odontoid tip through the foramen magnum. The PA projection will not demonstrate the foramen magnum, even with the excessive tube angle.

650. The answer is B. *(Ballinger, 7/e, vol 2, pp 217, 230–231. Bontrager, 3/e, p 328.)*   The AP axial projection of the skull best demonstrates the occipital bone. The AP position with sufficient flexion of the head (OML perpendicular to image receptor) places the occipital bone closest to the image receptor. The 30° caudal tube angle projects the anterior portion of the skull below and away from the occipital bone for improved visualization. For those patients with difficulty in achieving the desired level of flexion of the head, the IOML may be used instead. There is a 7° difference between the IOML and OML, which is accommodated for by increasing the tube angle to 37° caudad. Flexion of the head to place the glabellomeatal line at right angles with the image receptor is even more difficult than the OML flexion, especially in the AP position. If this line were used, less tube angle would be needed as there is a difference of about 8° between the OML and glabellomeatal line. The use of the acanthiomeatal line would raise the facial bones in respect to the occipital bone, requiring an even greater caudad tube angle to displace them. The use of a cephalad tube angle would project the facial structures upward, as in the AP acanthioparietal projection (reverse Waters).

651. The answer is D. *(Ballinger, 7/e, vol 2, pp 238–239. Bontrager, 3/e, pp 332.)*   The placement of the IOML parallel and the midsagittal plane perpendicular to the plane of the image receptor is required in positioning for the submentovertical projection of the skull. To achieve this, the patient must hyperextend the neck, moving the head backward. Sufficient support must be given to assist the patient with this position. The central ray is directed perpendicular to the IOML, midway between the mandibular angles. This projection provides a full basal projection of the skull. The PA and AP axial projections require the OML and midsagittal plane to be perpendicular to the image receptor. The lateral projection requires the interpupillary line to be perpendicular, the midsagittal plane to be parallel, and the head to be adjusted to place the IOML parallel with the transverse plane of the image receptor.

652. The answer is A. *(Ballinger, 7/e, vol 2, pp 230–231, 316–317. Bontrager, 3/e, pp 328, 371, 378.)*   The position described is that of the AP axial projection of the cranium, which will best demonstrate the occipital bone. This position places the occipital bone closest to the image receptor. The caudal tube angle will project the anterior skull structures below the occipital bone. Portions of the parietal bones are visible on this image, but they are best demonstrated by the lateral position. The AP axial projection is also used to demonstrate the zygomatic arches and mandibular rami. However, when these structures are of interest, the exit point of the central ray is lower than that described for the cranium. This also allows a specific entrance point to be identified. In order to place the zygomatic arches in the center of the field of view, the central ray should enter at a point 1 inch superior to the glabella. The image receptor is aligned to the central ray. When imaging the mandibular rami, the PA axial projection is preferred to minimize distance between the image receptor and rami. However, the AP version may need to be performed on trauma patients.

653. The answer is C. *(Ballinger, 7/e, vol 2, pp 238–239, 310. Bontrager, 3/e, pp 332, 369.)*   The submentovertical position of the skull may be used to demonstrate the zygomatic arches in profile. To do so, the skull is positioned with the IOML parallel and the midsagittal plane perpendicular to the image receptor. The central ray is directed perpendicular to the IOML and enters midway between the mandibular angles along a coronal plane that passes just posterior to the outer canthus. A reduction in exposure factors will be necessary to avoid overexposure of the zygomatic arches as commonly occurs when using this position to image the skull.

654. The answer is B. *(Ballinger, 7/e, vol 2, pp 296, 374. Bontrager, 3/e, pp 359, 402.)* The position described is that of the *parietoacanthial* projection of the skull. This position is used for examination of the facial bones and sinuses. When imaging the facial bones, this projection best demonstrates the orbits, zygoma, and maxillae. Of the paranasal sinuses, the maxillary sinuses are best seen by this projection. A distorted image of the frontal and ethmoid sinuses is also visible. It is preferred to have the patient erect for this projection, when the patient is able, in order to visualize air-fluid levels. To project the maxillary sinuses clear of other skull structures, the mentomeatal line is adjusted to be perpendicular to the image receptor. This position is also achieved by adjusting the orbitomeatal line 37° to the plane of the image receptor.

655. The answer is D. *(Ballinger, 7/e, vol 2, p 374. Bontrager, 3/e, p 402.)* The parietoacanthial projection demonstrates the maxillary sinuses by projecting the petrous ridges below the sinuses. This is achieved by extending the head and resting the chin on the image receptor. Proper extension is determined by aligning the orbitomeatal line to a 37° angle with the image receptor. This also places the mentomeatal line perpendicular to the image receptor. Placement of either the orbitomeatal or acanthiomeatal lines perpendicular to the image receptor would produce an insufficient amount of extension and the maxillary sinuses would not be cleared of the petrous ridges. Aligning the acanthiomeatal line to form a 37° angle with the image receptor would hyperextend the head and cause distortion of the sinuses.

656. The answer is B. *(Ballinger, 7/e, vol 2, p 300. Bontrager, 3/e, p 364.)* The acanthioparietal projection is the reverse of the parietoacanthial projection and is commonly performed on trauma patients. It may also be used with nontrauma patients who are unable to assume the prone position. For this situation, the head should be adjusted as for the prone version with the mentomeatal line, midsagittal plane, and central ray perpendicular to the image receptor. However, a patient in a neck brace or otherwise identified as having trauma to the cervical spine must not have the neck manipulated. The desired projection may be obtained by aligning the central ray parallel to the mentomeatal line (about 55° to the OML), entering at the acanthion. This method will demonstrate the maxillary sinuses free from superimposition by the petrous ridges. A modification of this projection is commonly used for imaging the facial bones. A reduced tube angle of approximately 30° cephalad directed toward the IOML (37° to the OML) will project the petrous ridges into the maxillary sinuses, but provide clear demonstration of the upper facial bones.

657. The answer is D. *(Ballinger, 7/e, vol 2, pp 308–309. Bontrager, 3/e, p 368.)* The superoinferior projection of the nasal bones provides an axial view of the nasal bones for evaluation of medial or lateral deviation from the normal position. The image receptor may be placed extending from below the mandibular symphysis (extraoral) or held between the teeth (intraoral). In order to demonstrate as much of the nasal bones as possible, the glabelloalveolar line must be aligned perpendicular to the image receptor. Improper adjustment of this line will cause superimposition of the nasal bones by either the frontal bone or the alveolar ridge of the maxillae.

658. The answer is B. *(Ballinger, 7/e, vol 2, pp 314–315, 320–321. Bontrager, 3/e, p 372.)* The tangential projection of a single zygomatic arch is achieved with the patient in either the supine or prone, erect or recumbent, position. The head is adjusted to place the infraorbitomeatal line as parallel as possible to the image receptor. The head is then rotated to place the midsagittal plane at a 15° angle with the image receptor. The direction in which the head is turned is determined by whether the AP or PA position is used. The *supine* position (AP) demonstrates the side *closest* to the image receptor, while the *prone* position demonstrates the *side away* (May method). For both options, the central ray is directed perpendicular to the IOML, "skimming" the zygomatic arch.

659. The answer is C. *(Ballinger, 7/e, vol 2, pp 332–337, 344. Bontrager, 3/e, pp 376, 379.)* The PA axial projection will best demonstrate the mandibular rami. This method requires the nose and chin to be placed against the image receptor (acanthiomeatal line perpendicular to image receptor) and the midsagittal plane perpendicular. The central ray is then directed at a 30° cephalad angle, entering midway between the TMJs. This tube angle will project the back of the skull upward to prevent it from being superimposed over the mandibular rami. The mandibular rami may also be demonstrated by placing the OML and the midsagittal plane perpendicular to the image receptor. The central ray is directed either perpendicularly or 20 to 25° cephalad. If the patient is in the supine position, these projections may also be obtained. However, a caudad tube angle would be used. The symphysis of the mandible is imaged by extending the patient's neck so that the inferior aspect of the chin rests on the image receptor. The central ray is angled 40 to 45° in a superoinferior direction toward the chin. The placement of the chin and nose on the image receptor and the central ray perpendicular would best demonstrate the body of the mandible. Positioning the head in the lateral position and directing the central ray 25° cephalad would provide an axiolateral projection of the rami closest to the image receptor.

660. The answer is A.   *(Ballinger, 7/e, vol 2, pp 338–341. Bontrager, 3/e, p 376.)*   The axiolateral projection may be performed with the head in various positions in relation to the image receptor, depending on the specific area of the mandible to be imaged. The patient may be in either the erect or recumbent position. With the head in the true lateral position, the chin extended, and the central ray directed 25° cephalad, the ramus closest to the image receptor will be best demonstrated. This projection should be performed on both sides to demonstrate the right and left rami. To demonstrate the body of the mandible, the head must be rotated about 30° from the lateral position toward the image receptor to place the body of the mandible parallel to the imaging surface. Even more head rotation (about 45°) is required to image the mandibular symphysis with this projection. The central ray angle remains the same. It should be directed just posterior to the mandibular angle for imaging the body and to the center of the symphysis when imaging that area.

661. The answer is D.   *(Ballinger, 7/e, vol 2, pp 348–353. Bontrager, 3/e, pp 383–385.)*   All the positions offered as answers may be used to demonstrate the TMJs. The axiolateral and axiolateral oblique positions require imaging of each TMJ separately. Additionally, two exposures are generally made of each side—one each with the mouth open and closed. The axiolateral places the patient's head in a true lateral position for imaging of the side closest to the image receptor. The central ray enters anterior and superior to the TMJ furthest from the image receptor. The axiolateral oblique position requires the patient's head to be rotated 15° toward the image receptor from the true lateral position. The central ray enters just superior to the TMJ furthest from the image receptor. The AP axial projection places the OML and midsagittal plane perpendicular to the image receptor, and the central ray enters about 3 inches above the nasion.

662. The answer is B.   *(Ballinger, 7/e, vol 2, pp 370–371. Bontrager, 3/e, pp 391, 400.)*   All four sets of paranasal sinuses are visible on a radiograph with the patient in the lateral position (see image below). The *frontal* (1) sinuses are the most superior and anterior set of sinuses. Just inferior to the frontals are the *ethmoid* (3) air cells. The *sphenoid* (2) sinuses are located just posterior to the ethmoid and the *maxillary* (4) just inferior to the ethmoid.

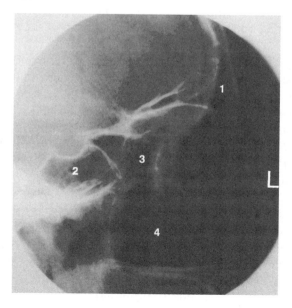

663. The answer is A. *(Ballinger, 7/e, vol 2, pp 364–365. Bontrager, 3/e, pp 390–391.)* The paranasal sinuses are air-filled cavities located within three of the cranial bones (frontal, ethmoid, and sphenoid) and one set of facial bones (maxillary). They begin development during fetal life, but are not completely formed until the late teenage years. The frontal sinuses, located within the vertical plates of the frontal bone, may be single, paired, or absent. The ethmoid sinuses are composed of air cells located in the lateral masses of the ethmoid bone on either side of the perpendicular plate. The sphenoid sinuses are located within the body of the sphenoid bone. The maxillary sinuses are considered to be the largest set and are located within the body of the maxillae.

664. The answer is D. *(Ballinger, 7/e, vol 2, p 370. Bontrager, 3/e, pp 329, 336, 400.)* The lateral position used for radiographing the paranasal sinuses is obtained by positioning the head in the true lateral position. The side of interest is placed closest to the image receptor with the midsagittal plane parallel and the inter-pupillary line perpendicular. Since the most posterior set of sinuses (sphenoid) is located anterior to the EAM, there is no need to include structures posterior to the EAM. The central ray should enter midway between the outer canthus of the eye and the EAM. The entrance point for the lateral cranium is 2 inches superior to the EAM; for the sella turcica it is 3/4 inch anterior and 3/4 inch superior to the EAM.

665. The answer is D. *(Ballinger, 7/e, vol 2, pp 368–369. Bontrager, 3/e, pp 400–401.)* In order to demonstrate air-fluid levels within the paranasal sinuses, the x-ray beam must be horizontal (parallel to the floor), the image receptor placed vertically to intercept the beam, and the patient erect (although with the patient recumbent, levels could still be demonstrated). The use of a tube angle will negate the desired effect; thus it is recommended that no angle be used on the PA axial projection if the image receptor holder can be angled the required 15° to project the petrous ridges below the frontal sinuses. Another important criterion to meet when attempting to demonstrate fluid levels is to allow time for the viscous material within the sinuses to settle out and form levels. This requires the patient to maintain each position for a few minutes before the exposure is made.

666. The answer is D. *(Ballinger, 7/e, vol 2, pp 373–374. Bontrager, 3/e, pp 401.)* The PA axial projection of the paranasal sinuses is used to demonstrate the frontal and anterior ethmoid sinuses. The head is adjusted to place the midsagittal plane and orbitomeatal line perpendicular to the image receptor. The central ray is then angled 15° caudad and centered to exit at the nasion. Since this method employs a tube angle, fluid levels will not be well demonstrated. If the vertical bucky can be angled (as on a head unit), it should be tilted 15° caudally and the central ray directed perpendicularly to exit at the nasion.

667. The answer is C. *(Ballinger, 7/e, vol 2, p 374. Bontrager, 3/e, pp 404.)* The basic parietoacanthial projection primarily demonstrates the maxillary sinuses. This projection will demonstrate the sphenoid sinuses by modifying the positioning routine to have the patient open his or her mouth. The other aspects of the procedure remain the same: OML placed to form a 37° angle (mentomeatal line perpendicular) with image receptor; midsagittal plane and central ray perpendicular and exiting at the acanthion.

668. The answer is B. *(Ballinger, 7/e, vol 2, pp 212–213. Bontrager, 3/e, pp 394–395.)* The eustachian (auditory) tube is located between the middle ear and the nasopharynx. Its function is to equalize the air pressure within the middle ear and the external atmosphere. This short passageway also allows the movement of germs between the nasopharynx and the middle ear, which leads to infections.

669. The answer is A. *(Ballinger, 7/e, vol 2, p 213. Bontrager, 3/e, pp 396–397.)* The semicircular canals, located within the internal ear, are considered to be organs of equilibrium. This structure consists of three enclosed canals configured at right angles to each other. They are referred to as the *superior, lateral,* and *posterior* semicircular canals and are responsible for maintaining balance in all three planes (vertical, horizontal, and transverse). The semicircular canals communicate with the vestibule (another organ of equilibrium) and the cochlea (organ of hearing) of the internal ear. The ossicles and tympanic membrane are organs of hearing located in the middle ear.

670. The answer is B. *(Ballinger, 7/e, vol 2, p 212. Bontrager, 3/e, pp 394–396.)*   The complex components of the ear are housed within the dense bony structure of the petrous portion of the temporal bone. Two temporal bones are included in the formation of the cranium. Each is located on the lateral aspect of the skull, making up a portion of the lateral, inferior wall and floor of the cranium. The temporal bone articulates with the sphenoid, parietal, and occipital cranial bones and the zygoma and mandible facial bones. This dense bone comprises four segments: the squamous, tympanic, petrous, and mastoid portions. The squamous and tympanic portions form the side wall of the skull and the outer aspect of the external auditory meatus, respectively. The petrous portion extends medially and anteriorly, forming a 45° angle with the midsagittal plane in the head with typical shape. The middle and inner auditory canals, containing the organs of hearing, are located in this portion. The mastoid portion extends from the inferoposterior portion of the temporal bone and contains air cells that communicate with the middle ear. The body of the sphenoid is located in the midline of the cranial base and houses the sphenoid sinus. The greater wings of the sphenoid bone project laterally from each side of the body and contribute to the formation of the orbits.

671. The answer is B. *(Ballinger, 7/e, vol 2, pp 392–393. Bontrager, 3/e, p 405.)*   The axiolateral oblique projection (Law method) of imaging the mastoid process originally used a dual angle on the x-ray tube while maintaining the position of the patient's head in a true lateral position. The central ray was directed 15° caudally and 15° anteriorly, entering the skull at a point 2 inches posterior and superior to the EAM. To accommodate the restrictions imposed by grids, the single angle method is frequently employed. This modification requires the patient's head to be rotated 15° toward the table (anteriorly) from the true lateral position. The central ray is then directed 15° caudad, entering 1 inch superior and posterior to the EAM furthest from the image receptor.

672. The answer is A. *(Ballinger, 7/e, vol 2, pp 420–421. Bontrager, 3/e, p 406.)*   The position described will best demonstrate a posterior profile (or anterior oblique) of the petrous portion of the temporal bone. The projection specifically images the internal acoustic canals. The shape of the average skull places the petrous ridge at an angle of 45° with the midsagittal plane. By rotating the head 45°, the long axis of the petrous ridge is placed parallel with the plane of the image receptor. The petrous ridge extends medially from the EAM; thus the centering point is midway between the EAM and outer canthus of the eye. This projection will also demonstrate the mastoid process in profile. The Arcelin method provides an anterior profile of the petrous portion and starts with the patient in the supine position to image the petrous ridge furthest from the image receptor, using a 10° caudad angle on the central ray. The Mayer method requires both the head to be rotated and the central ray to be angled 45° to produce an axioposterior oblique projection of the mastoid. The axiolateral oblique projection of the mastoid process is achieved by rotating the head 15° forward from a true lateral position and angling the central ray 15° caudad.

673. The answer is C. *(Ballinger, 7/e, vol 2, p 389. Bontrager, 3/e, p 405.)*   When preparing the patient for imaging of the mastoids, the radiographer must remove any item that may be in the area of interest, such as earrings or hair pins. Also, the auricles of the ears should be gently folded forward and taped in position to prevent their shadow from overlying the mastoid area. A patient's dentures are usually not of concern when imaging this area and therefore need not be removed. To further improve the quality of radiographic images of the mastoids, it is recommended that a small focal spot and a moderate level of kilovoltage (70 to 80) be used. High kilovoltage will overpenetrate the area and lower image contrast.

674. The answer is D. *(Ballinger, 7/e, vol 2, pp 396–397.)*   The AP tangential projection of the mastoid process is obtained by placing the patient in the supine position, either erect or recumbent. The head is rotated *away from* the side of interest, placing the midsagittal plane at a 55° angle with the image receptor. Flexion of the head is adjusted to place the IOML perpendicular to the image receptor. This position projects the mastoid process away from other bony structures of the skull. The central ray is then directed at a 15° caudal angle, entering at the union of the auricle with the skull and about 1 inch superior to the mastoid tip. If possible, angle the bucky 15° caudally and direct the central ray perpendicularly. This projection may also be obtained from the PA perspective. This method would require the side of interest to be closest to the image receptor. All other positioning factors would be the same.

675. **The answer is A.** *(Ballinger, 7/e, vol 2, pp 406–407, 415, 421. Bontrager, 3/e, pp 406, 409.)* Both petrous ridges are demonstrated on the submentovertex and AP axial projections of the cranium. The submentovertex projection may be positioned just as described for imaging the base of the cranium: IOML parallel and central ray (CR) perpendicular to the image receptor. According to Ballinger, however, the full extension of the head is not necessary when performing this position for demonstration of the petrous ridges. It is recommended to place the *OML* parallel and the CR perpendicular to the image receptor, or to place the supraorbitomeatal line parallel and angle the CR 15° cephalad to project the petrous ridges just posterior to the mandibular condyles. The AP or PA axial projection is positioned just as described for the cranium with the added recommendation of collimating to the petrous/mastoid area of the skull. The posterior profile of the petrous ridge demonstrates only one side, so that each side must be imaged separately.

676. **The answer is C.** *(Ballinger, 7/e, vol 2, pp 258–259. Bontrager, 3/e, p 374.)* The parieto-orbital oblique projection (Rhese method) is performed by placing the patient in the PA position with the midsagittal plane perpendicular to the image receptor. The head is rotated toward the side of interest, so the midsagittal plane forms a 53° angle with the image receptor. The chin is lifted to place the acanthiomeatal line perpendicular to the plane of the image receptor. The central ray is directed at right angles to the bucky at the level of the center of the dependent orbit. This should demonstrate a cross-sectional image of the optic canal projected in the lower outer quadrant of the orbit.

677. **The answer is D.** *(Ballinger, 7/e, vol 2, pp 258–259. Bontrager, 3/e, p 374.)* The parieto-orbital oblique projection for demonstration of the optic canal requires the head to be rotated from the PA position to place the midsagittal plane at a 53° angle with the image receptor. The head is further adjusted to rest on the nose, cheek, and chin with the acanthiomeatal line perpendicular to the image receptor. The central ray is then directed at right angles to the center of the orbit closest to the image receptor to demonstrate the optic canal on that side.

678. **The answer is A.** *(Ballinger, 7/e, vol 2, p 389. Bontrager, 3/e, pp 324, 330, 365, 371, 405.)* The anatomic structures of the skull have very fine details that require special consideration in order to image them properly. Any action to improve recorded detail should be taken. This includes cleaning screens and cassettes prior to use and using detail screens, maximum SID, and a small, undamaged focal spot. Proper immobilization techniques, such as short exposure times and head clamps, are needed. The bony structures of the skull do provide a higher level of contrast than do other areas of the body, but they are also small, thin structures. The kilovoltage range is generally between 60 and 80, depending on which bone is of interest and the desired level of image contrast.

679. **The answer is D.** *(Ballinger, 7/e, vol 2, p 257. Bontrager, 3/e, p 361.)* For a general survey of the cranium in the PA position, the central ray is directed perpendicular to the image receptor, exiting at the nasion. This will project the petrous ridges of the temporal bones within the orbital shadows. Modifications to this projection include various degrees of caudal tube angles to project the petrous ridges downward. An angle of 10 to 15° will demonstrate the petrous ridges in the lower third of the orbits, allowing the superior margin of the orbits to be visualized. A 20 to 25° angle will project the petrous ridges to the inferior margin of the orbits, but not clear of them. The 30° caudad tube angle is recommended to demonstrate the lower margin of the orbital rim clear of the petrous ridges.

680. **The answer is D.** *(Ballinger, 7/e, vol 2, pp 274–276.)* The process of localizing a foreign body within the eye requires careful positioning and exceptional recorded detail to image objects that often have poor radiation absorption. It is recommended that detail screens be used and that they be cleaned prior to the exam to eliminate dust particles, which would cause artifacts on the image. Once the patient is positioned, the head should be immobilized and the patient instructed not to breathe or move the eyes during the exposure. Finally, high-contrast images should be obtained, using low kilovoltage and close collimation to minimize scatter fog.

681. The answer is C. *(Ballinger, 7/e, vol 2, pp 274–277, 298.)* Radiographic images for the localization of a foreign body in the eye will commonly include the *PA axial, lateral,* and *parietoacanthial* projections. The submentovertex projection will not demonstrate the orbital area of the skull. The PA axial projection requires the placement of the patient's midsagittal plane and OML perpendicular to the image receptor and the central ray angled 30° caudad through the center of the orbits. The lateral projection is achieved with the patient in the true lateral position and the perpendicular central ray directed to the outer canthus of the eye. The beam should be tightly collimated to this area. The third common projection is a modified version of the parietoacanthial projection. The head is adjusted to place the OML at a 55° angle with the bucky, rather than the 37° angle recommended for imaging of the maxillary sinuses. This reduces the amount of flexion on the head, causing less distortion of the orbital shadows.

682. The answer is C. *(Ballinger, 7/e, vol 2, pp 26–27. Bontrager, 3/e, p 439.)* The process of imaging the soft tissue of the neck requires the use of low kilovoltage to enhance differential absorption of these low-density structures. With the patient in the lateral position, the central ray is directed at right angles to the neck, anterior to the cervical spine, and at the level of the laryngeal prominence (C6). The chin should be elevated slightly to avoid superimposition of the mandible over the neck. The shoulders should be depressed to improve visualization of the neck. The structures that will be best demonstrated include the larynx, trachea, and esophagus.

683. The answer is A. *(Ballinger, 7/e, vol 2, p 47. Bontrager, 3/e, p 487.)* The radiographic examination of the gallbladder is termed *cholecystography.* The term "chole" refers to *bile* and "cysto" refers to *bladder.* The gallbladder receives bile from the liver for storage and concentration until it is required in the digestion process. Upon stimulation, the bile is excreted into the duodenum via the common bile duct. *Cholangiographic* procedures image the biliary ducts only. The radiographic examination of both the gallbladder and biliary ducts is termed *cholecystocholangiography.* The blood vessels of the liver are imaged in the abdominal angiographic procedure known as *hepatoangiography.*

684. The answer is D. *(Ballinger, 7/e, vol 2, p 47. Bontrager, 3/e, p 495. Laudicina, pp 86–89.)* The biliary system may be opacified by the administration of contrast media in one of several methods. *Oral* administration is most commonly used for radiographic examination of the gallbladder (oral cholecystography). The patient ingests the contrast media several hours before the exam is scheduled, thus allowing time for the material to be picked up by the liver and concentrated in the gallbladder. The *intravenous* injection of the contrast medium will opacify the biliary ducts and eventually the gallbladder. This method requires a water-soluble, iodine-based material to be injected into the blood stream. The liver will extract it and then excrete it into the biliary ducts. The *direct* method of introduction of contrast media may be achieved through various means: percutaneous transhepatic, direct stick during operative procedures, T tube in postoperative devices, and endoscopic retrograde cholangiopancreatography (ERCP). The percutaneous transhepatic method requires the passage of a long, thin needle through the liver to directly puncture one of the biliary ducts to which the contrast is then injected. During surgery, the exposed biliary ducts may be injected with contrast media. Following surgery, a T-tube device is left in place to allow drainage. Contrast media may be directly injected into this tube for further evaluation of the bile ducts. ERCP requires the passage of an endoscopic tube down the esophagus, through the stomach, and into the duodenum. A fine cannula is then passed into the main pancreatic duct and contrast media injected to demonstrate the pancreatic and biliary ducts.

685. The answer is D. *(Ballinger, 7/e, vol 1, p 40. Bontrager, 3/e, p 486.)* The *asthenic* body type is characterized as being very thin with little or no muscle tone. Loosely attached organs, such as the stomach and gallbladder, will assume a low position close to the midline. This body type is commonly seen in elderly and emaciated patients. The gallbladder will be projected close to the spine and may even drop into the pelvic region on upright images. In order to effectively move the gallbladder away from the spine, the asthenic patient must be rotated to a greater degree (up to 40°) than the hypersthenic patient for the LAO projection. The radiographer will also need to center lower on the abdomen than with the huskier body type referred to as *hypersthenic.*

686. The answer is D. *(Ballinger, 7/e, vol 2, pp 75, 93. Bontrager, 3/e, p 494. Gray, 15/e, pp 947–948. Pansky, 5/e, pp 412–413.)* The endoscopic retrograde cholangiopancreatography (ERCP) procedure includes the introduction of contrast media into the biliary system via the hepaticopancreatic ampulla (union of common bile and pancreatic ducts). This procedure requires a fiberoptic endoscope to be passed down the esophagus, through the stomach, and into the duodenal loop. Utilizing the optics of the endoscope, the sphincter of Oddi (opening into the duodenum for the ampulla) is located and a small catheter introduced into the ampulla of Vater (hepaticopancreatic ampulla). Contrast media is then injected into the biliary ducts. An alternate method of opacifying the biliary ducts is via the transhepatic cholangiogram. During this procedure, the radiologist passes a long, thin needle across the liver until it intercepts a bile duct (as identified by the injection of small amounts of contrast media). The oral cholecystogram provides opacification of the gallbladder following the ingestion of contrast media in tablet or crystal form 10 to 12 h prior to the exam. The hypertonic duodenogram is an infrequently performed examination of the duodenum for the evaluation of the pancreas.

687. The answer is C. *(Ballinger, 7/e, vol 2, pp 53, 64. Bontrager, 3/e, p 500. Laudicina, pp 84, 95.)* In order to radiographically demonstrate the layering of calculi in the gallbladder, the patient must be in the right lateral decubitus or erect position. The right lateral decubitus position allows the gallbladder to fall away from the spine and iliac bone. A horizontal beam is used to demonstrate the calculi either above the bile within the gallbladder, if the stones are lighter than the bile, or in the most dependent part of the gallbladder, if they are heavy. The anterior oblique position is commonly used in obtaining preliminary radiographs of the opacifed gallbladder; specifically, the LAO will move the gallbladder away from the spine. The RAO and left lateral decubitus positions would cause the gallbladder to be superimposed over the spine.

688. The answer is B. *(Ballinger, 7/e, vol 2, p 53. Bontrager, 3/e, p 496. Laudicina, p 84.)* Preliminary radiographs are obtained as part of an oral cholecystogram to determine the level of contrast media in the gallbladder. A poorly functioning or nonfunctioning gallbladder may not be sufficiently opacified following a single dose of contrast tablets. The preliminary images are usually a PA of the abdomen and LAO of the right upper quadrant. The PA position places the gallbladder closer to the image receptor than does the AP position. For this reason the anterior oblique is preferred to the posterior oblique position. Placing the left side closest to the image receptor allows the gallbladder to move away from the spine, avoiding superimposition.

689. The answer is D. *(Ballinger, 7/e, vol 2, p 99. Bontrager, 3/e, pp 434, 442.)* The recumbent right lateral position of the stomach will best demonstrate the C loop of the duodenum in profile and the right retrogastric space. This position is more commonly performed than the left lateral, which best demonstrates the left retrogastric space. The RAO is the more commonly included projection in the oblique position. It will best demonstrate the pylorus, pyloric canal, and duodenal bulb, as well as the stomach and duodenum. The LPO projection is also frequently performed. This image will best demonstrate the fundus filled with barium and the air-filled duodenal bulb on profile.

690. The answer is B. *(Ballinger, 7/e, vol 1, p 38; vol 2, pp 94, 97. Bontrager, 3/e, pp 440–441.)* The PA and RAO projections are commonly obtained as part of an upper gastrointestinal (UGI) series. The central ray should be located at the level of L2 for these projections. This centering point is approximately midway between the xiphoid tip and umbilicus. The xiphoid tip is the landmark for T10, making it too high for these projections. The fourth lumbar vertebra is on a level with the umbilicus, making it too low for imaging of the stomach. The second sacral segment is too deep into the pelvis to be considered when positioning for radiographs of the stomach.

691. The answer is A. *(Ballinger, 7/e, vol 2, p 98. Bontrager, 3/e, p 443.)* The position described would satisfy the requirements for obtaining an LPO projection of the stomach. This is a frequently obtained radiograph for a UGI series. The posterior oblique position causes the stomach to move upward and away from the midline of the abdomen, thus requiring the high centering point (L1), whereas the anterior positions (PA or oblique) use L2 as the centering point. The LAO of the gallbladder is achieved with the patient in the prone position, as is the RAO of the esophagus. The centering point for the gallbladder is close to that of the stomach (about L2); however, for the esophagus it is much higher (about T6). The RPO of the colon is centered at the level of the iliac crest.

692. The answer is C. *(Ballinger, 7/e, vol 2, p 100. Bontrager, 3/e, p 444. Laudicina, p 98.)* The Trendelenburg position places the patient's head lower than the pelvis and legs. As part of the UGI series, this position may be used to demonstrate the presence of a hiatal hernia or esophageal reflux (which may or may not be associated with a hiatal hernia). In addition to having the patient's head low, the radiologist may instruct the patient to exert pressure on the abdomen in the form of a Valsalva maneuver. This added pressure may force a small hiatal hernia to present itself. The Trendelenburg position will also improve filling of the fundus of the stomach with barium, but will not improve visualization of the pyloric region.

693. The answer is A. *(Ballinger, 7/e, vol 2, p 92. Bontrager, 3/e, p 425. Ehrlich, 4/e, p 206.)* The advantage of the double contrast GI series (either upper or lower) is the ability to better visualize the mucosa of the GI tract and demonstrate smaller lesions within the mucosa. The technique requires the administration of thick barium and air (either directly introduced or through the use of air-producing tablets or crystals). In comparison with the single contrast GI or BE series, the double contrast exam may be more difficult for the patient to tolerate. The double contrast exam involves the administration of a small amount of thick barium to coat the mucosa, followed by the introduction of air to distend the stomach or colon. The patient is then instructed to roll around (supine to prone to supine) once or twice to completely coat the cavity. In the case of the UGI series, the double contrast exam requires the patient to be able to swallow the gas-producing material and avoid losing the air by suppressing the urge to belch. Generally, an increased number of radiographs are obtained to image the air-barium combination in both the UGI and BE series.

694. The answer is B. *(Ballinger, 7/e, vol 2, p 105. Bontrager, 3/e, p 470.)* The *terminal ileum* (TI) is the most distal portion of the small bowel. It opens into the colon at the cecum. This opening is protected by the *ileocecal valve*. The filling of this area with barium is commonly considered to be indicative of the completion of a small bowel series. When the barium reaches this point, the radiologist may fluoroscope the TI and obtain spot film images. The TI region may also be seen during the barium enema, when the barium refluxes into the small bowel. However, imaging of the TI is mostly associated with the small bowel series.

695. The answer is C. *(Ballinger, 7/e, vol 2, p 111. Bontrager, 3/e, p 460.)* Proper cleansing of the colon is important in order to obtain an accurate diagnosis. Retained fecal material will appear as an area of radiolucency, simulating a filling defect or polypoid lesion. Polyps are nodules of tissue attached to the mucosa and projecting into the colon. Since they are solid, they do not fill with barium and may move about their attachment from the force of the barium flow. Diverticula are outpouchings, or sacs, along the external aspect of the colon due to weakened areas in the mucosa. These sacs will fill with barium and thus have a radiopaque appearance. Colonic ulcers are small areas of erosion in the internal surface of the mucosa. These areas will also fill with barium, presenting a radiopaque appearance. Inflammation of the colon will appear as an irregular or ragged colonic wall radiographically; advanced conditions will manifest a lack of the normal haustral segments.

696. The answer is D. *(Ballinger, 7/e, vol 2, p 120. Bontrager, 3/e, p 480.)* The projection described in the question is the *PA axial* of the abdomen. This projection will specifically demonstrate the rectosigmoid region of the colon. The tube angle is required to elongate and open the colonic loops of this region. The reverse of this projection (AP axial) requires a 35° cephalad tube angle with the central ray entering about 2 inches inferior to the ASIS. The oblique positions are used to open the flexures. The anterior oblique position images the flexure closest to the image receptor, while the posterior oblique images the flexure furthest from the image receptor. The cecum is best demonstrated on the straight PA or AP projection of the colon.

697. The answer is B. *(Ballinger, 7/e, vol 2, pp 113, 115–116. Bontrager, 3/e, p 469.)* Although the specific routine for overhead radiography following the fluoroscopic portion of a barium enema is determined by each imaging facility, the inclusion of both lateral decubitus projections is most often limited to the double contrast study. This projection uses a horizontal beam for the demonstration of air-fluid levels, which are generally not present in the single contrast barium enema exam. However, both single and double contrast exams may require a PA or AP, both obliques (PA or AP), axial rectosigmoid, and lateral rectum projections.

698. The answer is B. *(Ballinger, 7/e, vol 1, p 38; vol 2, p 123. Bontrager, 3/e, p 473.)* The lateral rectum projection is obtained by positioning the patient on either the left (more common) or right side with the knees flexed and hips and shoulders superimposed. The central ray is directed perpendicular to the mid-axillary plane and enters at the level of the ASIS. This projection should include the entire rectum, anus and rectosigmoid region. Centering at the level of the iliac crest would cause the centering to be too high, while the symphysis pubis would be too low.

699. The answer is C. *(Ballinger, 7/e, vol 2, p 133. Ehrlich, 4/e, pp 203–205.)* Patients who have a colostomy have undergone a surgical procedure in which the colon was resected and the new terminal end of the colon was brought through the abdominal wall via a surgically created opening (stoma). A bag is placed on the external abdomen over the stoma to collect fecal material. A radiographic exam of the colon may be performed by retrograde administration of barium through the stoma. A smaller quantity of barium will be needed and care must be taken with the delicate tissues of the stoma. On occasion, it may be necessary to radiographically examine the unused section of colon via the rectum. A very small amount of barium may be needed to opacify this section, depending on the amount of colon remaining. Thorough cleansing of the distal colonic segment will also be required following the barium enema, since there is no natural ability for this structure to eliminate the barium.

700. The answer is D. *(Ballinger, 7/e, vol 2, pp 138–139. Bontrager, 3/e, p 507. Pansky, 5/e, p 422.)* The *hilum* of an organ is defined as a depression where the blood vessels, nerves, and other structures enter or exit the organ. This area is located on the medial border of the kidney. In addition to the vasculature and nerves entering and exiting, this area also includes the proximal portion of the ureter.

701. The answer is B. *(Ballinger, 7/e, vol 2, p 138. Bontrager, 3/e, p 505.)* The kidneys are located on each side of the vertebral column between T12 and L3 (on average), in the posterior aspect of the abdominal cavity. They lie at an oblique angle, following the curve of the spine, with the lower pole of the kidney anterior to the upper pole. The right kidney may be slightly lower than the left due to the area filled by the liver. Their medial-to-lateral dimension is parallel with the coronal plane. The upper poles are medial to the lower poles. See frontal (*A*) and lateral (*B*) diagrams below.

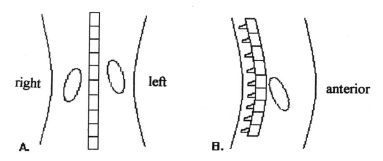

702. The answer is D. *(Ballinger, 7/e, vol 2, p 139. Bontrager, 3/e, p 507. Gray, 15/e, p 987. Pansky, 5/e, p 422.)* The medullary portion of the kidney contains the distal collecting tubules of the nephron and the macroscopic structures of the collecting system. These structures begin with the grouping of several fine tubules termed the *renal pyramids*, which receive the filtrate from the nephron. The pyramids empty into the *minor calyces*, which join together to form *major calyces* (two to three per kidney). The distal portion of the major calyces form the *renal pelvis* to which the ureter is joined.

703. The answer is B. *(Laudicina, pp 111–114.)*   Congenital conditions are present from birth. They may be life-threatening or asymptomatic. The condition described in the question is *horseshoe kidneys.* The lower poles of the two kidneys usually are located at the midline section of the body. This condition also results in the kidneys being turned, causing the renal pelves to be superimposed by the calcyes. Renal function is not usually affected. Polycystic kidneys present with numerous cysts within the renal parenchyma and may be highly life-threatening. Ectopic kidneys are those not in the usual location within the abdomen. Agenesis is complete absence of one or both kidneys.

704. The answer is B. *(Laudicina, pp 125–126.)*   *Benign prostatic hypertrophy* (BPH) is the enlargement of the prostate gland that commonly occurs in men over 50 years of age. The prostate gland is located inferior to the bladder and anterior to the rectum and surrounds the male urethra prior to its entrance into the penis. Although the prostate is best evaluated by physical exam, its presence can be demonstrated by intravenous urography (IVU). The enlarged gland causes pressure on the bladder, influencing how well it fills. The term *urinary tract infection* encompasses the kidneys, ureters, and bladder. A *bifid collecting system* is a congenital condition in which two collecting systems are present in a single kidney. This can be a unilateral or bilateral condition and has no negative effect on renal function. *Renal failure* is the inability of a kidney to function in its filtering capacity. This is frequently the end result of chronic renal disease.

705. The answer is A. *(Ballinger, 7/e, vol 2, p 151. Bontrager, 3/e, p 523.)*   The radiograph most frequently obtained as a scout film for an IVU exam is the routine AP abdominal or kidney, ureter, and bladder (KUB) projection. The patient must be flat, minimizing structural rotation, with the knees elevated to reduce the lordotic curve. Prior to this, the patient should have been instructed to empty the bladder. Retained urine in the bladder will dilute the contrast media and contribute to patient discomfort from a very full bladder later in the exam. This image is used to evaluate the patient for adequate preparation and to provide an overview of the structures of the abdomen. It also allows the radiographer to assess exposure factors and positioning of the patient. The AP position has the further advantage of minimizing the OID of the kidneys since they are posteriorly located organs. A prone projection may be requested as part of the exam, but not as the routine scout image. Some routines may also require a second scout image, collimated to the kidneys, which may be with or without tomography. The kidneys will move with the changing position of the diaphragm during respiration; therefore, all the images of the IVU series should be obtained during the same phase of respiration. Obtaining images on expiration will position the diaphragm at its most elevated level, allowing better visualization of the abdominal structures.

706. The answer is D (1, 2, 3). *(Ballinger, 7/e, vol 2, pp 150, 153. Bontrager, 3/e, pp 515–516, 527.)*   All three of the techniques listed as answer options will promote retention of contrast media in the renal pelves and proximal ureters. The compression band encompasses a balloon-type device that is positioned over the distal ureters with its uppermost border at the level of the iliac crest. These balloons are held in place with a radiolucent plate and velcro band wrapped about the patient's abdomen. When inflated, this device will exert pressure on the lower ureters, restricting the flow of contrast media out of the kidney. Some contraindications exist regarding the use of the compression band—specifically, when there is an increased potential of injury or rupture. The use of the prone position improves the filling of the renal pelvis because of its more dependent position as a result of the oblique angle at which the kidneys lie in the abdomen. The Trendelenburg position places the patient's head approximately 15° lower than the body and lower extremities. This position will retard the flow of contrast media out of the kidney and allow improved filling of the pelvicoureteral junction.

707. The answer is B. *(Ballinger, 7/e, vol 2, p 153. Bontrager, 3/e, p 525.)*   The oblique projection of the urinary system is commonly performed using the posterior (supine) oblique position. The patient's whole body is rotated about 30°. This method will demonstrate the kidney furthest from the image receptor in profile, but free of superimposition over the spine. However, this ureter will be projected over the spine. The ureter of the side closest to the image receptor will be visualized clear of the spine. The use of a steeper oblique angle will superimpose the kidneys and spine.

708. The answer is A. *(Ballinger, 7/e, vol 2, pp 164, 166–167, 170. Bontrager, 3/e, p 529.)* The position described by this question would best demonstrate the ureterovesical junction on the side furthest from the image receptor. Since the patient was rotated to the right, the left side will be visualized. The ureterovesical junction is located on the posterolateral aspect of the bladder (right and left sides). The steep oblique rotation is required to visualize this area. When imaging the bladder in the oblique position, both oblique projections are obtained. The radiographic imaging of the male urethra is obtained with the patient in a less steep oblique position (30°), usually an RPO. This will allow visualization of the entire male urethra without superimposition. The female urethra is imaged in AP position with the central ray centered at the symphysis pubis. A caudal tube angle of 5 to 15° may be employed to project the symphysis pubis away from the bladder. Additionally, a 30° RPO may also be obtained. When imaging the bladder or urethra in the oblique position, the legs should remain extended in order to prevent superimposition by the leg of the side elevated from the table.

709. The answer is A. *(Ballinger, 7/e, vol 2, p 151. Bontrager, 3/e, pp 505, 526.)* The kidney is encapsulated in a layer of adipose tissue and loosely attached within the retroperitoneal space by fascia. As a result there is normally some movement of the kidneys with the motion of the diaphragm during breathing, and they are in a slightly lower position in the abdomen when in the upright position compared to the recumbent position. In some cases, the kidneys may drop more than normal. This is referred to as *nephroptosis*. Therefore, the upright abdominal projection may be requested to evaluate this motility aspect of the kidneys. Since the suprarenal glands are not part of the urinary system, they are not imaged during the IVU exam. In order to visualize the vesicoureteral junction, either an oblique projection or Trendelenburg position is recommended. The oblique or lateral projection may be requested to demonstrate the area behind the kidney and in front of the vertebrae.

710. The answer is B. *(Ballinger, 7/e, vol 2, p 152. Bontrager, 3/e, pp 517, 524.)* The nephrotomogram provides sectional images of the kidneys and proximal ureters. These images must be obtained while the concentration of contrast media is at a peak level in the kidneys, which is during the first 5 min following injection of the contrast media. Most often, two to three images at various section levels are obtained at this time. The use of compression devices or techniques will help keep the contrast media in the calyces and renal pelvis longer, but the patient's condition may not allow these techniques.

711. The answer is B. *(Ballinger, 7/e, vol 2, p 141. Bontrager, 3/e, pp 91, 523.)* The structures of the abdomen are very similar in composition and result in low differential absorption of the x-ray beam. However, there are several anatomic structures that are generally visible because of the size or thickness differences relative to adjacent structures or because of the presence of high (calcifications) or low (fat, air) density structures around or within the organs of the abdomen. Thus, the structures identifiable without contrast media are the kidneys, psoas muscles, liver, full bladder, and bony structures of the pelvis and spine, as well as the stomach and colon if air is present within them and the gallbladder if it contains stones. Small structures that are invisible without contrast media include the ureters, urethra, calyces, renal pelvis, empty bladder, and GI tract when air is not present within it.

712. The answer is B. *(Ballinger, 7/e, vol 3, p 45. Bontrager, 3/e, p 524.)* The nephrogram should include the kidneys and proximal ureters, which are located in the upper half of the abdomen. An 11 by 14 or 10 by 12 inch image receptor, used crosswise, will be of sufficient size for this area. The patient is positioned supine with the midsagittal plane of the body centered to the midline of the image receptor. The perpendicular central ray enters midway between the xiphoid process and the iliac crest.

713. The answer is D. *(Ballinger, 7/e, vol 2, p 154. Bontrager, 3/e, pp 505, 526.)* The term *nephroptosis* indicates a dropping or forward displacement of the kidneys from their usual position. This condition is confirmed by the lower than usual position of the kidneys as demonstrated on an abdominal radiograph obtained in the upright position. It is normal for the kidneys to drop a bit (1 to 2 inches); however, for some persons the kidneys will drop to the level of the iliac crest or lower. This can cause urinary tract problems as a result of kinking of the ureters.

714. The answer is A. *(Ballinger, 7/e, vol 2, pp 184–185.)* The hysterosalpingogram is a retrograde study of the uterus and uterine tubes following opacification. It is considered to be retrograde because the contrast media is injected against the normal flow of material within this system (e.g., ova, menses). The contrast media is administered via a cannula placed at the cervix of the uterus. No contrast media should be injected into the vagina. Water-soluble iodinated contrast media is used because of its ability to be readily reabsorbed by the body. Generally a single radiographic projection is required to image these structures—an AP of the pelvis, centered at its midpoint, 2 inches above the symphysis pubis to ensure complete inclusion of the uterine tubes.

715. The answer is C. *(Ballinger, 7/e, vol 2, p 183. Ehrlich, 4/e, p 215.)* Hysterosalpingography is the radiographic exam of the uterus and uterine tubes following opacification. This exam uses a water-soluble iodine compound that can be readily absorbed by the body. The normal structure of the uterus and uterine tubes is open-ended. When contrast media is injected into the uterus, it flows into the uterine tubes and then spills into the peritoneum if the tubes are not blocked. This prevents the use of barium, which, if spilled into the peritoneum, would not be reabsorbed and would most likely become a hardened clump. Iodized oils were used prior to water-soluble iodine, but they too were poorly absorbed and thus remained in the peritoneum. Air was used to outline the female pelvic structures in an exam referred to as a *pelvic pneumogram*, which is not currently performed because of improved imaging with ultrasound.

716. The answer is B. *(Ballinger, 7/e, vol 2, pp 34–35. Bontrager, 3/e, p 91.)* The supine AP projection of the abdomen is achieved according to the following positioning instructions. The patient is recumbent in the supine position with the midsagittal plane centered to the midline of the image receptor. The patient's legs are extended with the knees slightly flexed and supported on a sponge or pillow. The center of a 14 by 17 image receptor is positioned at the level of the iliac crest with its bottom edge at the symphysis pubis for the average patient. This will ensure the urinary bladder is included. In the case of a hypersthenic patient, two crosswise image receptors may be needed to image the abdomen. The two images should overlap at the middle of the abdomen to correlate with each other.

717. The answer is D. *(Ballinger, 7/e, vol 2, pp 34–35. Bontrager, 3/e, p 94.)* The erect AP projection of the abdomen requires the central ray to be located higher than for the recumbent version. This is to ensure inclusion of the uppermost portion of the abdomen in order to demonstrate the presence of free air under the diaphragm. The midsagittal plane of the body is still centered to the midline of the image receptor. Centering at the ASIS would exclude the diaphragms and include useless area below the symphysis pubis.

718. The answer is B. *(Ballinger, 7/e, vol 2, pp 138, 156; vol 3, p 45. Bontrager, 3/e, pp 505, 517.)* The kidneys lie on an oblique angle, following the curve of the lumbar spine. This places the upper poles of the kidneys at a more posterior level than the lower poles. If a tomographic image obtained at the 8 cm fulcrum level shows the lower poles clearly, a lower or more posterior fulcrum setting will be required to demonstrate the posteriorly placed upper poles. The average kidney is about 3 cm thick, which indicates the 6 cm fulcrum as the most likely setting to image the upper kidneys. The 4 cm fulcrum level will most likely be too posterior to image the kidney. The higher fulcrum levels of 10 and 12 cm will image more anterior structures in the abdomen than the kidneys.

719. The answer is B. *(Ballinger, 7/e, vol 3, p 45. Bushong, 5/e, p 326.)* Nephrotomography is generally performed to provide images of the kidney parenchyma free of overlying structures such as loops of bowel. The average kidney is about 3 cm thick and a general tomographic survey may be conducted with two or three radiographs at varying levels of about 1.0 cm. Occasionally, 0.5 cm cuts may be requested to better define a suspicious area as identified on the initial images.

720. The answer is B. *(Bontrager, 3/e, pp 574–575.)* In tomography, the fulcrum level determines the level of the focal plane within the object. This focal (or object) plane defines that segment of the object that will be in maximum focus. The structures above and below this plane will be blurred. For the common variable fulcrum type of tomography unit, the table top is denoted as a fulcrum setting (level) of zero, with increasing values being used to indicate structures above the table top. Thus with the patient in the supine position, the fulcrum level increases from the posterior aspect of the patient to the anterior surface. The amplitude determines the thickness of the focal plane (section thickness), i.e., the amount of tissue in focus. As amplitude increases, the section thickness decreases (thinner focal plane). For this question, the problem is with the original fulcrum level setting rather than the amplitude. The transverse processes of the vertebrae are located at the posterior aspect of the vertebrae, while the kidneys are anterior to the vertebral body. Therefore, in order to better image the kidneys, the fulcrum level must be raised (to about 8 cm) to correspond with the more anterior region containing the kidneys. Lowering the fulcrum would image even more posterior vertebral structures. Changing the amplitude only would just provide increased blurring of the same region.

721. The answer is C. *(Ballinger, 7/e, vol 3, p 44. Bontrager, 3/e, p 575.)* The typical variable fulcrum device on a tomographic unit locates the zero mark at the level of the table top. In order to obtain a tomographic section, the fulcrum must be aligned with the level of interest within the body, and this level is denoted in ascending units of measurement (cm or mm) from the table top. Therefore, to properly align the fulcrum with the area of interest in this patient, the 16 cm mark is used, as indicated in the diagram below. The fulcrum positioned at the 10 cm level would image the body section 16 cm posterior to the sternum; the 20 cm level would image the body section 6 cm posterior to the sternum; and the 28 cm level would be above the patient altogether.

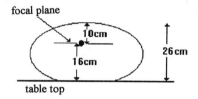

722. The answer is A (1, 2). *(Ballinger, 7/e, vol 3, pp 36–38.)* The tomographic imaging process allows an anatomic structure to be imaged in sections rather than as a whole. This technique provides a measure of depth to the usual radiographic images. The sectional images can thus better demonstrate small changes that may go unnoted by the usual imaging process. This includes the ability to evaluate a healing fracture and subtle or non-displaced fractures. The diagnosis of vasculature disease requires the use of contrast media to opacify the vessels. In order to achieve optimum visualization, the contrast media is injected under pressure to match the flow of blood in these vessels, and rapid serial imaging techniques are used. Tomographic imaging would be unable to meet this requirement.

723. The answer is A. *(Ballinger, 7/e, vol 2, pp 52–54, 66, 75–76; vol 3, pp 40, 45.)* Each of the procedures listed are exams of the biliary system. These exams are the oral cholecystogram (OCG), intravenous cholangiogram (IVC), percutaneous transhepatic cholangiogram (PTC), and endoscopic retrograde cholangiopancreatography (ERCP). Of these exams, only the IVC routinely employs tomography. This exam begins with the administration of contrast media via IV infusion. About 10 min after the end of the infusion, a non-tomographic image of the right upper quadrant is obtained in either the AP or RPO position to determine whether or not the contrast media is evident in the biliary ducts. Once full opacification is noted (about 30 to 40 min after infusion), tomographic images of the area are obtained at section intervals of 0.5 to 1.0 cm.

724. The answer is A. *(Ballinger, 7/e, vol 3, pp 44–45. Bushong, 5/e, pp 326, 328.)* The thickness of the tomographic cut is determined by the amplitude of the tomographic angle. The wider the amplitude, the thinner the section in focus will be. Small structures require wide-angle tomography in order to include their fine details. This is especially true when performing tomography of the cranial or facial bones. Thus, amplitudes of greater than 10° must be employed. The maximum amplitude of 50° will produce the thinnest cut at 1 mm thick.

725. The answer is C (1, 3). *(Ballinger, 7/e, vol 3, p 98. Bontrager, 3/e, pp 581, 585.)* The brainstem includes the *midbrain, pons,* and *medulla oblongata.* It is positioned so as to connect the cerebrum (forebrain) with the pons and cerebellum of the hindbrain and with the spinal cord. The medulla oblongata is the most inferior portion of the brainstem and continues directly with the spinal cord via the foramen magnum.

726. The answer is A. *(Ballinger, 7/e, vol 3, p 98. Bontrager, 3/e, p 582.)* The brain is divided into three sections: the forebrain, midbrain, and hindbrain. The forebrain is primarily composed of the cerebrum, the largest portion of brain tissue. The cerebrum is located in the most superior portion of the cranium. It is separated into two equal halves, the left and right hemispheres, by a structure termed the *longitudinal fissure.* Each hemisphere is further divided into five lobes, named for the region of the cranium in which they are situated. The midbrain is the smallest segment of the brain and is the most superior portion of the brainstem. It acts as a bridge between the forebrain and hindbrain. The hindbrain includes the pons, medulla, and cerebellum. The pons and medulla, along with the midbrain, compose the brainstem and are situated inferior to the cerebrum and anterior to the cerebellum. The cerebellum is the second largest segment of brain tissue and is located in the occipital fossa, inferior to the cerebrum. It too is separated into two hemispheres by a constricted area termed the *vermis.*

727. The answer is C. *(Ballinger, 7/e, vol 3, p 99. Bontrager, 3/e, p 244.)* The spinal cord is an extension of the brainstem and continues with the most inferior portion of the brainstem, the medulla oblongata. The cerebrum makes up the majority of the forebrain and the cerebellum is part of the hindbrain.

728. The answer is D. *(Ballinger, 7/e, vol 3, p 100. Bontrager, 3/e, p 583. Pansky, 5/e, p 122.)* The cerebrospinal fluid (CSF) originates in the choroid plexus located in the ventricles of the brain, primarily the lateral ventricles. The CSF flows from each of the lateral ventricles through the interventricular foramen (foramen of Monro) to the third ventricle. It then flows through the cerebral aqueduct (aqueduct of Sylvius) into the fourth ventricle, which then communicates with the subarachnoid space via the formina of Magendie and Luschka. The CSF then circulates around the cerebrum, cerebellum, and spinal cord.

729. The answer is C. *(Ballinger, 7/e, vol 2, pp 47–49, 78–83, 141–143. Bontrager, 3/e, pp 412, 446–449, 485–487, 510–511.)* The radiographic image in the figure demonstrates anatomic structures of the right upper quadrant of the abdomen. Some structures have been opacified with the use of contrast media. Made visible in this manner are the biliary, gastrointestinal, and urinary systems. The biliary system is demonstrated by the visualization of the hepatic, cystic, and common bile ducts. The small bowel and ascending colon are visible. Finally, the collecting systems of both kidneys are evident.

730. The answer is B. *(Ballinger, 7/e, vol 3, pp 134, 144. Bontrager, 3/e, pp 637, 639. Weir, p 105.)* The radiographic image in the question represents the arteries of the pelvis. These vessels are imaged as part of an angiographic study using the percutaneous method for catheterizing the aorta and administration of contrast media. This exam further requires the use of rapid serial imaging to capture the flow of contrast media through the vasculature. The structures identified on this image include the *(1) distal abdominal aorta, (2) right common iliac artery, (3) left external iliac artery, (4) left internal iliac artery, and (5) femoral artery.*

731–734. The answers are 731-C, 732-B, 733-A, 734-D. *(Ballinger, 7/e, vol 1, pp 75–77. Bontrager, 3/e, p 103.)* The radiographic images in the figure are the lateral (A), oblique (B), and PA (C) projections of the wrist. The labeled structures are as follows: *(1)* scaphoid (navicular), *(2)* lunate, *(3)* hamate, *(4)* ulnar styloids, *(5)* radial styloid, *(6)* trapezium, *(7)* capitate, *(8)* triquetrum, *(9)* pisiform, and *(10)* trapezoid.

735–737. The answers are 735-B, 736-B, 737-C. *(Ballinger, 7/e, vol 1, pp 53, 56, 92. Bontrager, 3/e, pp 106, 137. Weir, p 71.)* The lateral view of the elbow demonstrated in the figure is obtained by placing the humerus and forearm at right angles to each other, and the hand in a true lateral position. The elbow joint is composed of numerous articulations of the hinge and pivot types. The hinge joints exist as humeroulnar and humeroradial articulations. Specifically, these are between the *olecranon process (2), semilunar notch (3),* and the *coronoid process (5)* of the ulnar and the olecranon fossa, trochlea, and coronoid fossa of the humerus, respectively. The humeroradial articulation exists between the *radial head (4)* and the capitulum of the humerus. The pivot joint exists between the *radial tubercle (6)* of the radius and the radial notch on the ulnar. The superimposed *humeral epicondyles (1)* are also demonstrated.

738–739. The answers are 738-D, 739-C. *(Ballinger, 7/e, vol 1, pp 116, 128, 132. Bontrager, 3/e, pp 156, 158, 161.)* The figure demonstrates the AP position of the shoulder with external rotation. This is confirmed by the position of the *greater tubercle (4)* in profile by externally rotating the arm. In this position, the *lesser tubercle (8)* is projected onto the *humeral head (5)*. The other structures labeled on this figure include (*1*) acromial end of the clavicle, (*2*) coracoid process, (*3*) acromion process, (*6*) glenoid fossa, and (*7*) lateral border of the scapula.

740–741. The answers are 740-A, 741-B. *(Ballinger, 7/e, vol 1, pp 112–113. Bontrager, 3/e, p 148.)* The image in the figure represents a frontal view of the scapula. The labeled anatomic structures are as follows: (*1*) acromion process, (*2*) coracoid process, (*3*) spine of scapula, (*4*) superior angle, (*5*) glenoid cavity, (*6*) lateral (axillary) border, (*7*) medial (vertebral) border, (*8*) body of scapula, and (*9*) inferior angle.

742–744. The answers are 742-A, 743-C, 744-A. *(Ballinger, 7/e, vol 1, pp 162–163, 169, 177. Bontrager, 3/e, p 175.)* The image in the figure is of the medial oblique projection of the foot. The labeled anatomic structures are as follows: (*1*) first interphalangeal joint, (*2*) first metatarsophalangeal joint, (*3*) head of the third metatarsal, (*4*) fifth metatarsophalangeal joint, (*5*) base of the fifth metatarsal, (*6*) cuboid, (*7*) navicular, (*8*) medial (or first) cuneiform, (*9*) talus, and (*10*) calcaneus.

745–747. The answers are 745-D, 746-A, 747-C. *(Ballinger, 7/e, vol 1, pp 205. Bontrager, 3/e, pp 175, 200.)* The figure demonstrates the ankle in the lateral position. The image includes the superimposed ends of the distal tibia/fibula, all the tarsal bones, and the proximal ends of the metatarsals. The ankle joint is a hinge type that offers movement in the form of flexion and extension, primarily. There is a limited amount of rotation motion also. The lateral malleolus of the fibula articulates with the lateral surface of the distal tibia. The inferior surface of the tibia articulates with the superior aspect of the talus. The articulations between the tarsal bones provide a slight gliding motion. The structures identified on this image are (*1*) tibia, (*2*) lateral malleolus of fibula, (*3*) talus, (*4*) calcaneus, (*5*) navicular, (*6*) cuboid, (*7*) tibiotalar joint, (*8*) talonavicular joint, and (*9*) calcaneocuboid joint. The talocalcaneal joint is marked with a dashed line, but is not numbered.

748–749. The answers are 748-B, 749-A. *(Ballinger, 7/e, vol 1, pp 164–166, 216–217. Bontrager, 3/e, p 210.)* The lateral projection of the knee is demonstrated in the figure. The optimum image should demonstrate the femoral condyles superimposed, the patellofemoral space open, and the patella in lateral profile. The labeled structures on this image are as follows: (*1*) base of patella, (*2*) apex of patella, (*3*) tibial tuberosity, (*4*) head of fibula, (*5*) tibial spine, and (*6*) distal femur.

750–752. The answers are 750-C, 751-A, 752-B. *(Ballinger, 7/e, vol 1, pp 165, 204. Bontrager, 3/e, pp 174, 176. Weir, pp 167, 169.)* The radiographic image in the figure is the AP projection of the lower leg (tibia/fibula). The labeled structures are as follows: (*1*) head of the fibula, (*2*) lateral condyle of tibia, (*3*) medial condyle of tibia, (*4*) tibial spine, (*5*) shaft of fibula, (*6*) shaft of tibia, (*7*) lateral malleolus, (*8*) medial malleolus, (*9*) anterior tibial tubercle, and (*10*) tibiotalar joint.

753–756. The answers are 753-D, 754-A, 755-A, 756-C. *(Ballinger, 7/e, vol 1, p 242. Bontrager, 3/e, p 219. Pansky, 5/e, pp 488, 489, 492.)* The figure is a lateral projection of the hip bone, which includes the ilium, ischium, and pubis. The labeled structures on the diagram are as follows: (*1*) iliac crest, (*2*) anterior superior iliac spine, (*3*) anterior inferior iliac spine, (*4*) acetabulum, (*5*) obturator foramen, (*6*) pubis, (*7*) ischial ramus, (*8*) lesser sciatic notch, (*9*) ischial spine, (*10*) greater sciatic notch, (*11*) posterior inferior iliac spine, and (*12*) posterior superior iliac spine.

In this view, the greater sciatic notch is located on the posterior aspect of the hip bone, just at the beginning of the ischium. It is a large cut-away (notch) just above the ischial spine.

The ischial spine is a small projection off the superior portion of the ischium and lies between the greater and lesser sciatic notches. It serves as an attachment point for the sacrospinous ligament, which extends between the ischium and sacrum/coccyx.

The acetabulum provides the "socket" component for the hip's ball-and-socket type of joint. It is made up of portions of all three of the hip bones: the ilium, ischium, and pubis. On the lateral view of the hip bone, the acetabulum is located in the anterior inferior area. Four bony prominences are evident on the ala of the ilium bone: the anterior superior iliac spine (ASIS), anterior inferior iliac spine (AILS), posterior superior iliac spine (PSIS), and posterior inferior iliac spine (PIIS). These landmarks are used for palpation and location of other anatomic structures. The ASIS is the most prominent and commonly used in radiographic positioning. The names of each of these prominences identify their location on the ilium, and these prominences may be seen on both lateral and AP projections of the ilium.

757–758. The answers are 757-D, 758-B. *(Ballinger, 7/e, vol 1, pp 370–371. Bontrager, 3/e, pp 298–299, 306.)* The image displayed in the figure is that of the sternum in the RAO projection. This projection is commonly used to image the sternum projected away from the thoracic spine. To further improve visualization, a long exposure time (at low milliamperage) is used with the patient breathing during the exposure. This will cause blurring of the ribs and better viewing of the sternum. The breathing technique is a form of tomography referred to as *autotomography.* It is also commonly used for imaging the thoracic spine in the lateral position and the transthoracic projection of the upper humerus. A long exposure of several seconds will enhance the effectiveness of this technique. The anatomic structures demonstrated on this image include the uppermost portion of the sternum, the *manubrium (2),* the *jugular notch (1),* and the *clavicular notches (3);* the latter are part of the sternoclavicular joints. The *body (5)* of the sternum, also known as the *gladiolus,* is the largest portion of the sternum. The junction of the body and manubrium is termed the *sternal angle (4).* The most distal portion of the sternum is the *xiphoid process (8).* The curved structures along the borders of the sternum are the chondral facets, which provide attachment sites for the seven pairs of true ribs *(6).* Also visible on this image is the *inferior angle* of the scapula *(7).*

759–761. The answers are 759-B, 760-D, 761-C. *(Ballinger, 7/e, vol 1, p 281. Bontrager, 3/e, p 251. Pansky, 5/e, p 191.)* The figure is a lateral projection of a typical vertebra. The labeled structures are as follows: *(1)* vertebral body, *(2)* pedicle, *(3)* inferior articular facet, *(4)* superior articular facet, and *(5)* spinous process.

Two pedicles are located on each vertebra (C2–L5). Each arises from the posterior aspect of the vertebral body and projects posteriorly and laterally, forming the anterior lateral portion of the neural arch. The pedicles join with the laminae and give rise to the superior and inferior articular facets and ultimately end in the formation of the transverse processes. On the inferior and superior surfaces of the pedicle is a notch that forms the intervertebral foramina.

One spinous process is located at the most posterior aspect of the vertebra (with the exception of C1, which has a posterior tubercle instead of a spinous process). This process originates at the junction of the two laminae (which form the posterior portion of the neural arch). The spinous process projects posteriorly and caudally on the cervical and thoracic vertebrae and projects posteriorly and horizontally on the lumbar vertebrae.

Each vertebra is connected at three articulation points: the intervertebral disk and two zygapophyseal joints. The intervertebral junction is the anterior union of the spinal column between two vertebral bodies (one above the other) and the disk material between them. Posteriorly, the vertebrae connect together at the zygapophyseal joints, one on each side of the neural arch. The zygapophyseal joints are the union between an inferior articular facet of one vertebra with the superior articular facet of the vertebra below it. Both the inferior and superior articular facets arise from the pedicle at the point of its union with the lamina. These joints are of the diarthrodial (gliding) type. Their specific location on the vertebra varies between the cervical, thoracic, and lumbar regions of the spine, requiring different positions in order to demonstrate them radiographically.

762–765. The answers are 762-D, 763-C, 764-A, 765-C. *(Ballinger, 7/e, vol 1, pp 340–343. Bontrager, 3/e, p 262.)* The radiographic image in the figure represents the left posterior oblique projection of the lumbar spine. This position best demonstrates the zygapophyseal joint on the side closest to the image receptor (in this case the left side). The patient is positioned supinely and rotated 45° toward the left. The hips and shoulders should be supported to ensure the patient's position. The central ray is then directed perpendicular to L3 and enters approximately 1 inch above the iliac crest and 2 inches to the right side of the patient's midline. Since there are two sets of zygapophyseal joints at each junction of vertebrae, the patient should be radiographed from both oblique positions (right and left). The joints closest to the image receptor will be demonstrated when performing posterior (supine) oblique projections.

The correctly positioned oblique image of the lumbar spine portrays vertebral structures in the image of a "scotty dog." The *inferior articular facet of L2 (2)* forms the front leg of the scotty dog. It articulates with the *superior articular facet of L4 (1),* which forms the ear of the scotty dog. Also visible on this radiograph are the *pedicle of L3 (3),* which is the eye of the dog, the *transverse process of L3 (4),* which is the nose, and the *lamina* (unmarked), which is the body of the dog. The body of L4 is labeled *5.*

766–768. The answers are 766-B, 767-A, 768-D. *(Ballinger, 7/e, vol 1, p 303. Bontrager, 3/e, pp 277, 289. Weir, p 53.)* The lateral projection of the cervical spine is demonstrated in the figure. As required, all seven cervical vertebrae are visible without superimposition by the mandible or shoulders. This position best demonstrates the zygapophyseal joints, intervertebral disk spaces, vertebral bodies, and spinous processes. Specific to the first cervical vertebra, this position demonstrates the anterior and posterior arch with the odontoid process of C2 projecting upward through the ring of C1. The labeled structures are *(1)* anterior arch of C1, *(2)* body of C3, *(3)* superior articular facet of C3, *(4)* inferior articular facet of C3, *(5)* spinous process of C6, *(6)* zygapophyseal joint of C5–6, and *(7)* intervertebral joint (disk space) of C5–6.

769–772. The answers are 769-C, 770-D, 771-C, 772-B. *(Ballinger, 7/e, vol 2, pp 225–229. Bontrager, 3/e, p 322.)* The labeled structures as demonstrated on the lateral projection radiograph of the skull are as follows: *(1)* parietal bone, *(2)* frontal bone, *(3)* greater wing of the sphenoid bone, *(4)* sella turcica (pituitary fossa), *(5)* anterior clinoid processes, *(6)* dorsum sella, *(7)* mastoid portion of the temporal bone, *(8)* occipital bone, *(9)* lambdoidal suture, and *(10)* coronal suture.

The frontal and parietal bones compose the major portion of the anterior and lateral aspects of the skull. Their union is formed by the *coronal suture.* The sphenoid bone contains the greater and lesser wings, which make up a portion of the orbits, and the housing for the pituitary gland, formed by the *anterior clinoid processes, sella turcica, dorsum sella,* and *posterior clinoid processes.* The ethmoid is the smallest of the cranial bones. It is located in the anterior aspect of the cranium, making up a portion of the cranial floor and orbital and nasal cavities. Each temporal bone is divided into squamous, zygomatic, petrous, and mastoid portions. The *petrous portion* houses the auditory canals and organs of hearing and balance. The *mastoid portion* contains the air cells. The occipital bone is the most posterior bone, composing the back of the skull. The union of the occipital bone with the parietal bones is formed by the *lambdoidal suture.*

773–776. The answers are 773-D, 774-B, 775-D, 776-A. *(Ballinger, 7/e, vol 2, p 35. Bontrager, 3/e, p 91. Weir, p 109.)* The correct way to view this radiograph of the abdomen is as if the patient were facing the viewer, i.e., patient's left on viewer's right and vice versa. The structures are *(1)* stomach outlined with air, *(2)* transverse colon outlined with air, *(3)* left kidney, *(4)* left psoas muscle, *(5)* liver, *(6)* right kidney, *(7)* right psoas muscle, *(8)* iliac crest, and *(9)* spleen. The ability to visualize sections of the upper or lower GI system on the plain film KUB depends on the presence of air in the system to act as a contrast agent.

777–778. The answers are 777-C, 778-B. *(Ballinger, 7/e, vol 1, p 412. Bontrager, 3/e, p 56.)* The figure demonstrates the PA projection of the chest. This radiographic exam is primarily performed for visualization of the lungs; however, other thoracic structures are also visible. An optimum chest radiograph should demonstrate a nonrotated view of the full lung fields to include the *apices (1)* and the *costophrenic angles (6 and 8).* The air-filled *trachea (2)* is frequently visible, contrasted against the thoracic spine. A small portion of the *aortic arch (3)* is demonstrated on the left side of the upper mediastinum. The *cardiac shadow (4)* extends from just to the right of midline well into the left side of the thorax. The *diaphragms (5)* mark the inferior aspect of the thorax and *bronchiopulmonary markings (7)* are visible to varying degrees throughout the lungs.

779–781. The answers are 779-D, 780-A, 781-C. *(Ballinger, 7/e, vol 2, pp 78–79. Bontrager, 3/e, p 418. Pansky, 5/e, pp 394, 406, 407. Weir, p 121.)* The radiograph in the question demonstrates an RAO projection of the stomach, opacified with barium. The *cardiac orifice (1)* is the opening into the stomach that accommodates the esophagus. This upper portion of the stomach is referred to as the *fundus (2)* of the stomach. The *body* of the stomach *(3)* curves to the right, across the midline of the body. The medial aspect of the stomach is termed the *lesser curvature (4)* while the lateral aspect is termed the *greater curvature (5)*. The most distal portion of the stomach is the *pylorus (6)*, which connects with the duodenum of the small bowel. The *duodenal loop (7)* curves around the head of the pancreas, forming a C shape.

782–785. The answers are 782-B, 783-D, 784-C, 785-C. *(Ballinger, 7/e, vol 2, pp 81, 135. Bontrager, 3/e, pp 448–450. Pansky, 5/e, p 414. Weir, p 123.)* The radiograph is that of the abdomen in the LPO position to demonstrate the large intestine opacified with barium. The LPO projection requires the patient to be rotated 45° toward the left from the supine position. This projection opens the hepatic flexure for better visualization. The colon extends from the small intestine at the ileocecal junction. The *ileum (8)* of the small intestine joins with the *cecum (9)* of the colon. The colon then continues with the *ascending colon (5)* on the right side of the abdomen and the *hepatic flexure (1)*, which then turns horizontally to form the *transverse colon (4)*. On the left side is the *splenic flexure (2)*, which turns inferiorly to form the *descending colon (3)*. The end portion of the colon becomes the very twisted *sigmoid colon (6)* before terminating with the *rectum (7)*.

786–787. The answers are 786-C, 787-D. *(Ballinger, 7/e, vol 3, p 100. Bontrager, 3/e, p 583.)* The diagram depicts a lateral view of the ventricular system of the brain. The structures identified are as follows: *(1)* anterior horn of the lateral ventricle, *(2)* body of the lateral ventricle, *(3)* posterior horn of the lateral ventricle, *(4)* cerebral aqueduct (communication channel between the third and fourth ventricles), *(5)* fourth ventricle, *(6)* interventricular foramen (communication channel between the lateral and third ventricles), *(7)* third ventricle, and *(8)* inferior horn of the lateral ventricle.

788–791. The answers are 788-C, 789-A, 790-D, 791-B. *(Ballinger, 7/e, vol 1, pp 281–282. Bontrager, 3/e, pp 274–275. Pansky, 5/e, p 190.)* Each vertebra, with the exception of C1, has an anterior portion, *the body,* and a posterior portion, *the vertebral arch.* The vertebral arch is formed by the two pedicles' joining with the two laminae. Together, these two portions of the vertebra form an opening called the *vertebral foramen.* The stacked cervical, thoracic, and lumbar vertebrae form a spinal canal, which conveys the spinal cord from the brainstem to the sacrum and continues with the sacral canal.

The most posterior structure of the vertebral arch is the *spinous process.* It is most prominent on the seventh cervical vertebra, which is thus termed the *vertebra prominens.*

The *zygapophyseal joints* are formed by the articulations between inferior articular facets of one vertebra and the superior articular facets of the vertebra immediately below it. This union causes the alignment of the vertebral notches (located on the superior and inferior aspects of the pedicles) of each of the vertebrae, which form openings at the lateral aspect of the vertebral arch. These openings between vertebrae are called *intervertebral foramina* and allow the passage of nerves and blood vessels.

The junction of the pedicle and lamina gives rise to the *transverse process.* These processes are found on all vertebrae of the true vertebral column. The transverse processes of the cervical vertebrae each contain an opening termed a *transverse foramen.* A rib facet is included on the transverse process of each thoracic vertebra. The lumbar vertebrae include two additional processes as part of each transverse process: a mammillary process on the superior aspect and an accessory process on the inferior aspect.

792–799. The answers are 792-E, 793-A, 794-D, 795-B, 796-C, 797-C, 798-D, 799-E. *(Ballinger, 7/e, vol 2, pp 204–210. Bontrager, 3/e, pp 318–321.)* The frontal bone supports the supraorbital margin, glabella, and part of the nasion. The occipital bone has the external occipital protuberance (inion), foramen magnum, and lateral condyles. Each temporal bone has a tympanic portion, styloid process, zygomatic process, petrous portion, and mastoid process. The sphenoid bone has two greater and lesser wings, the sella turcica, dorsum sella, posterior and anterior clinoid processes, and pterygoid processes. The ethmoid bone contains a crista galli, cribriform plate, perpendicular plate, the lateral masses containing the air cells, and the superior and middle conchae.

800–804. The answers are 800-B, 801-A, 802-D, 803-E, 804-C. *(Ballinger, 7/e, vol 2, p 217. Bontrager, 3/e, pp 314–316.)* The landmarks on the face and skull are frequently used to identify centering points and in positioning of the head for imaging of the cranium, paranasal sinuses, and facial bones. The *glabella* is the most superior landmark, being located at the midpoint on the inferior portion of the frontal bone. Just below the glabella is the *nasion*, which is located at the union of the nasal bones with the frontal bone. The *acanthion* is located at the junction of the nose with the upper lip (also a midline point). The most inferior midline landmark is the *mental point*. This is the tip of the chin. From the lateral perspective of the head, additional landmarks can be located. The *inner* and *outer canthi* are located at the junction of the upper and lower eyelids (at the inner and outer aspects of the eye). The *infraorbital margins* mark the lowermost border of the orbit. The *external auditory meatuses (EAM)* are the openings into the auditory canals. The *gonion* (angle of the mandible) is the most inferior lateral landmark on the head. The *inion* (external occipital protuberance) is the most posterior landmark.

805–809. The answers are 805-C, 806-A, 807-B, 808-B, 809-C. *(Ballinger, 7/e, vol 2, pp 214–216. Bontrager, 3/e, pp 347–348.)* The only facial bone that contains a paranasal sinus is the maxillary bone. This large bone forms the anterior portion of the upper face and a portion of the oral, nasal, and orbital cavities. The inferior border of the maxilla is referred to as the *alveolar process* and supports the upper teeth. The mandible is a large single bone that forms the lower portion of the face. The articulation between the *coronoid process* of the uppermost portion of the mandibular rami and the mandibular notch of the temporal bone forms a hinge type of diarthrodial joint. The only other unpaired bone is the vomer, located along the midsagittal plane and forming the floor of the nasal cavity. The vomer articulates with the perpendicular plate of the ethmoid bone, forming the nasal septum. The zygoma bones form the lateral posterior aspect of the face and articulate with the maxilla (anteriorly) and temporal and sphenoid bones (posteriorly). The zygomatic arch is formed by the articulation between the zygoma and zygomatic process of the temporal bone.

810–813. The answers are 810-B, 811-A, 812-C, 813-D. *(Ballinger, 7/e, vol 2, pp 370, 373, 374, 377. Bontrager, 3/e, pp 400–403.)* Although more than one set of sinuses may be visible by these projections, a primary set or sets of sinuses are best demonstrated. On the PA axial projection, the frontal sinuses are best seen. A portion of the anterior ethmoid sinuses is also visible. The maxillary sinuses are best seen on the parietocanthial projection. However, the frontal and ethmoid are also partially evident. The submentovertex projection demonstrates only the sphenoid and ethmoid sinuses. All paranasal sinuses are visible with the patient in the lateral position.

814–817. The answers are 814-C, 815-D, 816-B, 817-A. *(Ballinger, 7/e, vol 2, pp 223–224, 250–251, 374. Bontrager, 3/e, pp 328–330, 333, 359.)* The anatomic structure of interest should always be centered to the middle of the image receptor. Whether an entrance or exit point for the central ray is stated depends on the relevant anatomic structures, especially with cranial anatomy. When an angle is applied to the central ray, its entrance will vary above or below the area of interest in order for it to be projected into the center of the image receptor. Therefore, the exit point will more commonly be stated. The numerous structures of the skull require the use of various tube angles and adjustment of the skull position to demonstrate structures of interest. A radiograph demonstrating the lateral projection of the cranial bones must include from the most anterior anatomy (all the frontal bone) to the most posterior (the occipital bone). No tube angle is used for this projection and the midpoint is identified as the point 2 inches above the EAM, which is where the central ray should enter/exit. This remains true regardless of whether the exam is performed in the erect or recumbent positions or with a horizontal beam. The axial projection (AP or PA) will project either the dorsum sella or sella turcica within the foramen magnum, depending on how much tube angle is used. For either structure, the foramen magnum is identified as the exit point. In the parietoacanthial projection, the x-ray beam enters via the parietal bones and exits at the acanthion, which is at the level of the maxillary sinuses. The PA projection of the frontal sinuses generally employs a caudally directed central ray that exits at the nasion.

818–825. The answers are 818-C, 819-B, 820-A, 821-E, 822-C, 823-D, 824-C, 825-D. *(Ballinger, 7/e, vol 2, pp 141–143; vol 3, p 168. Bontrager, 3/e, pp 514, 517–519. Laudicina, pp 106–109.)* The examination procedures of the urinary system are strictly radiologic exams or urologic exams with radiographic assistance. The basic radiographic exam of the urinary system is the *excretory* or *intravenous urogram (IVU)*. This procedure is a functional as well as structural exam of the kidneys, ureters, and bladder. Contrast media is intravenously injected by either bolus or infusion method. The contrast media is then filtered from the blood into the collecting system. Variations on the exam routine are made to best demonstrate specific conditions. The *hypertensive IVU* is one such variation that requires numerous (three to five) radiographs (straight or tomographic) of the kidneys to be obtained immediately following a bolus injection of the contrast media. This routine will demonstrate renal function for comparison between the two kidneys. Any differences noted may be indicative of a narrowed renal artery, which may be the source of a patient's high blood pressure (hypertension).

The *percutaneous antegrade urogram* allows the injection of contrast media directly into the renal pelvis and calyces through a nephrostomy tube. This is generally performed for the patient with an obstruction and suspected hydronephrosis, which would impair the concentration of contrast media if it were administered intravenously. The nephrostomy tube is primarily inserted to drain the urine from the obstructed kidney, thus avoiding significant renal damage. Evaluation of the hydronephrosis and the collecting system can be made by this method of direct opacification.

The examination of the lower urinary system (distal ureters, bladder, and urethra) is performed as a retrograde study in either the radiology or urology department. The contrast media is introduced via a urinary retention catheter placed in the patient's bladder. The bladder is filled with contrast media contained in an IV package suspended above the exam table. This procedure may be limited to the examination of the bladder and distal ureters, which is properly termed a *cystogram*. When the exam is extended to include imaging of the opacified urethra during voiding of the contrast media, the exam is termed a *voiding cystourethrogram*. In addition to evaluating the structure and function of the bladder and urethra, this exam is also performed to determine the presence and extent of ureteral reflux before and during voiding.

The *retrograde urogram* is a urologic exam with radiographic assistance. As such, it is performed in a specially designed room to satisfy urology and radiography requirements. The contrast media is injected against the flow of urine (retrograde) through catheters positioned within the ureters (close to the renal pelvis) by the urologist. These catheters enter the distal end of the ureters via the vesicoureteral orifices. This exam is a nonfunctional procedure, demonstrating only the structure of the collecting system and ureters. One or both sides may be examined.

826–828. The answers are 826-C, 827-D, 828-A. *(Ballinger, 7/e, vol 2, pp 138–139. Bontrager, 3/e, p 507.)* The structure of the kidney contains various macroscopic and microscopic components responsible for its primary function, which is to filter waste products from the blood. The most external portion of the kidney is termed the *renal cortex (1)*, which contains the microscopic structures of the filtering process (the nephrons). Medial to the cortex is the *medullary portion (7)*, which contains some of the microscopic and all the macroscopic functional structures of the kidney. Only the macroscopic structures are included on this diagram. The smallest of these are the renal *pyramids (6)*, which are the distal portion of the macroscopic renal structures. These structures convey the waste material (urine) into the *minor calyces (2)*, which join together to form a *major calyx (3)*. Each kidney has two to three major calyces, which communicate with the *renal pelvis (4)*. This dilated portion of the collecting system drains into the *ureter (5)*.

829–833. The answers are 829-B, 830-E, 831-C, 832-A, 833-A. *(Bontrager, 3/e, p 514. Laudicina, pp 112–126.)* Abnormal conditions of the urinary system can involve individual sections or the total system. Congenital conditions can be life-threatening or asymptomatic, as with an ectopic kidney. The kidneys usually ascend to the normal abdominal location during fetal development. When this does not occur, the kidney will be located in the lower abdomen or pelvic region. In the absence of an inflammatory condition, ectopic kidneys do not present a major finding. Infections within the urinary system can occur in the kidney, the bladder, or the entire urinary tract (UTI). Cystitis is commonly the result of a bacterial infection in the bladder. The short urethra in females allows the easy transmission of bacteria into the bladder. Another source of bladder infection is due to a fistulous communication between the bladder and the vagina (vesicovaginal) or the rectum (vesicorectal). An infection within the kidney and renal pelvis is termed *pyelonephritis*. Hydronephrosis is the accumulation of urine in the renal pelvis and calyces that causes dilatation of those structures. This condition is frequently the result of an obstruction or stricture in the ureter, causing a "backup" of urine flow.

834–838. The answers are 834-D, 835-C, 836-A, 837-D, 838-B. *(Ballinger, 7/e, vol 2, pp 152–155. Bontrager, 3/e, pp 525–526.)* The erect AP bladder may be requested toward the end of an IVU exam in order to document a prolapsed (forward displacement or "dropped") bladder. This suspected condition requires the radiographer to center lower than is usual for bladder imaging. The postvoid bladder image will best demonstrate an enlarged prostate gland and may likely demonstrate incomplete emptying of the bladder due to constriction caused by the enlarged gland. The Trendelenburg position places the patient's head about 15° lower than the horizontal plane. This position delays the emptying of the contrast media from the renal pelvicalyceal system. It also causes the fundus of the bladder to move forward, thus providing better visualization of the vesicoureteral junctions. The RPO projection of the abdomen will demonstrate the entire left ureter, free from superimposition over the spine, including the left vesicoureteral junction.

839–843. The answers are 839-B, 840-E, 841-A, 842-C, 843-B. *(Ballinger, 7/e, vol 2, pp 3, 80. Bontrager, 3/e, pp 485–486. Pansky, 5/e, pp 412–413.)* The ducts listed as answer options are those of the salivary glands and the biliary system. The three sets of salivary glands are the parotid, which is drained by *Stensen's duct*; the submandibular, from which *Wharton's duct* extends; and the sublingual gland, which has numerous ducts referred to as the *ducts of Rivinus*. The biliary system conveys secretions from the liver, gallbladder, and pancreas to the duodenum. The diagram below shows the biliary ducts. The main ducts from the liver are the right (*1*) and left (*2*) hepatics, which combine to form the *common hepatic duct (3)*. The *cystic duct (7)* arises from the gallbladder and joins with the common hepatic duct to form the *common bile duct (4)*. The main *pancreatic duct (5)* extends from the pancreas and joins with the common bile duct to form the *ampulla of Vater (6)*, a small, dilated segment of duct that is protected by the *sphincter of Oddi* as it empties into the duodenum.

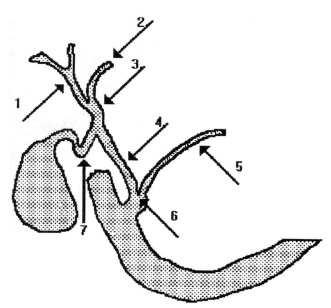

844–850. The answers are 844-B, 845-C, 846-A, 847-C, 848-E, 849-D, 850-D. *(Bontrager, 3/e, pp 427, 431, 455, 459, 487. Eisenberg, pp 135–137, 140–142, 150–152. Laudicina, pp 53, 64, 69, 75, 79, 94–95.)* Each of the exams listed as choices are performed with the assistance of fluoroscopy in order to allow the radiologist to observe the dynamic function of the GI system and to record the images in serial format as needed. The *esophagram* (barium swallow) is the radiographic study of the esophagus and a patient's ability to swallow. The common complaints leading to this exam include dysphagia (difficulty swallowing), such as that due to an obstruction, and heartburn as a result of reflux of gastric juices into the esophagus. The esophagram requires the patient to swallow thick or thin barium, depending on the suspected problem, with the patient in the erect and recumbent positions.

The *oral cholecystogram* allows for the examination of the gallbladder following the patient's ingestion of water-soluble iodine contrast media 10 to 12 h prior to the exam. Common complaints that would suggest the need to evaluate the gallbladder are right upper quadrant pain, especially after eating certain foods, or jaundice. Cholelithiasis refers to the presence of stones in the gallbladder. These stones may move out of the gallbladder into the biliary ducts, causing an obstruction and jaundice. Preliminary scout films are obtained to determine the level of concentration of the contrast media. If satisfactory, the radiologist will image the gallbladder fluoroscopically. The frequency of this exam is currently being reduced because of the practice of evaluating the gallbladder with ultrasound imaging.

The *upper gastrointestinal series* (UGI) provides a radiographic exam of the esophagus, stomach, and duodenum. Patients with complaints of dyspepsia (indigestion) or epigastric or abdominal pain may have such conditions as gastritis, gastric or duodenal ulcers, or cancer. The UGI series requires the patient to swallow barium, which coats the gastrointestinal mucosa. The radiologist uses fluoroscopy to follow the movement of the barium and varies the patient's position in order to visualize all aspects of the anatomy under observation.

The radiologic exam of the colon is referred to as a *lower gastrointestinal series* (barium enemas). This exam is frequently performed on patients who are experiencing blood in their stool, diarrhea, lower abdominal pain, and weight loss. These complaints may be indicative of such conditions as colitis, diverticulitis, obstruction, or cancer. Diverticulosis is the presence of outpouchings of the mucosa at any point along the GI tract. These outpouchings are most frequently found in great number on the colon, specifically on the descending or sigmoid portions. Inflammation of these pouches (*diverticulitis*) causes lower abdominal pain and may be due to dietary irritants or changes in bowel patterns. The barium enema exam involves the retrograde administration of barium into the colon. Using fluoroscopy, the radiologist follows the flow of barium, rotating the patient into various positions to visualize the entire colon.

The *small bowel series* is commonly combined with the UGI in order to radiograph the small bowel. Patient complaints of dark, tarry stools, abdominal pain, and weight loss may indicate bleeding within the small bowel or enteritis (inflammation of the small intestines). Crohn's disease (localized or regional enteritis) is most frequently associated with the small bowel. This condition is usually located at the most distal end of the small bowel, the terminal ileum. The small bowel series requires the ingestion of additional barium following the UGI series and follow-up abdominal radiographs at timed intervals until the entire small bowel is opacified.

Patient Care

DIRECTIONS: Each numbered question or incomplete statement below contains lettered responses. Select the **one best** response.

851. Informed consent documentation indicates that:
1. The exam procedure was explained to the patient (parent/legal guardian of minor or mentally incompetent)
2. The risks associated with the procedure were fully explained
3. The hospital/clinic takes no responsibility for the possible negligence of an employee performing or assisting with the procedure

(A) 1 & 2
(B) 2 & 3
(C) 1 & 3
(D) 1, 2, & 3

852. To ensure the legitimacy of an informed consent document, when should the procedural explanation and patient signature take place?

(A) While the patient is being given anesthesia
(B) At the conclusion of the procedure
(C) During the procedure
(D) Prior to beginning the procedure

853. A patient's right of privacy includes which of the following elements?
1. Protecting patient's modesty
2. Explaining the exam and its potential risks
3. Obtaining patient's permission to allow student health care professionals to attend the exam

(A) 1 & 2
(B) 2 & 3
(C) 1 & 3
(D) 1, 2, & 3

854. A "do not resuscitate" (DNR) order or other request for minimal medical treatment may be made via

(A) the patient through a living will
(B) the family members of a competent patient
(C) the medical and nursing staff
(D) any member of the health care team

855. Ethical behavior on the part of a radiographer includes:

1. Respectful and competent interaction with patients, fellow employees, and visitors
2. Careful handling of hospital equipment
3. Proper utilization of hospital supplies

(A)   1 & 2
(B)   2 & 3
(C)   1 & 3
(D)   1, 2, & 3

856. "Failure of a radiographer to provide reasonable care or caution" is a description of

(A)   assault
(B)   negligence
(C)   libel
(D)   battery

857. Which of the following actions are forms of communication between a radiographer and a patient?

1. Verbalization
2. Appearance
3. Touch

(A)   1 & 2
(B)   2 & 3
(C)   1 & 3
(D)   1, 2, & 3

858. What is the *best* way of communicating with a patient who does not speak the same language as the radiographer?

(A)   Use of patient's family members
(B)   Use of an interpreter
(C)   Use of pictures and demonstrations
(D)   Talking louder to the patient

859. What is the most appropriate way for a radiographer to communicate with a patient with hearing loss?

(A)   Increase both the pitch and volume of speech
(B)   Look directly at the patient when speaking
(C)   Request an interpreter
(D)   Talk as little as possible as the patient will not be able to understand anyway

860. How should the radiographer communicate with unconscious patients?

(A)   Instruct and explain to these patients as if they were conscious
(B)   Do not attempt any form of communication
(C)   Do not be concerned with what is said around the unconscious patient
(D)   Talk loudly to overcome their unconsciousness

861. What is the most common source of fire in a radiology department?

(A)   Open flames
(B)   Cigarettes
(C)   Spontaneous combustion
(D)   Electrical components

862. When possible, what is the best way to move a heavy object?

(A)   Push
(B)   Lift
(C)   Pull
(D)   Drag

863. Movement of heavy objects, such as assisting patients, requires an adequate base of support that is achieved by which body position?

(A)   Standing with legs apart, knees bent
(B)   Standing with legs apart, knees straight
(C)   Standing with legs together, knees bent
(D)   Allowing as much distance as possible between object and lifter

864. The use of proper body mechanics is essential in order to minimize

(A)   the number of persons needed to lift
(B)   personal injury as a result of lifting
(C)   the need for accessory equipment to assist in lifting
(D)   complaints by the patient regarding difficulty getting on and off x-ray tables

865. When a patient arrives in the radiology department on a stretcher, all the following statements are true EXCEPT

(A) the stretcher wheels should be locked before transferring patient to x-ray table
(B) the patient should be assisted off stretcher and use a footstool to get onto the x-ray table
(C) one person may guide patients who can move themselves from the stretcher to the table
(D) more than one person should assist patients who cannot move themselves

866. Which of the following methods may be used to move a patient from a stretcher to the x-ray table?
    1. Slider board
    2. Draw sheet
    3. Log roll

(A) 1 & 2
(B) 2 & 3
(C) 1 & 3
(D) 1, 2, & 3

867. Why is it recommended that a pillow or sponge be placed under a supine patient's knees?

(A) To improve circulation in the lower limbs
(B) To keep patients from rolling off the table
(C) To relieve stress on patient's lower back
(D) To keep legs together when patient is being moved

868. What immediate action should be taken for a patient who suddenly appears pale and complains of weakness?

(A) Stand the patient up
(B) Send the patient back to his or her room
(C) Sit the patient down with the head back
(D) Lay the patient down

869. Which of the following locations are common sites to evaluate a patient's pulse rate?
    1. Carotid artery
    2. Brachial artery
    3. Radial artery

(A) 1 & 2
(B) 2 & 3
(C) 1 & 3
(D) 1, 2, & 3

870. The average respiration rate for the average adult is

(A) 6 to 10 times a minute
(B) 8 to 16 times a minute
(C) 12 to 20 times a minute
(D) 18 to 26 times a minute

871. When a patient hyperventilates, why is it recommended to have the patient breathe into a paper bag?

(A) It forces slower breathing
(B) It forces faster breathing
(C) It helps elevate the carbon dioxide level in the blood
(D) It helps to lower the carbon dioxide level in the blood

872. A sphygmomanometer is used to evaluate a patient's

(A) body temperature
(B) respiration rate
(C) pulse rate
(D) blood pressure

873. When should one evaluate a patient's respiration rate?

(A) While explaining the exam to the patient
(B) While listening to the patient describe the complaint
(C) While taking the patient's blood pressure
(D) At the conclusion of taking the patient's pulse

874. A *nosocomial* infection is one that

(A) interferes with sleep patterns
(B) is acquired during hospitalization
(C) occurs primarily in young children
(D) requires isolation in order to treat it

875. The hepatitis B virus is primarily transmitted by

(A) blood
(B) air
(C) food
(D) water

876. How is the human immunodeficiency virus (HIV) transmitted?
  1. Air
  2. Body fluids
  3. Contaminated objects

(A) 1 & 2
(B) 2 only
(C) 1 & 3
(D) 3 only

877. A contaminated object that may act as a source of disease transmission is termed a

(A) host
(B) fomite
(C) vector
(D) spore

878. The basic principle of the "universal precautions" policy recommended by the Centers for Disease Control (CDC) requires the

(A) wearing of gloves, a mask, and a protective apron when interacting with all patients
(B) disclosure of all persons infected with HIV
(C) testing of all health care providers for HIV infection
(D) treatment of all patients as a potential source of infection

879. Which of the following are components of a universal precautions policy?
  1. Wash hands between patients
  2. Isolate HIV-infected patients
  3. Use a barrier (e.g., gloves, mask) whenever contact with body substances is probable

(A) 1 & 2
(B) 2 & 3
(C) 1 & 3
(D) 1, 2, & 3

880. How frequently should radiographic tables be cleaned to reduce the potential of disease transmission?

(A) After each patient
(B) Only if the surface is soiled by the patient
(C) Three times a day, regardless of conditions
(D) Never, these surfaces do not act as a source of disease transmission

881. If there is a potential for the radiographer to be splashed by body fluids during a procedure, what precautions should be taken?
  1. Wear gloves
  2. Wear mask and eye protection
  3. Ask patient if he or she is HIV-infected

(A) 1 & 2
(B) 2 & 3
(C) 1 & 3
(D) 1, 2, & 3

882. Mosquitoes and ticks can be a source of disease transmission known as

(A) fomites
(B) hosts
(C) vectors
(D) pathogens

883. The human immunodeficiency virus (HIV) is the cause of which infectious disease?

(A) Hepatitis B
(B) Acquired immunodeficiency syndrome (AIDS)
(C) Pneumonia
(D) Malaria

884. Which aseptic technique is required for surgical procedures and equipment?

(A) Cleanliness
(B) Disinfection
(C) Sterilization
(D) Immunization

885. What procedure should be followed regarding reuse of disposable equipment or supplies?

(A) Thoroughly wash the used items between patients
(B) Sterilize disposable materials after use
(C) Be sure all disposable items are used by the same patient
(D) Do not reuse disposable materials

886. What method of disease transmission is responsible for infection of a radiographer following an accidental needle stick?

(A) Fomite
(B) Vector
(C) Direct contact
(D) Air-borne transmission

887. The sterilization process considered most effective is

(A) moist heat applied through boiling
(B) steam heat under pressure
(C) dry heat
(D) freezing

888. Which of the following is the most effective aseptic technique that all health care providers should employ?

(A) Use of a mask when in contact with any patient
(B) Frequent, thorough hand washing
(C) Employment of isolation techniques at all times
(D) Use of eye protection when in contact with any patient infected with hepatitis B

889. What should you do if you suspect a sterile field has been contaminated?

(A) Cover the contaminated area with a sterile cloth
(B) Record the event on an incident report
(C) Discard the old field and set up a new one
(D) Nothing, sterile fields cannot be contaminated

890. Proper hand-washing technique includes which of the following steps?
  1. Wet hands, apply soap, rub hands together vigorously
  2. Keep hands higher than elbows while washing and drying
  3. Use paper towels to turn faucets off when finished

(A) 1 & 2
(B) 2 & 3
(C) 1 & 3
(D) 1, 2, & 3

891. When a patient with a chest tube arrives for a chest x-ray procedure, what precaution must be taken?

(A) Maintain tension on the tube extending from the patient's chest
(B) Keep the drainage system higher than the patient's chest
(C) Keep the drainage system lower than the patient's chest
(D) Remove the tube from the patient before making exposure

892. What action should be taken by the radiographer if a patient's IV fluid runs out while the patient is in the radiology department?

(A) Turn IV off
(B) Remove IV from the patient
(C) Call for nursing assistance
(D) No action is necessary

893. What precautions must be taken when dealing with a patient with a Foley catheter in place?

(A) Disconnect the drainage bag from the catheter
(B) Maintain the position of the drainage bag lower than the bladder
(C) Maintain the position of the drainage bag higher than the bladder
(D) Maintain the position of the drainage bag level with the bladder

894. If an intensive care patient equipped with an endotracheal tube, chest drainage tube, and Foley catheter is scheduled for a chest radiograph, which objects may be identified on the image?

      1. Endotracheal tube
      2. Chest tube
      3. Foley catheter

(A) 1 & 2
(B) 2 & 3
(C) 1 & 3
(D) 1, 2, & 3

895. Which of the following steps are routinely included in the preparation of a patient for a barium enema?

      1. Clear liquid diet for a 24-hour period before the scheduled exam
      2. Administration of laxatives the day before the exam
      3. Administration of muscle relaxants prior to beginning the exam

(A) 1 & 2
(B) 2 & 3
(C) 1 & 3
(D) 1, 2, & 3

896. What instructions should be given to a patient following an exam using barium sulfate?

(A) Increase fluid intake
(B) Decrease fluid intake
(C) Remain NPO until all barium is eliminated
(D) Use a cleansing enema

897. Patients who experience cramping during an enema procedure should be instructed to

(A) hold their breath and bear down (Valsalva)
(B) take slow, deep breaths
(C) increase their breathing rate
(D) curl into a fetal position on their side

898. What action, if any, should the radiographer take to ease a patient's cramping during an enema procedure?

(A) Raise the enema bag
(B) Lower the enema bag
(C) Stop the flow of liquid
(D) No action taken by the radiographer will relieve cramps

899. Which of the following steps are routinely included in the preparation of a patient for an upper gastrointestinal series?

      1. Clear liquid diet and laxatives the day before the scheduled exam
      2. NPO for 8 to 10 h before the exam
      3. No smoking or gum chewing 8 to 10 h before the exam

(A) 1 & 2
(B) 2 & 3
(C) 1 & 3
(D) 1, 2, & 3

900. The basic instructions for preparation of a patient for an intravenous urogram (IVU) include:

      1. Clear liquid diet the day before the exam
      2. Administration of diuretic drugs the day before the exam
      3. Administration of laxatives or cleansing enemas

(A) 1 & 2
(B) 2 & 3
(C) 1 & 3
(D) 1, 2, & 3

901. If the following series of radiologic exams are to be performed on the same patient, in what order should they be scheduled?

      1. UGI
      2. BE
      3. IVU

(A) 1, 2, 3
(B) 2, 3, 1
(C) 3, 1, 2
(D) 3, 2, 1

902. Which of the following patients should be scheduled to have the first radiographic exam?

(A) Elderly patient for a chest radiograph
(B) Diabetic patient for an IVU
(C) Child for a UGI
(D) Adult for a UGI

903. Which of the following is an advantage of using a nonionic, water-soluble iodinated contrast medium over its ionic counterpart?

(A) It is less expensive
(B) It is less likely to cause an allergic reaction
(C) It may be injected IM as well as IV
(D) It has higher osmolality

904. The likelihood of an allergic reaction is greatest following the administration of

(A) barium sulfate
(B) nonionic, water-soluble iodine
(C) ionic, water-soluble iodine
(D) oil-based iodine

905. A patient with a contrast medium reaction presents with symptoms of nausea and vomiting and a warm sensation. This would be classified as what type of reaction?

(A) Mild
(B) Moderate
(C) Severe

906. What characteristic of barium and iodine contributes to their effectiveness as contrast agents?

(A) Low atomic number
(B) High atomic number
(C) Low molecular density
(D) High molecular density

907. For which radiographic procedure would an iodized oil be the only type of contrast medium used?

(A) Myelography
(B) IVU
(C) Angiography
(D) Lymphangiography

908. Which drug would be administered to a patient having a contrast media reaction that manifests as widespread or giant hives?

(A) Anticoagulant
(B) Antihistamine
(C) Anesthetic
(D) Bronchodilator

909. For which symptom would epinephrine (Adrenalin) be the drug of choice?

(A) Hives
(B) Nausea or vomiting
(C) Bleeding
(D) Respiratory distress

910. What type of medical intervention should be applied if a patient has a contrast media reaction involving dizziness, nausea, and vomiting?

(A) Reassure patient, observe for other changes
(B) Call physician for administration of medications
(C) Call for immediate emergency assistance (i.e., code blue)
(D) Instruct patient to breathe into a paper bag

911. How can a radiographer assess a patient for the probability of having a contrast media reaction?

(A) Note the patient's general health status
(B) Ask how much the patient weighs
(C) Ask the radiologist
(D) Ask the patient for a history of allergies

912. Each of the following questions would be useful in assessing a patient for potential allergic reaction to iodine contrast media EXCEPT:

(A) Do you have allergies to foods?
(B) Do you have hay fever?
(C) Are you pregnant?
(D) Have you had an iodine type of contrast medium previously?

913. *Extravasation* refers to

(A) a syndrome involving nausea and vomiting, dizziness, and weakness
(B) respiratory and cardiac arrest
(C) leakage of contrast media from a vein into the tissues
(D) a nose bleed

914. Which of the following methods of administering medications require the use of a needle and syringe?
   1. Sublingual
   2. Subcutaneous
   3. Intravenous

   (A) 1 & 2
   (B) 2 & 3
   (C) 1 & 3
   (D) 1, 2, & 3

915. The *gauge* of a hypodermic needle refers to

   (A) its length
   (B) its diameter
   (C) its strength
   (D) the number of times it can be used

916. If, during intravenous injection, the patient complains of pain and swelling is observed at the needle site, what has most likely occurred?

   (A) Vasovagal reaction
   (B) Extravasation
   (C) Venipuncture
   (D) Allergic reaction

917. How is a bolus intravenous injection of contrast media administered?

   (A) Slowly over a specified period of time
   (B) Rapidly in quarters of the total dose
   (C) Rapidly in a single dose
   (D) By the drip infusion method

918. Before any IV injection is administered, what must be verified?
   1. Verify the contents of the syringe
   2. Verify the patient identification
   3. Verify the physician's order

   (A) 1 & 2
   (B) 2 & 3
   (C) 1 & 3
   (D) 1, 2, & 3

919. What factors should be examined on the label of a solution to be given via an intravenous injection?
   1. Name of the medication
   2. Possible side effects
   3. Expiration date

   (A) 1 & 2
   (B) 2 & 3
   (C) 1 & 3
   (D) 1, 2, & 3

920. When transferring a patient from a portable oxygen source to a fixed wall outlet in the radiographic room, what factor must be determined?

   (A) Patient's need to be suctioned first
   (B) The type of oxygen appliance to change to
   (C) Quantity of oxygen available from the wall source
   (D) Oxygen flow rate set on portable tank

921. When it appears that a patient may need cardiopulmonary resuscitation, the first step a rescuer should take is to

   (A) determine if there is a pulse
   (B) open the airway
   (C) check for injuries to the arms and legs
   (D) establish unresponsiveness in the patient

922. When performing CPR, the proper site to palpate for a pulse in an adult victim is the

   (A) antecubital fossa
   (B) carotid artery
   (C) radial artery
   (D) femoral artery

923. The correct method for performing cardiac compressions during CPR requires the

   (A) rescuer to straddle the victim's supine body
   (B) rescuer's hands to be positioned one on top the other on the victim's upper sternum
   (C) rescuer to lean directly over victim with arms extended and elbows locked
   (D) rescuer to press down on victim's sternum in a rapid, jerky motion

924. In comparison to an adult, chest compressions on a child or infant should

(A) be performed at a slower rate
(B) be performed from the prone position
(C) compress the sternum less deeply
(D) compress the sternum more deeply

925. The Heimlich maneuver should be employed when

(A) the victim has no pulse or breathing
(B) the victim has an obstructed airway
(C) the victim has a pulse but is not breathing
(D) responsiveness in the victim must be established

926. Under what conditions should CPR be discontinued?

1. When rescuer is too tired to continue
2. When so instructed by a physician
3. When a pulse is reestablished

(A) 1 & 2
(B) 2 & 3
(C) 1 & 3
(D) 1, 2, & 3

927. Incorrectly performed CPR can cause

(A) the blood to flow in the wrong direction
(B) the patient to go into shock
(C) injuries to the thorax or abdomen
(D) an increase in intracranial pressure

928. Which type of surface is appropriate for performing effective CPR on an adult victim?

(A) Very soft
(B) Moderately soft
(C) Very firm
(D) Any type of surface is appropriate

929. Before initiating chest compressions, a rescuer should check for the absence of a pulse for

(A) 2 to 5 s
(B) 5 to 10 s
(C) 10 to 20 s
(D) 20 to 30 s

930. The correct cycle of chest compressions and ventilations for one person performing CPR on an adult would be

(A) 5 compressions, 1 breath
(B) 5 compressions, 2 breaths
(C) 15 compressions, 1 breath
(D) 15 compressions, 2 breaths

931. A patient who is experiencing syncope has

(A) a nosebleed
(B) a faint
(C) dizziness
(D) uncontrolled bleeding

932. The protective garments that should be routinely worn by a radiographer when radiographing a patient on respiratory precautions include

(A) gown and mask
(B) gloves and gown
(C) gloves only
(D) mask only

933. The minimum number of persons required to perform a radiographic exam on a patient in strict isolation is

(A) one
(B) two
(C) three
(D) four

934. A blood pressure of 130/80 mmHg specifically indicates a

(A) diastolic pressure of 130
(B) diastolic pressure of 80
(C) diastolic pressure of 50
(D) systolic pressure of 80

935. A slower than average pulse rate is termed

(A) bradycardia
(B) tachycardia
(C) hypertension
(D) hypotension

936. The type of fracture most likely to occur following blunt trauma to the skull is

(A) transverse
(B) spiral
(C) impacted
(D) depressed

937. A Colles' type of fracture would be revealed during a radiographic exam of the

 (A) ankle
 (B) hip
 (C) wrist
 (D) shoulder

938. Which of the following is the correct description of the type of fracture known as an *avulsion*?

 (A) Bone shatters into multiple fragments
 (B) One part of the bone is forced into the other part
 (C) Bone is incompletely fractured
 (D) Bone pieces are pulled away from the main bone

939. For which type of medical emergency should a pillow be placed under the patient's head?

 (A) Patient in need of rescue breathing
 (B) Patient in need of CPR
 (C) Unconscious patient with an obstructed airway
 (D) Patient having a seizure

940. If a trauma patient arrives for a radiographic procedure wearing a splint or other temporary immobilization device, how should the radiographer proceed to perform the required exam?

 (A) Completely remove the immobilization device for the exam
 (B) Partially remove the immobilization device for the exam
 (C) Leave the immobilization device in place for the exam
 (D) Ask the supervisor for instructions

941. How should proper positioning of the lower limb be handled when positioning a trauma patient for hip radiographs?

 (A) No one should attempt to manipulate the affected limb
 (B) Slowly and gently rotate the affected limb medially
 (C) Slowly and gently rotate the affected limb laterally
 (D) A physician should manipulate the affected limb

942. For the patient with an injury to the cervical spine, what radiographic exam should be performed first?

 (A) Supine chest radiograph
 (B) Supine AP cervical spine, including C1–7
 (C) Erect lateral of cervical spine with weights to depress shoulders
 (D) Lateral projection of cervical spine with horizontal x-ray beam

943. Which of the following correctly states the method for obtaining images of the cervical spine in the oblique position on a patient with injury to the cervical spine?

 (A) From the supine recumbent position, rotate the patient's whole body 45° and direct the central ray 15° caudad to C4
 (B) From the prone recumbent position, rotate the patient's whole body 45° and direct the central ray 15° cephalad to C4
 (C) With the patient in the supine recumbent position, direct the central ray 45° medially and 15° cephalad to C4
 (D) With the patient in the prone recumbent position, direct the central ray 45° medially and 15° caudad to C4

944. Which rule must be applied when radiographing an extremity on a trauma patient?

 (A) Obtain two projections at right angles to each other
 (B) Remove immobilization devices to prevent superimposition
 (C) Obtain images of the opposite extremity for comparison
 (D) Include the joint furthest from injury on long bones

945. Which statement expresses the optimum method for palpation during patient positioning?

 (A) Use both hands to ensure accuracy
 (B) Use the palmar surface of one hand only
 (C) Use the second through fifth fingers of one hand only
 (D) Use 1 or 2 fingers of one hand only

946. Characteristics that apply to *negative* types of contrast media include:
  1. May be administered intravenously
  2. Easily penetrated by x-rays
  3. Appear as areas of increased density

  (A) 1 & 2
  (B) 2 & 3
  (C) 1 & 3
  (D) 1, 2, & 3

947. Diabetic patients who have fasted for a radiologic procedure may suddenly exhibit symptoms of excessive sweating, nervousness, and weakness that indicate

  (A) diabetic coma
  (B) hypoglycemia
  (C) hyperglycemia
  (D) anaphylactic shock

948. Which medical emergency is most likely occurring when a patient is seen clutching his or her throat?

  (A) Heart attack
  (B) Obstructed airway
  (C) Vertigo
  (D) Syncope

949. The correct method for administering rescue breathing to an adult victim is to deliver a

  (A) forceful, quick breath every 5 s
  (B) forceful, quick breath every 3 s
  (C) gentle, slow breath every 5 s
  (D) gentle, slow breath every 3 s

950. Which of the following are types of immobilization devices?

  (A) Tape, compression bands, grids
  (B) Compression bands, sandbags, velcro straps
  (C) Sandbags, slider boards, tape
  (D) Cassette holder, slider board, head clamps

951. Which of the following are useful in immobilizing infants or very young children for a radiographic exam?
  1. Stockinette
  2. Sheets
  3. Provision of clear instructions

  (A) 1 & 2
  (B) 2 & 3
  (C) 1 & 3
  (D) 1, 2, & 3

952. Who should sign an informed consent form for a radiologic procedure?
  1. Patient or responsible person
  2. Referring physician
  3. Witness

  (A) 1 & 2
  (B) 2 & 3
  (C) 1 & 3
  (D) 1, 2, & 3

953. Which of the following procedures require the use of surgical aseptic techniques?
  1. Myelography
  2. Barium enema
  3. Angiography

  (A) 1 & 2
  (B) 2 & 3
  (C) 1 & 3
  (D) 1, 2, & 3

954. How should a radiographer verify a patient's identity prior to performing a radiologic exam?

  (A) Check the chart that arrived with the patient
  (B) Check the patient's wrist band
  (C) Call out the patient's name
  (D) Check the label on the patient's IV medication

955. Which of the following conditions may require protective isolation precautions due to the patient's reduced immune status?

    1. Burn patients
    2. Organ donors
    3. Chemotherapy patients

(A) 1 & 2
(B) 2 & 3
(C) 1 & 3
(D) 1, 2, & 3

956. When putting on sterile gloves, what part of the glove, if any, may be touched by the ungloved hand?

(A) The palmar surface of the glove
(B) Under the folded cuff of the glove
(C) The inside surface of the glove
(D) No part of the glove may be touched

957. What action should a radiographer take to reduce the occurrence of postural hypotension?

(A) Keep patient's head lower than feet
(B) Keep patient's head higher than feet
(C) Sit patient up slowly from a recumbent position
(D) Stand patient up quickly from a recumbent position

958. Which of the following procedures employs the *Seldinger* technique for catheterization?

(A) Percutaneous transhepatic cholangiography
(B) Cystography
(C) Endoscopic retrograde cholangiopancreatography (ERCP)
(D) Angiography

959. The BUN and creatinine levels in a patient's blood will provide an indication of what physiologic function?

(A) Liver function
(B) Renal function
(C) Coagulation factor
(D) Pulmonary function

960. What types of contrast media are commonly used for enhancement during CT imaging?

    1. Barium sulfate
    2. Air
    3. Oily iodine
    4. Water-soluble iodine

(A) 1 & 2
(B) 2 & 3
(C) 3 & 4
(D) 1 & 4

961. Which imaging modalities do NOT employ ionizing radiation?

(A) Nuclear medicine and ultrasound
(B) Magnetic resonance imaging and single photon emission computed tomography
(C) Single photon emission computed tomography and nuclear medicine
(D) Ultrasound and magnetic resonance imaging

962. What instructions, if any, should be given to a patient following a myelogram in which water-soluble iodine contrast media were used?

(A) Remain in a completely supine position
(B) Remain seated in a completely upright position (upper body at 90° angle to lower body)
(C) Remain in a semierect position, head elevated 20 to 30°
(D) No specific instructions regarding position are required

963. Which of the following is true regarding myelography using water-soluble iodinated contrast media?

(A) The contrast medium must be removed at the conclusion of the exam
(B) The contrast medium begins to be absorbed within 30 min following injection
(C) This medium provides poor visualization of the nerve roots compared with oily iodinated agents
(D) This procedure requires the patient to remain in a completely supine position following the exam

964. Which radiographic procedure may be performed for its *therapeutic* value as well as its *diagnostic* capability?

(A) Myelography
(B) Hysterosalpingography
(C) Arthrography
(D) Lymphography

965. Arthrography is performed on which of the following types of joints?
    1. Synarthrotic
    2. Amphiarthrotic
    3. Diarthrotic

(A) 2 only
(B) 1 & 2
(C) 2 & 3
(D) 3 only

966. The preferred method for imaging joints such as the knee and shoulder is

(A) discography
(B) MRI
(C) CT
(D) arthrography

967. A patient who is showing "cyanotic" changes is most likely experiencing

(A) a lack of oxygen
(B) increased BP
(C) a rapid pulse
(D) a need to void

DIRECTIONS: Each group of questions below consists of lettered headings followed by a set of numbered items. For each numbered item select the **one** lettered heading with which it is **most** closely associated. Each lettered heading may be used **once, more than once, or not at all**.

Questions 968–970

Identify the type of unethical behavior or violation of a patient's rights that would occur as a result of the actions stated in each question.

    (A)   Invasion of privacy
    (B)   False imprisonment
    (C)   Failure to provide informed consent
    (D)   Battery on a patient

968.   Performing an exam on the wrong patient

969.   Breach of patient confidentiality

970.   Detaining or inhibiting a patient from departing the department or hospital

Questions 971–976

Identify the patient position described in the following questions.

    (A)   Fowler position
    (B)   Sims position
    (C)   Trendelenburg
    (D)   Ventral decubitus

971.   The patient's head is positioned about 30° lower than the body and legs

972.   The patient is in the left lateral position with the right leg flexed and placed in front of the left leg

973.   This position should be used when a patient feels faint

974.   The patient's head and knees are elevated from the completely flat supine position

975.   This position should be used when a patient is having difficulty breathing

976.   The position used for the insertion of an enema tip

Questions 977–981

Identify the most appropriate type of contrast medium for the radiologic procedures stated in each question.

    (A)   Barium sulfate
    (B)   Water-soluble iodine
    (C)   Air
    (D)   Iodized oils

977.   Angiography of any blood vessel

978.   Routine upper gastrointestinal series

979.   Lymphography

980.   Radiolucent effect on double-contrast lower gastrointestinal series

981.   Upper gastrointestinal series on a patient suspected of having a perforated ulcer

Questions 982–986

For each of the stated physiologic conditions, indicate the level of severity, if any, it presents as a possible allergic reaction to the IV administration of water-soluble iodine contrast media.

    (A)   Mild
    (B)   Moderate
    (C)   Severe
    (D)   Not an allergic reaction

982.   Anaphylactic shock

983.   Sweating

984.   Hemorrhage

985.   Tachycardia

986.   Convulsion

Questions 987–990

Identify the type of emergency medical situation described in each question.

(A) Shock
(B) Cardiac arrest
(C) Respiratory distress
(D) Head injury

987. Increased intracranial pressure

988. Drop in blood pressure due to extensive blood loss

989. Partial or complete obstructed airway

990. Lack of a pulse

Questions 991–996

Identify the imaging modality described in each question.

(A) Ultrasound
(B) Nuclear medicine
(C) Magnetic resonance imaging
(D) Computed tomography
(E) Mammography

991. The procedure that requires dedicated equipment to image the subtle differences of soft tissue structures

992. The procedure that is frequently employed to determine fetal gestational age

993. The technique that employs ionizing radiation to obtain cross-sectional images

994. The modality that employs nonionizing radio frequencies to stimulate a tissue sample to generate a signal in the same electromagnetic frequency range

995. The modality that uses equipment capable of detecting ionizing radiation rather than emitting it

996. The modality that primarily records the image directly on film rather than via computer-assisted imaging techniques

Questions 997–1000

Indicate the radiologic procedure most accurately referred to by each of the statements.

(A) Sialography
(B) Myelography
(C) Arthrography
(D) Lymphography
(E) Hysterosalpingography

997. The exam that requires the use of a true "dye"

998. The exam that requires the removal of the contrast media from the opacified structure at the conclusion of the exam

999. The exam that is most commonly performed using double-contrast media (positive and negative types)

1000. The exam that begins in a fluoroscopic room with the introduction of the contrast media and preliminary filming and then frequently is concluded with CT imaging before the contrast media is lost

Patient Care

Answers

851. The answer is A (1, 2). *(Adler, pp 350–351. Ehrlich, 4/e, p 17.)* The purpose of an informed consent document is to protect patients from being subjected to medical procedures of which they were not thoroughly informed. The components of informed consent include a complete explanation of the procedure to be performed, including the possible risks associated with the exam, and an opportunity for the patient to ask questions or consult other family members before the onset of the exam. This document does not, however, relieve the hospital of responsibility for any negligent action or malpractice on the part of employees attending the patient.

852. The answer is D. *(Adler, pp 350–351. Ehrlich, 4/e, p 17.)* The intention of the consent form is to document that the coherent patient has had the procedure explained and was allowed an opportunity to ask questions before the exam was initiated. Patients are instructed to read all parts of the consent form and then sign it as a means of verifying that they have been informed of the actions that will take place and any possible risks associated with the procedure. The patient may decide against having the exam at any time before or after completing the consent form.

853. The answer is C (1, 3). *(Adler, pp 327–329. Ehrlich, 4/e, p 17.)* A patient's right to privacy while having a medical exam includes such issues as protecting a patient's modesty before, during, and after a procedure; providing health care professionals of the same sex as the patient, especially if the patient requests such, during exams that may be of a sensitive nature; obtaining the patient's permission to have any unnecessary personnel attending the exam, including students of any type; and ensuring confidentiality in regard to a patient's personal information of any type. Explaining the exam and its risk factors is considered part of the patient's right of informed consent for medical procedures.

854. The answer is A. *(Ehrlich, 4/e, p 18.)* The decision to limit medical treatment, particularly in the case of a terminally ill patient, may be made by the patient and conveyed to all parties involved through a living will. This type of action is generally made by a competent adult to ensure that his or her wishes are met. Family members may make the decision to limit treatment for those patients who are incompetent (e.g., unconscious). The medical staff may be consulted in the decision-making process, but may not make such a decision on their own.

855. The answer is D. *(Bontrager, 3/e, p 43. Ehrlich, 4/e, pp 10–11, 18.)* The code of ethics for the radiographer as developed by the American Society of Radiologic Technologists addresses not only patient safety issues, but the proper use and care of equipment provided by the hospital/clinic for the purpose of performing radiographic procedures. This includes appropriate utilization of radiographic equipment as well as supplies, all of which are hospital property.

856. The answer is B. *(Adler, p 349. Ehrlich, 4/e, p 21.)* The radiographer (or any health care professional) is responsible for providing reasonable care and caution to each patient in his or her charge. Failure to do so is the basis for a charge of negligence and may also constitute malpractice. The term "reasonable" is used to indicate the expected action by a radiographer in a similar situation. The code of ethics published by the American Society of Radiologic Technologists may be used to indicate the expected level of behavior for radiographers.

857. The answer is D (1, 2, 3). *(Adler, pp 123–125. Ehrlich, 4/e, pp 29–31.)* The radiographer communicates with the patient in a variety of ways, including the three mentioned in the question. Good verbal communication skills are important for instructing and reassuring the patient throughout the course of an exam. Nonverbal communication must also be considered. The radiographer should face and look at patients while talking to them and present a calm, pleasant manner toward them. Included in this is the manner in which a patient is touched by the radiographer. Whether as part of positioning the patient for the exam or when offering comfort and reassurance, the patient should not be subjected to roughness or inappropriate touching. The appearance of the radiographer and the exam/waiting rooms to which the patient is exposed is another form of communication. Disorderly facilities or persons do not instill a sense of confidence; an organized and clean environment and staff do.

858. The answer is B. *(Adler, pp 127–128. Ehrlich, 4/e, p 36.)* The assistance of an interpreter would be the best way of communicating with a patient who does not speak the same language as the radiographer. Trained interpreters are particularly helpful and will translate what is being said most accurately. Family members may be helpful and should be asked to assist if no interpreter is available; however, they may have language difficulties themselves or may not repeat the instructions as accurately as they should. The use of pictures or demonstrations by the radiographer is useful when interpreters are not available, but may be time-consuming and limited by the nature of the patient's condition. Talking louder is completely illogical when a language difference is the problem.

859. The answer is B. *(Adler, p 127. Ehrlich, 4/e, p 38.)* Successful communication with patients who are hearing-impaired requires that the speaker be sure to have the patient's attention and face the patient when speaking. The radiographer should also speak clearly so that words do not run together. The loss of hearing is generally in the upper registers of sounds, so lowering the pitch while speaking louder may also be successful. Hearing-impaired persons need to be fully informed as to the procedure and possible risks involved; therefore, it is just as important to communicate with them as with any other patient. Be patient and open to trying various methods of communication with all patients.

860. The answer is A. *(Adler, p 127. Ehrlich, 4/e, p 40.)* Unconscious patients may be able to hear and remember what is said while they are in an unconscious state, even though they are unable to respond. For this reason, it is important to treat all patients with respect and dignity. When performing radiographic procedures on these patients, continue to use their name and explain what is being done to them. Speak to the patient in a normal voice.

861. The answer is D. *(Ehrlich, 4/e, pp 54–55.)* The large quantity of electrical equipment found in the typical radiology department provides the most common source for the outbreak of fire in the department. There is no reason for the existence of an open flame in the radiology department. More and more health care facilities are becoming "smoke-free" as a means of promoting healthier life styles, thus reducing the likelihood of fires being caused by smokers. Spontaneous combustion most commonly is caused by improper storage of flammable materials, such as cleaning or paint products. Regardless of the source of fire, prevention and readiness policies are commonplace in radiology departments. All personnel must be aware of proper procedures in the event of a fire. Departments should also contain the appropriate fire-fighting equipment, such as class C extinguishers, which contain carbon dioxide or Halon for handling electrical fires. Regular fire drills and annual inservice programs on the facility's fire safety policy are recommended.

862. The answer is A. *(Ehrlich, 4/e, pp 62–63.)* The use of proper body mechanics to move heavy objects or persons is necessary to avoid personal injury or injury to a patient. When possible, a heavy object should be pushed, using the strong muscles of the thighs. This technique is not useful for patient transfers as it would most likely be uncomfortable or injurious for the patient.

863. The answer is A. *(Adler, pp 143, 148. Ehrlich, 4/e, pp 61–62.)* Proper body mechanics for the safe lifting of heavy objects requires a wide base of support for the lifter and the center of gravity of the object close to the lifter's base of support. To achieve the best base of support, the lifter should stand with legs apart and knees slightly bent. This position improves stability. The center of gravity is an imaginary point within the person or object that represents the greatest concentration of mass. The lifter must stand as close as possible to the person or object in order to align the center of gravity over the base of support. The lifting should then be done using the leg muscles and keeping the back straight.

864. The answer is B. *(Adler, p 143. Ehrlich, 4/e, pp 61–71.)* The use of proper body mechanics is recommended in order to reduce the chance of personal injury from lifting patients. Many patients require assistance in getting onto or off an x-ray table or even in lying down and getting up again. Radiographers are at risk for back injury if they do not use their body correctly. They also risk injury to the patient. Before lifting any patient, the radiographer should talk with the patient and assess the patient's chart for the possibility of the patient's moving without assistance. Some patients may only require minimal assistance in terms of guidance or assurance against falls during the move. If a patient requires more assistance than a single person can provide, the radiographer should enlist the aid of other personnel.

865. The answer is B. *(Adler, pp 153, 157. Ehrlich, 4/e, pp 67–71.)* The transfer of a patient from the stretcher to the x-ray table may be done by one person who can guide the ambulatory patient, with the assistance of an accessory moving device, or by the lifting of the patient by more than one person or with a mechanical device. In order to safely transfer a patient, the stretcher must be positioned alongside and against the x-ray table, and the wheels locked. For patients able to move themselves, the radiographer may assist by acting as a guide or by helping to move a restricted part of the patient, e.g., a casted extremity. Two or more people should be available if the patient must be lifted. A transfer device, such as a slider board or mechanical lift device, may also be available to assist in moving patients. Patients arriving on a stretcher should not be allowed to get off the stretcher even if they think they are up to it.

866. The answer is A (1, 2). *(Adler, pp 153, 157. Ehrlich, 4/e, pp 67–71.)* The use of a slider board is an acceptable means of transferring a patient from the stretcher to the x-ray table. This device is made of plastic and is positioned under a sheet that is under the patient. It provides a bridge between the stretcher and the table, and the movers are able to push/pull the patient, using the sheet, across the slider board and safely onto the table. The slider may then be removed or left in place during the radiographic exam. When a slider board is not available, the patient must actually be lifted by two or more persons using the draw sheet under the patient's chest and abdomen. With movers on both sides of the table, the draw sheet is rolled up close to the patient's body. One person should indicate the appropriate time for movement of the patient and the lifters should act as a unit. Proper care must be taken with the patient's head, neck, and legs. Transfer of a patient by means of a log roll (patient rolls or is rolled onto the stomach then back from stretcher to table) is not recommended as it can be hard on the patient and further limited if an IV line, oxygen support, or catheter is in place.

867. The answer is C. *(Ehrlich, 4/e, pp 71–74.)* When a patient is lying in a supine position on the x-ray table with the legs extended, the lordotic curve of the lower back is accentuated. Most patients would find this position very uncomfortable, especially elderly or heavily arthritic persons. Providing relief from this stress will aid in the patient's ability to tolerate and cooperate during the exam. The few minutes it takes to be sure the patient is comfortable will make the exam go smoother for all parties. Patients who are restless or uncooperative may need to be restrained to keep them from rolling off the table.

868. The answer is D. *(Adler, p 269. Ehrlich, 4/e, p 85.)* A patient who suddenly becomes weak and pale may be close to fainting and should be placed in a recumbent position as quickly as possible. This will prevent more significant injury should the patient fall as a result of fainting. In addition, the patient's feet should be elevated to assist in increasing blood flow to the brain. The application of a cool, wet cloth to the forehead will also assist in comforting the patient. These patients should not be left alone and must be carefully monitored for further changes in their condition.

869. The answer is D (1, 2, 3). *(Adler, pp 183–184. American Red Cross, p 119. Ehrlich, 4/e, pp 89–90.)* Evaluation of a patient's pulse rate is readily possible by palpating a superficial artery for the presence of a pulsed wave as blood is pumped from the heart through the arteries. For the average healthy person, this pulse wave is easily felt at the radial, carotid, and brachial arteries. The radial artery is located on the radial (thumb) side of the distal forearm. The carotid pulse may be found just below the angle of the mandible on either side of the trachea. The less often used brachial artery may be palpated in the antecubital fossa of either arm for the adult and on the underside of the upper arm, midway between the elbow and shoulder, on an infant. In emergency situations, two other locations for pulse evaluation are the femoral artery, located in the groin, and the apical pulse (using a stethoscope to listen to the heart itself).

870. The answer is C. *(Adler, p 181. Ehrlich, 4/e, pp 93–94.)* The average respiration rate for the healthy adult is in the range of 12 to 20 times a minute. One respiration is considered one inspiration and expiration. A lower than average breathing rate is termed *bradypnea*, while *tachypnea* refers to a rapid rate of breathing. The average respiration rate for young children is higher than adults, in the range of 20 to 30 respirations per minute. Monitoring of a person's respiration rate is done by discretely observing and counting the number of times the chest and abdomen rise and fall for a minimum period of 30 s (multiplied by 2 to equal the respiration rate). It is important to determine the patients' true respiration rate without alerting them and causing them to alter their breathing rate. Usually this is done at the conclusion of pulse taking, while still holding the patient's wrist. Patients with a shallow respiration pattern may be difficult to observe. In this case, the radiographer may need to place a hand on the patient's diaphragm to feel it rise and fall.

871. The answer is C. *(Ehrlich, 4/e, p 94. Mosby, 3/e, p 592.)* During normal respiration, a balanced exchange of oxygen and carbon dioxide gases is maintained as needed for metabolic activity. Hyperventilation (an increased rate of breathing) results in an increased intake of oxygen and a loss of carbon dioxide. If this condition is prolonged, the patient will become dizzy and may faint. To counter the effects of hyperventilation, the patient is instructed to breathe into a bag at a slow rate, thus rebreathing carbon dioxide and restoring the proper balance of these blood gases. There are many possible causes of hyperventilation, including emotional as well as physiologic factors.

872. The answer is D. *(Adler, pp 185–186. Ehrlich, 4/e, p 94.)* A person's blood pressure is determined with the use of a sphygmomanometer, also known as a *blood pressure cuff*, and a stethoscope. The sphygmomanometer includes an inflatable cuff that is wrapped around an arm or leg. A bulb is attached to the cuff to pump air into it, causing pressure on the artery underlying the cuff. A gauge is also connected. When the cuff is properly positioned on the upper arm, the stethoscope is placed over the brachial artery in the area of the antecubital fossa, and the cuff is inflated. The air is then slowly released from the cuff while one listens for a pulse. The point at which the pulse is first noted is correlated with the reading on the gauge to determine the systolic pressure. As the air in the cuff continues to be released, there will come a point when the pulse is no longer heard. The reading on the gauge is again noted and represents the diastolic pressure. The final result is stated in ratio form to indicate systolic pressure over diastolic pressure.

873. The answer is D. *(Adler, p 182. Ehrlich, 4/e, p 93.)* The monitoring of the patient's respiration rate should be done without the knowledge of the patient, so that the breathing will not be altered. Since this type of monitoring is generally achieved by watching the rise and fall of the chest and abdomen, it is easily performed after taking the patient's pulse. If you continue to hold the patient's wrist while observing the chest, the patient will assume the pulse is still being monitored. Patients who have a shallow breathing pattern may be hard to adequately observe. For these occasions, a hand may be placed on the diaphragm to feel for the rise and fall of the chest.

874. The answer is B. *(Adler, pp 203–204. Ehrlich, 4/e, p 103.)* *Nosocomial* infections are those acquired from the hospital or other health care facility. The fact that hospitals house a wide variety of patients with a wide variety of illnesses, including infectious diseases, means there is an increased likelihood of exposure to infections. The weakened condition of most patients' immune systems further increases the likelihood of acquiring such an infection. To reduce the transmission of infection within the hospital, particular attention to cleanliness of the facility is required. Also required is the knowledge and implementation of universal precautions by all personnel. Nosocomial infections can be caused by the transmission of bacteria, viruses, protozoa, or fungi and can manifest as such common illnesses as an upper respiratory infection, urinary tract infection, or the more serious conditions of infection caused by the hepatitis B or human immunodeficiency viruses. Patients and health care providers are equally at risk for nosocomial infections.

875. The answer is A. *(Adler, pp 204–205. Ehrlich, 4/e, pp 103–104. Laudicina, pp 90–91.)* The hepatitis B virus (HBV) is a blood-borne pathogen and is transmitted by direct contact with a contaminated blood source, such as transfusions, needle sticks, or wounds. Recent Occupational Safety and Health Administration (OSHA) regulations require health care workers to be vaccinated against hepatitis B in order to reduce their risk of infection. Further protection can be gained by implementation of the guidelines for universal precautions from the Centers for Disease Control (CDC), which are intended to reduce exposure to any blood-borne pathogen, including HBV and HIV.

876. The answer is B (2). *(Adler, p 204. American Red Cross, p 9. Ehrlich, 4/e, p 106. Mosby, 3/e, pp 1577–1579.)* HIV is a blood-borne pathogen and is transmitted by direct contact with infected body fluids during sexual contact, transfusion of contaminated blood, or sharing of contaminated needles or from mother to fetus in utero. Testing of blood and blood products has been available for some time, effectively reducing transfusions as a source of infection. Since no vaccine is presently available, the only way to prevent disease transmission is through the practice of universal precautions and avoidance of unsafe behavior (e.g., unprotected sex, sharing of hypodermic needles).

877. The answer is B. *(Adler, p 203. Ehrlich, 4/e, pp 103–105.)* Three indirect means of disease transmission are possible. These methods are *air-borne* transmission and transmission through carriers known as *fomites* and *vectors*. A fomite is any object or surface that has been contaminated with an infectious microorganism, such as utensils, catheters, the x-ray table, or faucets on a sink. To prevent objects from becoming fomites, proper storage, usage, disposal, and cleaning (sterilizing) of all materials that are likely to be contaminated must be done. A second type of carrier includes insects and animals that are referred to as vectors. Examples of vectors are raccoons, skunks, or dogs carrying rabies and deer ticks, which cause Lyme disease. A *host* is an animal or plant that provides favorable conditions for the growth of infectious organisms. The *spore* is a protective stage of the life cycle of an infectious microorganism that allows it to live outside the host in a dormant phase. It can easily revert to its active cycle of growth when returned to a favorable host environment.

878. The answer is D. *(Adler, pp 209–210. Ehrlich, 4/e, pp 106–107.)* "Universal precautions" is a plan of action recommended by the Centers for Disease Control (CDC) for the reduction of nosocomial infections by assuming all blood and body fluids are infected with a blood-borne pathogen. The specifics of this policy require the use of a barrier (e.g., gloves, masks, shields, aprons) whenever one is likely to be exposed to bodily substances. Health care providers must evaluate each patient with whom they come in contact to determine how extensive a barrier is needed for a particular exam. To approach every patient fully covered with gloves, mask, and apron may be overreactive and hinder the performance of the exam. Universal precautions further require the proper separation, identification, and disposal of any hazardous materials. A simple and primary practice of universal precautions is that of thorough and frequent hand washing. At this time, confidentiality rights of patients and health care workers prohibit the disclosure of an HIV or HBV diagnosis without the person's approval. Therefore, the likelihood of being exposed to an infected person within the health care setting should be considered high, further supporting the need for universal precautions.

879. The answer is C (1, 3). *(Adler, pp 209–210. Ehrlich, 4/e, pp 107–108. Mosby, 3/e, pp 1577–1586.)* The recommendations of the CDC for the implementation of universal precautions in the presence of blood and body fluids are meant to protect patients and personnel from accidental exposure to blood-borne pathogens. The specifics of this policy include the use of barriers (e.g., gloves, masks, shields, aprons) when body substances are present. The degree of barrier use is dependent on the quantity and type of body substance present. Also, health care providers are required to wash their hands before and after working with each patient. The correct and thorough compliance with these precautions precludes the need to isolate patients with known blood-borne pathogens. To isolate patients out of fear or prejudice is a violation of their right to fair and equal medical care.

880. The answer is A. *(Ballinger, 7/e, vol 1, p 7. Ehrlich, 4/e, p 111.)* Radiographic tables and upright film stands should be cleaned after each patient. Contaminated table surfaces can act as a fomite in the transmission of infectious microorganisms. Disinfectant cleaning products should be used to effectively eliminate the presence of any pathogens.

881. The answer is A. *(Mosby, 3/e, p 1578. Ehrlich, 4/e, p 108.)* Personnel involved in any procedure in which body fluids may be splashed into the mucous membranes of the mouth, nose, or eyes must wear a mask and eye protection or a face shield. These barriers are in addition to the gloves that must be worn any time body fluids are present. Patients and physicians will determine the extent of maintaining the confidentiality of the patients' HIV status. If it is not noted on any of the documents pertaining to the exam, the radiographer should not breach that confidentiality. If universal precautions are followed, there should be no need for any health care provider to be concerned.

882. The answer is C. *(Adler, p 203. Ehrlich, 4/e, p 105.)* The transmission of infectious pathogens can occur through direct contact with the microorganisms or indirectly via air-borne droplets of infectious material or via carriers. Two types of carriers are fomites and vectors. A fomite is any object contaminated by infectious material. Vectors are animals or insects that become infected and then pass it on to humans through bites. Dogs, skunks, and raccoons are likely vectors of rabies, while mosquitoes can transmit microorganisms that cause malaria and encephalitis. Bites from an infected deer tick are the source of Lyme disease.

883. The answer is B. *(Adler, pp 199, 204–205. Ehrlich, 4/e, p 106. Mosby, 3/e, pp 719, 933, 1577.)* The human immunodeficiency virus (HIV) has been identified as the cause of acquired immunodeficiency syndrome (AIDS). After a person is infected with HIV, the virus may have a latent period for as long as 10 years before symptoms appear. The virus is transmitted by the exchange of body fluids, such as through sexual contact or by contaminated blood as occurs with the sharing of used needles. To date, no effective cure or vaccine is available. Mortality is about 90 percent once symptoms begin to manifest. Prevention is the best advice. Health care workers are at risk for infection and should follow universal precautions to minimize their risk. Hepatitis B (caused by the hepatitis B virus) is another blood-borne pathogen for which health care workers are at risk and for which universal precautions should be applied. Vaccinations and treatments are available for hepatitis B. Malaria is an infectious disease transmitted by a bite from an infected mosquito or through infected blood. The actual source of the disease is a protozoan of the *Plasmodium* species. Pneumonia is an inflammation of the lungs due to infectious microorganisms (bacteria, viruses, or fungi). The pneumococcal bacterium is the most common source of pneumonia and is transmitted via ingestion of air-borne droplets.

884. The answer is C. *(Adler, pp 206-207. Ehrlich, 4/e, p 124.)* Aseptic techniques reduce or eliminate the presence of infectious microorganisms. Two types of asepsis are applied in the health care environment: medical and surgical. Medical asepsis is the reduction of microorganisms through such practices as cleaning and disinfection. General cleaning practices include dusting, floor washing, and trash disposal. Disinfection is achieved through the use of chemical agents capable of killing microorganisms and is part of the general cleaning process. These techniques are applied throughout a medical facility in an effort to minimize nosocomial infections. Surgical asepsis is the complete elimination of any pathogens through the process of sterilization. The open wounds present in the surgical environment allow for easy entrance of microorganisms into the body. Sterilization techniques are applied to the surgical room, equipment, and clothing of the personnel to prevent such easy transmission. The various methods of sterilization include boiling, dry heat, steam under pressure, gas, and chemical agents. The autoclaving process (steam under pressure) is the most widely used method.

885. The answer is D. *(Ehrlich, 4/e, pp 111–112.)* Disposable equipment and supplies are meant to be discarded after use. These materials are commonly used in health care facilities in order to reduce the transmission of infectious disease. Commonly available disposable items include needles, syringes, catheters, gloves, urinals, bedpans, emesis basins, and so on. Many items are supplied in packaging that maintains the sterility of the contents. Some nonsterile items, such as bedpans and emesis basins, may be reused by the same patient after cleaning, but should then be discarded.

886. The answer is A. *(Adler, pp 202–203. Ehrlich, 4/e, pp 104–105. Mosby, 3/e, pp 1582–1583.)* A used needle can act as a fomite if it contains infected blood and is accidentally stuck into any other person. For this reason, universal precautions recommend that needles be discarded along with the syringe in an approved puncture-resistant container rather than recapped. Accidental needle sticks can be a source of HIV or HBV infection for health care workers. If a needle stick should occur, an incident report must be filed. The CDC further recommends that health care facilities develop a policy for follow-up of workers who have been exposed to blood or body fluids. This should include identifying and testing (if permitted) of the patient; if testing is not possible, the worker should be monitored for HIV or HBV infection.

887. The answer is B. *(Adler, p 208. Ehrlich, 4/e, pp 125–126.)* The application of heat is the most common method of sterilization, with moist heat being more effective than dry heat. Moist heat can be applied through boiling objects or through steam. Autoclaving is the process of applying steam heat under pressure and is considered the most efficient method of sterilization for items that can tolerate it. This method is further preferred because it allows application of a reactive adhesive tape that acts as an indicator of sufficient temperature by changing color during the autoclaving process. Such indicators are not available for boiled or dry-heated materials. Sterilization by means of freezing can effectively kill pathogens, but not in a reliable manner.

888. The answer is B. *(Adler, p 217. Ehrlich, 4/e, p 108.)* The simplest and most effective means of minimizing the transmission of pathogens is the practice of frequent and thorough hand washing. Proper handwashing technique requires the hands to be wet before application of a liquid soap product. The hands should be vigorously rubbed together and the areas between the fingers and under the nails should be included in the washing. The hands are then rinsed, keeping them lower than the wrists and allowing the water to run down. The faucets should be turned off using paper towels to avoid recontamination from that source. Further protection practices require the wearing of gloves whenever one is likely to come in contact with body fluids. A mask and eye protection should be worn if the possibility of being splashed by body fluids exists. Isolation techniques are applied for certain illnesses likely to be transmitted by air-borne or direct contact, but these techniques cannot be applied to all patients. Knowledge of body substance precautions is important, but the actual implementation of the policy is required to be effective. All personnel must be informed and willing to practice universal precautions.

889. The answer is C. *(Adler, pp 217–219. Ehrlich, 4/e, pp 129–131.)* If a sterile field is suspected of being contaminated, it must be discarded and a new sterile field set up. A sterile field becomes contaminated when any nonsterile item touches it. Therefore, to reduce the chance of clothing coming in contact with it, one must be careful when walking by the tray and avoid reaching across a sterile field. There is no need to complete an incident report as long as the correction is made.

890. The answer is C (1, 3). *(Adler, pp 208–209. Ehrlich, 4/e, pp 108–110.)* To reduce the chance of disease transmission, health care workers must wash their hands before and after they come in contact with each patient. Proper hand-washing technique must be applied to be effective. The recommended process is as follows: Avoid contact of clothing and body with the sink as it should be considered contaminated. If knee or foot controls are not available, use paper towels to operate the faucets. The water should not splash out of the sink. Wet hands and apply a soap product (preferably a liquid type); rub hands together vigorously, being sure to clean between the fingers, backs of hands, and under the nails. Keep hands lower than elbows to allow water to flow from wrists to fingers. Rinse hands and dry with paper towels. Again use paper towels to turn faucets off.

891. The answer is C. *(Adler, pp 231–232. Ehrlich, 4/e, p 262.)* Chest tubes and drainage systems are used to remove blood, other fluids, or air from the pleural cavity and allow reexpansion of the collapsed lung. These systems employ a tube placed in the patient's pleural cavity and attached to a suction-operated drainage container. When these patients are radiographed, careful attention must be paid to avoid interruption or disruption of the system. Proper operation requires the container portion to be kept lower than the patient's chest. If the container is placed higher than the chest, the contents of the container may return to the pleural cavity, causing a reversal of the patient's condition. The tube should *never* be removed for any reason.

892. The answer is C. *(Ehrlich, 4/e, p 160.)* Patients who arrive in the radiology department with an IV set-up must be monitored for the status of the set-up. Moving the patient can cause the flow of the IV contents to be disrupted. The radiographer should also note the quantity of IV solution available. If it appears to be low, or the exam is lengthy, steps should be taken to notify the patient's nursing staff of the need for additional IV material. This action should be taken prior to the solution's running out. If this should occur, the nursing staff should be notified immediately in order to ensure that correct treatment is followed. The radiographer should not just ignore this situation. Nor should the radiographer disengage the IV set-up.

893. The answer is B. *(Adler, pp 233–234.)* The Foley catheter is placed into the patient's urinary bladder via the urethra. The external portion of the catheter is attached to a drainage bag for collection of urine. This system functions by way of gravity, and thus the drainage bag should always be lower than the bladder. If it is placed above the bladder, the urine could flow back into the bladder and may be a cause of bladder infection.

894. The answer is A (1, 2). *(Adler, pp 231–237. Ehrlich, 4/e, pp 260–264. Mosby, 3/e, p 427.)* The endotracheal tube is used as a temporary means of maintaining a patent airway in the critically ill or injured patient. This plastic tube is inserted into the oral cavity and down into the trachea. On the chest radiograph, the distal end of the endotracheal tube may be visualized in the distal trachea, just above the bifurcation into the main stem bonchi. The chest drainage tube may be placed in the pleural cavity to remove blood, other fluid, or air that has collapsed the lung. The tip of the tube is visible on the radiograph and may be located at any point in the pleural cavity. The Foley catheter is inserted into the urinary bladder for the purpose of emptying it. It will not be evident on the chest radiograph.

895. The answer is A (1, 2). *(Ballinger, 7/e, vol 2, pp 110–111, 114. Ehrlich, 4/e, pp 193–197.)* The preparation of the patient for a barium enema is for the purpose of completely emptying and cleansing the large intestine. This process will allow for unimpaired visualization of the intestine. The actual process varies with the requirements of each imaging center, but some common aspects include dietary restrictions, the use of laxatives or cleansing enemas or both, and the maintenance of NPO status for 8 to 12 h before the exam. Muscle relaxants are not required for this exam. Occasionally glucagon will be administered during the exam to relax colonic spasms.

896. The answer is A. *(Adler, pp 253, 306. Ehrlich, 4/e, pp 208–209.)* Following the administration of barium, the patient should be instructed to increase fluid intake in order to assist in the complete elimination of the barium. Barium sulfate is a suspension, which means the barium does not dissolve into the water. If left to stand, a barium mixture will separate with the barium sulfate settling at the bottom of the container. Since the primary function of the colon is the absorption of water, it is possible that the barium would become hardened within the colon. This may be avoided by maintaining the water content of the barium and hastening its elimination from the body. Some department protocols may also include instructing patients to follow another course of laxatives. Patients may resume a normal diet following these exams, assuming no other exams requiring fasting are to be done. The use of a cleansing enema is not generally recommended.

897. The answer is B. *(Adler, p 252.)*   During an enema procedure (either cleansing or barium), the patient may experience intestinal cramps. The patient should be instructed to breath slowly and deeply through the mouth. This will help relax the abdomen and allow the contractions to pass. The flow of the enema liquid should also be stopped until the cramps subside. Holding of breath or breathing fast may contribute to increased anxiety rather than relaxation.

898. The answer is C. *(Adler, p 252.)*   When a patient experiences cramping during an enema procedure, the radiographer should interrupt the flow of liquid into the patient until the cramp passes. The patient should also be instructed to breathe slowly and deeply through the mouth. Raising the enema bag will cause the liquid to flow faster, aggravating the spasms. Lowering the bag will slow the flow and cause a back flow into the bag, emptying the colon. This may be necessary in cases when the patient's discomfort is excessive.

899. The answer is B (2, 3). *(Ballinger, 7/e, vol 2, p 90. Bontrager, 3/e, p 432. Ehrlich, 4/e, pp 80, 206.)*   The upper gastrointestinal series primarily images the stomach. For this reason, the routine patient preparation requires steps to empty the stomach prior to the exam. This is achieved by requiring the patient to refrain from eating or drinking for 8 to 10 h before the exam. This order is stated as NPO ("nihil pro ora" or "nothing by mouth") from midnight on. Most imaging centers also prohibit smoking and gum chewing during the NPO period as these actions can stimulate gastric secretions. The clear liquid diet and laxatives are required if the UGI is to include evaluation of the small bowel.

900. The answer is C (1, 3). *(Ballinger, 7/e, vol 1, p 147. Bontrager, 3/e, p 515. Ehrlich, 4/e, pp 193–197, 220.)*   The patient preparation for an intravenous urogram requires clearing of the colon in order to improve visibility of the kidneys, ureters, and bladder. Fecal material or gas in the colon can obscure these structures. Therefore, the general routine of a low-residue diet, laxatives the day before the exam, and a cleansing enema the morning of the exam will sufficiently clear the colon. Also, the patient is instructed to remain NPO from midnight the night before the exam. This will maintain the clear colon and more importantly reduce the chance of aspiration of vomitus should the patient have a reaction to the IV contrast media used. Since diuretic drugs are used to promote fluid excretion, their use would tend to prohibit the desired concentration of the contrast media needed for optimum imaging. Diuretic drugs should be withheld during the 24-h period before the scheduled exam.

901. The answer is D (3, 2, 1). *(Adler, p 320. Ehrlich, 4/e, pp 191–192.)*   The proper scheduling of radiologic procedures, including nuclear medicine exams, requires consideration of patient preparation and the type of contrast media or radioisotope likely to be used. For example, nuclear medicine procedures of the thyroid should be performed before the introduction of any iodine-based contrast media. Since water-soluble iodine contrast media are readily absorbed and excreted by the urinary system, exams using this type of contrast (IVU, angiography) should be performed before the introduction of barium-based contrast media. Barium sulfate is eliminated from the body via the gastrointestinal system, which may take a day or two, depending on the route of administration and the patient's system. Barium will clear from the colon following a BE exam faster than from the system following a UGI series. Therefore, the BE should be scheduled before a UGI or small bowel series.

902. The answer is B. *(Adler, p 317.)*   The order in which patients are scheduled for their radiologic exams should be influenced by the degree of discomfort the patient may experience in being prepared for the exam. Therefore, exams that require fasting should be performed first. Since many fasting patients may be scheduled, further consideration must be given to those who would have the greatest difficulty tolerating fasting. Priority should be given to the elderly and diabetic patients, then children, and finally adults. The proper scheduling for the patients listed as the answer options would be (B) diabetic patient for IVU, (C) child for UGI, (D) adult for UGI, and (A) elderly patient for chest exam.

903. The answer is B.   *(Adler, pp 310, 314. Ehrlich, 4/e, pp 215, 218.)*   *Nonionic* iodinated contrast media has proved to be less likely to cause an allergic reaction than *ionic* iodinated contrast media. Nonionic contrast media do not dissociate into ionic particles when introduced to the blood stream as do the ionic types of iodine contrast media. This results in a lower osmotic effect on the cells (less movement of water from the cells). This reduced disruption of the cells lessens the occurrence of allergic reactions. Thus the nonionic contrast media can be used more readily, especially in patients identified as having a higher likelihood of a reaction to IV contrast media. Unfortunately, the cost of nonionic contrast media is significantly more than for the ionic form, making it necessary for imaging centers to decide if the nonionic form will be offered to all patients. Many imaging centers have established criteria for the required use of nonionic contrast media for patients who are more susceptible to a contrast media reaction. Water-soluble contrast media are administered by ingestion, the intravenous route, or by direct injection into a body cavity. There is no advantage in injecting any contrast media intramuscularly.

904. The answer is C.   *(Adler, pp 306–308, 314–317. Ehrlich, 4/e, pp 198–200, 218–220.)*   Allergic reactions to contrast media are most likely to occur when the media are introduced directly to the circulatory system (IV administration), as the water-soluble iodine types (ionic and nonionic) are. Of the two types, the ionic iodine contrast media are most likely to cause an allergic reaction. This is due to the fact that they form large particles (ions) in the blood stream and have a high osmotic effect, disrupting the cells and promoting an allergic reaction, which can be mild, moderate, or severe. Barium is administered orally or rectally and eliminated from the body as is, with only some removal of water from the barium suspension by the colon. Side effects are associated with the leakage of barium into the peritoneum through a perforation in the GI system. Other contraindications to barium use relate to the ability of the patient to eliminate the barium or the existence of a disease process that may be aggravated by the barium. Oil-based iodine contrast media have a very restrictive use in radiography due to the advantages offered by the newer nonionic, water-soluble iodine. The iodized oils are not rapidly absorbed and excreted and thus may be present within the body for many years before they are eliminated. When they are used, efforts should be made to remove the material from the system at the end of the exam. This was commonly done in myelography, sialography, and bronchography. If these exams are performed today, nonionic, water-soluble media are used. Like barium, iodized oils have contraindications to use, but do not cause allergic reactions.

905. The answer is A.   *(Adler, p 318. Bontrager, 3/e, p 513. Ehrlich, 4/e, p 183.)*   The intravenous administration of water-soluble, iodine-based contrast media carries the potential for an allergic reaction. The reactions can range from very mild irritations to life-threatening conditions, such as cardiac arrest. The radiographer must be aware of the possible symptoms, which are categorized as mild, moderate, or severe. The symptoms of nausea, vomiting, and a warm or flushed feeling are examples of a mild reaction. This is one reason for requiring patients to be NPO the night prior to the exam. If the patient should have an episode of vomiting, having an empty stomach will decrease the chance of aspiration of the vomitus. Some patients may exhibit these mild symptoms and nothing else. For others, more serious reactions may follow or occur without these warning symptoms.

906. The answer is B.   *(Bushong, 5/e, pp 184–185. Carroll, 5/e, pp 153–154.)*   Contrast media are employed to enhance x-ray differential absorption in adjacent structures that are similar in makeup. Barium sulfate- and iodine-based agents fulfill this requirement because of their high atomic number relative to the structures to which they are added. The atomic number for soft tissue is about 7.4; for iodine it is 53; and for barium it is 56. This difference in atomic number (soft tissue to barium) increases the probability of photoelectric interactions, producing an area of low radiographic density. For this reason, these agents are referred to as *positive* contrast media. Since the atomic number for soft tissue structures is so low, a contrast medium with a similar atomic number, such as air (Z = 7.2), would provide little enhancement. Air works as a contrast medium because of its low molecular density as compared with soft tissue or bony structures. This low density results in few x-ray/matter interactions, producing high radiographic density, and air is referred to as a *negative* contrast medium.

907. The answer is D.   *(Adler, pp 308–309, 315–316. Bontrager, 3/e, p 676. Ehrlich, 4/e, pp 213–214, 233.)* Iodized oils used to be more widely used in the radiographic exams than they are currently. Such exams as bronchography (replaced by CT or bronchoscopy), myelography, and sialography (which currently use non-ionic, water-soluble iodinated contrast media) used iodized oils such as dionosil, pantopaque, and ethiodol. The lymphangiogram still uses the slow introduction of iodized oils into the small lymphatic vessels of the foot for opacification of the lymph vessels. Since this contrast medium is not quickly absorbed from the body, delayed imaging may be conducted on the day following the initial exam. At that time the contrast medium will be concentrated in the lymph nodes. Angiography has always employed water-soluble iodine-based contrast media.

908. The answer is B.   *(Adler, pp 283–284. Ehrlich, 4/e, pp 136, 138, 183.)*   Hives over a large area is classified as a moderate type of reaction to the IV administration of iodine-based contrast media. This may require treatment with an antihistamine. Therefore, diphenhydramine (Benadryl) is commonly included in an emergency treatment kit wherever iodine-based contrast media are used. Anticoagulant drugs are used to reduce blood clotting. Anesthetics promote the loss of feeling. Bronchodilators work to relieve bronchial spasms and increase the diameter of bronchioles, thereby easing breathing.

909. The answer is D.   *(Adler, pp 282–284. Ehrlich, 4/e, pp 135, 138.)*   Epinephrine (Adrenalin) is classified as a bronchodilator and is used to ease respiratory distress. It acts to relieve spasms of the bronchioles and thereby increase their diameter for more efficient air flow. Respiratory distress is a possible severe reaction to the IV administration of iodine-based contrast media. Epinephrine should be included in the emergency drug kit available wherever iodine-based contrast media are used.

910. The answer is A.   *(Adler, pp 318–319. Ehrlich, 4/e, p 183.)*   There is a wide range of symptoms that may indicate a patient's allergic reaction to iodine contrast media. The radiographer must be aware of what these symptoms are and what type of medical response is required. A mild reaction, such as nausea, vomiting, and dizziness, requires the radiographer to reassure the patient that these reactions are common and that they are generally short-lived. Further assistance with an emesis basin or cool cloth on the forehead will comfort the patient. The radiographer must also continue to observe the patient for persistence of these symptoms or worsening of the situation.

911. The answer is D.   *(Bontrager, 3/e, p 512. Ehrlich, 4/e, p 219.)*   Before administration of any iodine-based contrast media (especially intravenously), the patient's allergy history must be obtained and documented. This is commonly done while explaining the exam and obtaining informed consent. The history taking should include questions regarding any type of allergy the patient may have. Patients should also be asked whether they have received contrast media previously, what their response to it was, and whether any treatment was required. Those patients with a previous reaction to contrast media or who have general hypersensitivity are at greater risk for a current reaction.

912. The answer is C.   *(Bontrager, 3/e, p 512. Ehrlich, 4/e, p 219.)*   Prior to beginning a radiographic exam, the radiographer should explain the exam and obtain a history as to why the exam is being performed and whether or not allergic reaction to the contrast media is probable. The questions listed in the answer options should be asked and answered with the exception of the reference to pregnancy. While it is true this question must be asked, it is in reference to whether the exam should be performed from the standpoint of radiation safety, not in relation to a possible reaction to contrast media.

913. The answer is C. *(Adler, pp 260, 268–269, 292. Bontrager, 3/e, p 513. Ehrlich, 4/e, pp 156, 183, 186.)* *Extravasation* (or *infiltration*) is the leakage of any material from a vessel into the surrounding tissues. This is a possible occurrence during intravenous injection of any fluid, including contrast media. The signs of an extravasation are swelling at the needle site and pain or discomfort. Should this condition occur, the IV injection should be stopped, the needle removed, and pressure applied to the site. Warm, moist compresses will aide in relieving the discomfort. An episode of nausea, vomiting, dizziness, and weakness is termed a *vasovagal response* and may result from anxiety or a mild allergic reaction. Respiratory and cardiac arrest is a severe anaphylatic response that may occur following contrast media administration. A nose bleed is referred to as *epistaxis* and is not associated with iodine-based contrast media.

914. The answer is B (2, 3). *(Adler, p 290. Ehrlich, 4/e, pp 142–143.)* Medications may be administered via oral, topical, or parenteral methods. Oral medications are available in pill, capsule, or liquid form and are absorbed into the bloodstream through the gastrointestinal tract. Topical applications of medications are applied to the skin or administered under the tongue (sublingual) for absorption into the blood stream. Parenteral methods of administration require the use of a needle and syringe to introduce the medication directly into the bloodstream. Various routes may be used with this method, including intravenous (within a vein), intramuscular (within a muscle group), subcutaneous (under the skin), or intradermal (within the layers of skin).

915. The answer is B. *(Adler, pp 287–288. Ehrlich, 4/e, p 147.)* The needle used in the parenteral method of drug administration comes in a variety of sizes to fit the type of injection to be made. Needle sizes are stated in terms of their diameter (the gauge) and length. The gauge of a needle is stated as a numerical value and is inverse to its diameter. For instance, a 23 gauge needle has a smaller diameter than an 18 gauge. Small gauge needles are most commonly used for patient injection, while very large gauge needles are used to "draw up," or fill, a syringe with the desired fluid. The length of a needle is stated in terms of inches and indicates the distance between the hub and the tip of the needle. All needles are made of stainless steel and should be disposed of after a single use.

916. The answer is B. *(Adler, p 292. Bontrager, 3/e, p 513. Ehrlich, 4/e, pp 156, 183–184.)* A possible problem that may arise during intravenous injection as described in this question is termed *extravasation*, or *infiltration*. This situation results in the leakage of the material being injected from the vein into the surrounding tissues. Swelling at the injection site will be noted and the patient may experience pain or discomfort. When this situation occurs, the injection should be terminated and the needle removed. Pressure should be applied to the swelling as well as a warm, moist compress.

917. The answer is C. *(Adler, pp 292–293. Ballinger, 7/e, vol 2, p 156. Ehrlich, 4/e, pp 148–149.)* The bolus method of injection of contrast media requires the rapid delivery of the fluid in a "push" of the entire dose. This method is commonly employed in IVU procedures in order to avoid dilution of the quantity of contrast media used. It provides rapid, but temporary opacification of the collecting system of the kidneys. The alternate method for intravenous introduction of fluids is via a drip infusion. This method delivers the fluid at a slower rate, determined by the instructions of the physician. The contents of the IV bag are delivered slowly via gravity rather than pushed in. The IV drip set-up includes a means for setting and controlling the desired flow rate.

918. The answer is D (1, 2, 3). *(Adler, p 286. Ehrlich, 4/e, pp 133, 141, 157.)* Although not all radiographers perform venipuncture, they will be required to prepare materials for others to inject into a patient. Therefore, the radiographer has a role in the process of ensuring that medications and contrast media are administered properly. This includes understanding the physician's order by checking the patient chart or rephrasing the physician's oral instructions as given. Before, during, and after the preparation of the material to be injected, the label of the solution must be checked to verify that it is the correct solution and that it has not exceeded its expiration date. This verification should also include showing the bottle from which the material came to the person who will be doing the injection, prior to the injection. Finally, the patient's identification should be checked, prior to injection, to verify that the right patient will receive the right medication or contrast medium.

919. The answer is C (1, 3).   *(Adler, p 286. Ehrlich, 4/e, p 144.)*   The preparation of a drug or contrast medium for intravenous injection requires careful evaluation of the label of the solution to be used. The label should be read to verify the name of the medication or contrast medium, the strength of the solution, and its expiration date. It is recommended that the label be checked three times before administering the injection to the patient. It should also be shown to the person doing the injection for that person's verification. Specific information regarding the side effects of or contraindications to the use of a drug is generally found on the crimp sheet, which is packaged in the box with the bottled solution.

920. The answer is D.   *(Adler, pp 187–188. Ehrlich, 4/e, p 164.)*   When patients arrive in the radiology department connected to a portable source of oxygen, the radiographer may need to transfer the oxygen connection to the wall source available in the radiographic room. This is especially necessary if the procedure will be fairly long and may deplete a portable source that will be needed to return the patient to his room. Before disconnecting the patient from the portable oxygen, the radiographer must note the designated flow rate. This rate is then set at the wall source. This outlet is connected to a large source of oxygen for which one need not be concerned as to its contents. No other changes need to be made. Whatever type of oxygen appliance the patient has should be used. There is no need to suction the average patient prior to administering oxygen.

921. The answer is D.   *(Adler, p 264. American Red Cross, pp 15, 28. Ehrlich, 4/e, p 169.)*   Before any action is taken, the rescuer must first determine the responsiveness of the person. It is vital to be sure CPR is needed before it is actually performed. Checking the responsiveness of a patient is done by gently shaking the patient by the shoulder and shouting something like "Are you okay?" If no response is given, it is assumed the patient is unconscious and in need of further medical assistance. Once this is established, the airway should be opened to determine the patient's breathing status. If the patient is not breathing, artificial ventilation is applied and the pulse is checked to determine circulatory function. Checking for injuries on the arms and legs is done only after the life-threatening conditions have been resolved.

922. The answer is B.   *(Adler, p 265. American Red Cross, p 30.)*   According to accepted practice recommended by the American Red Cross and the American Medical Association, the carotid artery should be palpated to determine the presence of a pulse in an adult or child. This large artery lies on each side of the trachea. If a pulse is felt, cardiac function is continuing, even if breathing is not present. This condition can rapidly change and thus the pulse needs to be routinely evaluated. Assessment of a pulse on an infant should be made on the brachial artery, located on the medial aspect of the upper arm, midway between the shoulder and elbow.

923. The answer is C.   *(Adler, p 265. American Red Cross, pp 64, 66.)*   The correct method for performing cardiac compressions during CPR is as follows:
  1. Victim is supine on a hard surface with rescuer kneeling on one side of the victim.
  2. Rescuer finds the correct hand position by locating the xiphoid of the sternum and placing the middle finger of one hand on the xiphoid. The heel of the other hand is then placed beside the index finger of the first hand, along the length of the sternum. This should position the hand over the lower half of the body of the sternum, but not on the xiphoid. The heel of the second hand is placed on top of the first, keeping the fingers of both hands off the patient's thorax.
  3. Rescuer then leans directly over the victim, arms extended and elbows locked.
  4. Compression is made by using one's weight to lean into the victim's chest, pushing the sternum down about 1.5 to 2 inches on the adult, then releasing the pressure to allow the sternum to rise up, without removing the hands from their correct position. The movement should be smooth and avoid bouncing or jerky movements.
  5. Compressions are applied at a rate of about 80 to 100 per minute.

924. The answer is C. *(Adler, p 265. American Red Cross, pp 66, 89, 103, 119.)* The difference in performing chest compressions on an adult versus a child or infant is in terms of the pressure needed to compress the chest and the maximum depth of compression. For the adult, two hands are used to compress the sternum 1.5 to 2 inches. The child between the ages of 1 and 8 years requires less pressure and thus only one hand is needed. The sternum should be displaced downward 1 to 1.5 inches. In the infant, minimal effort is needed to compress the sternum. It is recommended that only two fingers (second and third fingers) should be used to compress the chest by 0.5 to 1 inch. In all cases, the compressions are applied with the victim in the supine position and at a rate of 80 to 100 per minute.

925. The answer is B. *(Adler, p 262. American Red Cross, p 44. Ehrlich, 4/e, p 176.)* The Heimlich maneuver is employed for victims with an obstructed airway. This technique may be performed on the conscious or unconscious patient. When apparent choking and respiratory distress are noted, a rescuer should confirm the suspected problem by asking the victim if he or she is choking. Upon an affirmative response, the rescuer stands behind the victim and reaches around the victim's abdomen. One hand is closed into a fist with the thumb protruding and placed on the abdomen between the navel and xiphoid process. The other hand grasps the fist, and with the victim held tight against the rescuer's body, the rescuer pulls the fist into the victim's abdomen in a forceful upward motion. This causes an altered intrathoracic pressure to dislodge and force the object up and out of the throat. A modification of this technique can be used on unconscious and infant victims.

926. The answer is D (1, 2, 3). *(Adler, p 265. American Red Cross, p 64.)* Once CPR has been initiated, it should be continued until additional emergency medical services are available. Once a code blue team or EMTs arrive, additional strategies can be employed to increase the patient's chance of survival. However, after a while, the physician in charge of the emergency may need to decide that all reasonable efforts have been made and call for an end to the CPR. The exhausted lone rescuer may need to end the CPR attempt before the arrival of assistance. Once a patient's pulse and breathing are reestablished, the artificial ventilation and chest compressions may be stopped.

927. The answer is C. *(Adler, pp 265, 268.)* Using the correct technique when performing CPR will increase the effectiveness of the artificial cardiopulmonary system being established and decrease the risk of further injury to the victim. Incorrect hand position can lead to fractures of the ribs or sternum. These can then cause laceration of the liver, lungs, or spleen, adding further risk for the patient's survival. Incorrect CPR will not cause blood to flow in the wrong direction. Victims may go into shock during CPR attempts, but it will be due to injuries rather than incorrect CPR techniques. An increase in intracranial pressure may result from head trauma, but not from incorrect CPR.

928. The answer is C. *(Adler, p 264. American Red Cross, pp 63–64.)* In order for the chest compressions to be effective, the patient must be supine on a firm, level surface. The radiographic table is a very good surface to use. If the patient is on a bed with a mattress, the compressions will push the whole patient into the mattress, rather than squeeze the heart between the sternum and spine. Either the patient should be moved onto the floor or a board placed under the patient's back. Backboards used by EMTs are also effective.

929. The answer is B. *(Adler, p 265. American Red Cross, pp 30, 33.)* When checking an unconscious victim, the first item to be attended to is to open the airway and see if the patient is breathing. If the patient is not breathing, two full breaths are delivered, then the presence of a pulse is determined. If the patient is breathing, there will be a pulse and there is no need to check it. For adults and children the pulse is evaluated by palpating the carotid artery in the neck. This may be felt on either side of the trachea. The brachial pulse, located in the upper arm, is used on infants. The presence of a pulse indicates the heart is still beating and chest compressions will *not* be necessary. It is important that the pulse be sufficiently checked so as to prevent one from applying chest compressions when they are not needed. The pulse should be evaluated for 5 to 10 s before beginning chest compressions.

930. The answer is D.   *(Adler, p 265. American Red Cross, pp 68, 102–103, 119.)*   For the single rescuer with an adult victim, the ratio of chest compressions to ventilations should be 15:2. This means that upon determining that the victim is not breathing and has no pulse, the rescuer should apply 15 chest compressions, then deliver two slow breaths, then repeat with the chest compressions. After performing this cycle repeatedly for 1 min, the rescuer should reevaluate the patient by rechecking the patient's pulse and breathing. If there is still no response, CPR should be continued for several minutes before rechecking for pulse and breathing again. If the victim is a child or infant, the cycle is 5 chest compressions to 1 breath.

931. The answer is B.   *(Adler, pp 269–270. Ehrlich, 4/e, pp 184–185.)*   *Syncope* is the medical term for fainting. The correct medical terms to express the other conditions listed in the answer options are *epistaxis* for a nosebleed, *vasovagal reaction* for dizziness (which may lead to syncope), and *hemorrhage* for uncontrolled bleeding.

932. The answer is D.   *(Adler, p 210. Ehrlich, 4/e, p 287.)*   Respiratory precautions are applied to a patient with an infectious disease that is transmitted by airborne material as a result of coughing or sneezing. Health care workers who must interact with these patients should wear a mask to avoid inspiring the airborne particles. Some institutions will also have the patient wear a mask as a double precaution. If the exam requires contact with oral or nasal secretions from such a patient, gloves should also be worn.

933. The answer is B.   *(Adler, p 211. Ehrlich, 4/e, p 117.)*   Strict isolation precautions are applied to those patients with an infectious disease that may be transmitted by air or direct contact. Radiographic procedures for these patients require two persons, one to handle the items that come into contact with the patient ("dirty tech") and the other to handle the radiographic equipment ("clean tech"). Both persons must wear a protective gown, mask, and gloves before entering the patient's room. The cassettes must be placed in protective plastic or cloth bags. When in the room, the radiographer touching the patient will position the protected cassettes under the patient. The other radiographer will manipulate the radiographic equipment. After the exposure, the dirty tech will remove the cassette package and pull back the cover for the clean tech to withdraw the cassette. Upon exiting the patient's room, both persons remove the protective garments without touching the outside of the garments and dispose of them appropriately. Also, both persons must thoroughly wash their hands.

934. The answer is B.   *(Adler, pp 185–186. Ehrlich, 4/e, p 94.)*   The blood pressure indicates the force on the arterial walls as the heart pumps the blood through the circulatory system. The reading is given in the form of a ratio that compares the force exerted on the heart during contraction (systolic pressure) with the relaxation force following contraction (diastolic pressure). Therefore the ratio is stated as the systolic to diastolic pressures. In the reading stated in the question, 130 indicates the systolic pressure, while 80 indicates the diastolic pressure. The normal range of blood pressure is from 95 to 140 systolic and 60 to 90 diastolic. Hypertension, a condition of above-normal blood pressure, causes the heart to work harder and may lead to damage of the heart muscle. Hypotension is a below-normal blood pressure which may be effectively normal for some people or may be caused by the loss of fluid volume, causing dizziness, confusion, and even loss of consciousness.

935. The answer is A.   *(Adler, pp 180, 185. Ehrlich, 4/e, pp 90, 185. Mosby, 3/e, p 166.)*   The term *bradycardia* refers to a slower than average pulse rate. This may occur in the exceptionally fit person whose "normal" heart rate is slow (less than 60 beats per minute). It may also be a pathologic condition that may manifest as dizziness due to insufficient circulation. The opposite of this condition is termed tachycardia, which exhibits a "racing" heart. *Hyper-* and *hypotension* refer to high and low blood pressure, respectively.

936. The answer is D.   *(Ehrlich, 4/e, pp 180–181. Laudicina, pp 173, 215.)*   Fractures of the skull may be linear, comminuted, or depressed. Blunt trauma to the skull generally causes a depressed fracture. Transverse, spiral, and impacted types of fractures are common to long bones.

937. The answer is C. (*Laudicina, pp 179, 182–183.*)   The fracture of the distal radius and a chip fracture of the ulnar styloid are characteristics of a Colles' type fracture. This injury is generally the result of trying to break one's fall by landing on an outstretched hand. Fractures involving the hip are commonly of the intertrochanteric, transcervical, and subcapital types. The Pott's type of fracture is common to the distal tibia and fibula. The impacted type of fracture is common to the shoulder.

938. The answer is D. (*Laudicina, pp 168–169, 174, 176.*)   The term *avulsion* means "to pull away from." Avulsion fractures generally occur at the point of a ligament or tendon attachment with a bone. The trauma results in a small piece of bone being pulled away from the main bone. A comminuted type of fracture results in the bone shattering into many pieces. The type of fracture in which one portion of a bone is driven into another portion of the same bone is termed *impaction*. This is common with long bones. The simplest of all fractures is the greenstick type, which is an incomplete break through the bone. This type is most commonly found in children.

939. The answer is D. (*Adler, pp 269–270. Ehrlich, 4/e, pp 185–186.*)   In the case of a patient having a seizure, the radiographer should respond by protecting the patient from injury during the event. Seizures are generally characterized by spastic movements of the limbs and body. The patient should be helped into a recumbent position and a pillow provided to protect the head from being banged. Attempts to immobilize the patient should not be made as this, too, may cause more damage than assistance. Those emergency situations in which the patient's airway is compromised require the head to be extended in the head-tilt, chin-lift manner to open the airway. To achieve this, there should be no pillow under the patient's head.

940. The answer is C. (*Adler, pp 167–170. Ballinger, 7/e, vol 1, p 474. Ehrlich, 4/e, p 180.*)   Trauma patients should have their radiographic exams performed with the immobilization devices in place. This is especially true for the initial set of images obtained on a patient. After screening a patient for life-threatening injuries with the devices in place, the physician may request additional images with the devices removed. Many current immobilization devices are constructed of radiolucent material, which does not hinder the x-ray beam. However, even if the device is radiopaque, it must be left in place.

941. The answer is D. (*Ballinger, 7/e, vol 1, pp 256–260. Bontrager, 3/e, p 225.*)   Optimum radiographs of the pelvis or hip require internal rotation of the lower limb to overcome anteversion of the femoral neck. Failure to do this results in a distorted image of the femoral neck. In the case of patients with suspected or healing hip fractures, only a physician should attempt the necessary manipulation of the affected limb. If a physician is not available, the radiographer should obtain AP and cross-table lateral projections with the patient's limb positioned as it is.

942. The answer is D. (*Ballinger, 7/e, vol 1, p 316. Bontrager, 3/e, p 294.*)   The trauma patient with a suspected injury to the cervical spine should not be moved until the status of the cervical spine has been evaluated. To achieve this, a horizontal beam is used to obtain a lateral projection of the cervical spine without moving the patient. Any immobilization device on the patient should be left in place. If patients are able, they should be instructed to depress their shoulders by reaching for their feet. If they are unable, an assistant may be needed to provide traction on the arms. A trauma patient, especially with injury to the cervical spine, should *never* be moved into an erect position until the patient has been sufficiently evaluated and a physician has given permission.

943. The answer is C. (*Ballinger, 7/e, vol 1, p 317. Bontrager, 3/e, p 295.*)   Radiographs of the cervical spine should be obtained without moving the patient. This may be achieved by using a horizontal beam for the lateral projection and a double tube angle for the oblique projection. The AP projection in the supine recumbent position does not require the patient to be moved and thus may be obtained using the usual methods. The oblique projection is performed by positioning the image receptor under the patient's neck with its midpoint corresponding with the angled central ray. A double angle is applied to the central ray so that it is directed 45° medially and 15° cephalad to C4. The opposite side must also be imaged in order to demonstrate both sets of intervertebral foramina. Trauma patients should not be turned prone during the initial evaluation of the cervical spine.

944. The answer is A. *(Ballinger, 7/e, vol 1, p 474. Bontrager, 3/e, pp 109–110.)* Radiography of the trauma patient will often require the radiographer to modify the exam routine to accommodate the limitations of the patient. However, it is important to obtain images of high quality and as close to the nontrauma routine as possible. Many radiologic exams of the extremities can be performed with the patient on the stretcher or wheelchair, rather than requiring them to move to the radiographic table and risk further injury or pain. At a minimum, it is important to obtain at least two images of the injured part in projections that are at right angles to each other: AP/PA and lateral. If an immobilization device is in place, it should not be removed unless so directed and supervised by a physician. Many immobilization devices are constructed of radiolucent materials to minimize their impact on the image. It is not generally the routine to obtain comparison images of the noninjured extremity because this will increase radiation exposure. However, it may be requested. When long bones, such as the lower and upper arm or leg, are to be imaged, the optimum goal would be to include both joints involving the injured bone on the same image. If this is not possible, due to the size of the bone or limitations of the patient, the joint closest to the injury should be included. An alternative would be to obtain two images, one including the proximal joint and as much shaft as possible and the other including the distal joint and shaft, creating an overlapped effect of the bone shaft.

945. The answer is D. *(Adler, p 125.)* The correct patient positioning and centering of the x-ray beam require touching of the patient to locate anatomic landmarks. This is referred to as *palpation.* Some patients are less comfortable than others when it comes to being touched; therefore, it is important to let the patient know you will be touching them and why and to do so in an appropriate and efficient manner. To do this, palpation should be performed with a gentle, yet firm touch using the tip of the index or middle finger or both.

946. The answer is B (2, 3). *(Adler, pp 302–303. Ehrlich, 4/e, p 212.)* Contrast media are categorized as being either *positive* or *negative*, depending on their ability to absorb x-ray photons. Negative contrast media do not absorb x-rays (easily penetrated) and thus are considered radiolucent. Conversely, positive contrast media are radiopaque, providing an increase in the number of photoelectric interactions and resulting in low density areas on the image. The introduction of materials with low molecular density creates the negative contrast effect. Such materials include room air or carbon dioxide gas. These agents are introduced into body cavities such as the gastrointestinal tract and joint spaces. They are never used intravenously because they could cause life-threatening air emboli.

947. The answer is B. *(Adler, p 261. Ehrlich, 4/e, pp 187–188.)* Diabetes is the condition whereby the body is unable to correctly metabolize blood sugar. The condition may be one of two types: hypoglycemia (low blood sugar as a result of too much insulin in the blood) or hyperglycemia (high blood sugar). The condition described in the question is that of hypoglycemia resulting from taking the required dose of insulin, but not having the appropriate level of carbohydrates for metabolism because of the fasting requirements. Diabetic patients should be scheduled to have exams early in the day when their exams require fasting. If the symptoms described in the question are noted, some source of sugar will need to be administered, usually sweetened orange juice or a glucose product kept with emergency supplies in the department. Hyperglycemia is the opposite condition and has a more gradual onset, but it can be just as life-threatening if left untreated. The symptoms include hyperventilation, excessive thirst and urination, and a sweet or fruity smell to the breath. These symptoms can lead to a diabetic coma if not treated. Anaphylactic shock is generally a severe allergic reaction that manifests with difficulty breathing, drop in blood pressure, and respiratory and cardiac arrest if not treated.

948. The answer is B. *(Adler, p 262. American Red Cross, p 43. Ehrlich, 4/e, pp 173, 176.)* A person who is clutching at the throat is demonstrating the universal sign for choking and may require assistance in clearing the airway. A person who is choking, yet is able to cough forcibly, should just be watched and encouraged to continue coughing. If the condition deteriorates so that coughing is not possible, the victim will need assistance such as the Heimlich maneuver. A person who is having a heart attack generally complains of chest or arm pain and may clutch at the chest. Vertigo is dizziness and syncope is fainting. Both of these may cause a patient to hold his or her head.

949. **The answer is C.** *(American Red Cross, p 47.)* Rescue breathing is performed on unconscious victims who are not breathing on their own but have a pulse. This is done by opening the airway using the head-tilt, chin-lift method to pull the tongue away from the back of the throat. The rescuer then pinches the victim's nose closed and completely covers the victim's mouth with the rescuer's mouth, forming a tight seal to prevent air from escaping. A full, gentle breath is then delivered to the victim at a relatively slow rate, lasting 1 to 1.5 s for each breath. Upon initial response to the victim, two breaths are given and then, after establishing that a pulse is present, the rescue breathing is continued at a rate of one breath every 5 s for the adult victim. The rate is increased to one breath every 3 s for a child or infant.

950. **The answer is B.** *(Adler, pp 153, 164–166. Ehrlich, 4/e, pp 74–75.)* Immobilization devices are used to assist patients to hold still during radiographic procedures, thereby minimizing the chance of motion artifacts and the need for repeat exposures. Devices such as sandbags, tape, and velcro straps can stop the trembling of an extremity that has been traumatized and also assist the patient in maintaining a somewhat difficult position. Compression bands will also assist a patient to hold position, as will head clamps. Grids are used to improve image quality, but are not immobilizers. Cassette holders are useful in maintaining the correct position of the cassette when the bucky tray is not used. Slider boards are used to assist in the transfer of a patient from a stretcher to the radiographic table.

951. **The answer is A (1, 2).** *(Adler, pp 171, 173–174. Ehrlich, 4/e, p 75.)* Infants and very young children will most often need to be immobilized during radiography procedures. This is for their safety as well as obtaining quality images with minimal exposure. Many materials and devices are available as restraints. Some are readily available, such as a sheet in which to wrap the child or a stockinette for keeping the arms or legs together. Tape may be used, but sparingly, as young skin can be very sensitive to the adhesive material. Commercial devices are also available, such as the Pigg-O-Stat or positioning boards equipped with velcro straps. Explaining the exam to children or asking them to hold still is not usually helpful. However, an appropriate level of communication and taking time to develop a rapport with older children (about age 4 or more) can result in sufficient cooperation to eliminate the need for immobilization devices.

952. **The answer is C (1, 3).** *(Adler, p 351. Ehrlich, 4/e, pp 15, 17, 275.)* Part of the general informed consent form is the inclusion of a signature. This requires the signature of the patient having the exam or a person responsible for an incapacitated patient. There may be more than one area for the patient's signature, relative to various components of information provided to the patient. The form should also be signed by a witness, preferably someone not associated with the patient or the exam procedure. This signature verifies that the patient or the patient's representative received the information and signed the form. These signatures must be obtained at the time the information is provided and prior to performing the exam.

953. **The answer is C (1, 3).** *(Ehrlich, 4/e, pp 124, 201, 233, 238.)* Myelography and angiography require the introduction of a needle or catheter into the subarachnoid space and vascular system, respectively. This action provides a means of infection transmission and therefore requires the implementation of sterile asepsis. This would specifically require the radiologist to wear sterile gloves, to clean and drape the area to be invaded, and to administer contrast media under sterile conditions. Further protection is required for the angiography exam, including wearing sterile gowns, caps, and masks, because of the increased invasiveness of the procedure. Barium enemas are performed under clean, but nonsterile conditions. However, the disposable enema tubes are packaged as sterile and should remain so packaged until used.

954. **The answer is B.** *(Adler, p 286.)* In order to ensure patient safety, careful steps must be taken to ensure the correct identity of the patient. The patient's name band, usually located on the patient's wrist, should be matched with the information on the exam requisition. Patients able to comprehend should also be asked to state their name. Patients may answer to the wrong name due to confusion in the waiting room, apprehension about the pending exam, or misunderstanding of what was said. Having patients state their own name eliminates this conflict. Using the patient's chart as identification is not always possible as it is not always transferred with the patient. Also, it may possibly be the wrong chart. A patient will not always have an IV and it is generally not labeled with patient information.

955. The answer is C (1, 3). *(Adler, p 204. Ehrlich, 4/e, p 122.)* Patients with a reduced immune status are said to be *compromised* or *immunosuppressed*. Such patients would include neonates, burn victims, patients being treated with chemotherapy, and patients who have received organ transplants. These patients have had their immune systems compromised by their conditions or as a side effect of drugs administered for their conditions. In the case of transplant patients, the administration of antirejection drugs causes suppression of the immune system. The organs *donors* do not need this immunosuppression, but must be as carefully treated as any postsurgical patient.

956. The answer is C. *(Adler, p 226. Ehrlich, 4/e, pp 129–130.)* Sterile gloves are packaged with the cuff of the glove partially folded inside out. This permits the wearer to pick up the first glove while only touching the inside surface at the cuff. By only touching this cuffed area, the glove is pulled onto the hand, leaving the cuff folded. To put on the second glove, the fingers of the gloved hand are inserted *under* the cuff, touching only the outside of the glove. The glove is pulled onto the hand and each of the cuffs unfolded by touching the outside of the glove only.

957. The answer is C. *(Adler, p 145. Ehrlich, 4/e, p 185.)* When patients are in the recumbent position for a period of time and then are moved to an upright position, they may experience dizziness and light-headedness to the point of fainting. This change in position causes a decrease in blood supply to the brain and a drop in blood pressure (hypotension). When assisting patients to an upright position, have them move slowly and allow them to sit for a while before standing up. If these precautions are not taken, patients may fall and injure themselves unnecessarily.

958. The answer is D. *(Ballinger, 7/e, vol 3, p 131. Bontrager, 3/e, p 644. Ehrlich, 4/e, p 238. Snopek, 3/e, p 175.)* The Seldinger technique is employed in the process of catheterizing a blood vessel for angiographic exams. This technique provides an opening into a vessel for the introduction of a catheter. A compound needle with a removable inner stylet is used to pierce both walls of the selected vessel. The needle is then slowly withdrawn into the vessel until a steady blood return is achieved. The inner core of the needle is then removed and a flexible guide wire inserted through the needle into the vessel. The remainder of the needle is then withdrawn over the guide wire. The catheter is placed over the guide wire and fed into the vessel. Finally the guide wire is removed and the vessel is catheterized. Percutaneous transhepatic cholangiography is achieved by passing a long, thin needle through the liver into an enlarged bile duct. Once in place, the needle remains in position until the exam is complete. Catheterization of a patient for a cystogram is performed by the direct introduction of the catheter into the bladder via the uretha. The ultimate goal of an ERCP exam is to catheterize the pancreatic duct through the assistance of an endoscope positioned within the duodenum at the ampulla of Vater.

959. The answer is B. *(Adler, pp 313–314. Ehrlich, 4/e, pp 218–219. Mosby, 3/e, pp 271, 700, 987.)* The BUN (blood urea nitrogen) and creatinine levels found in a patient's blood are indicators of renal function. Elevated levels of these substances may contraindicate the use of intravenous contrast media, which could cause further stress on renal function. The radiographer should check a patient's chart for this information and bring it to the attention of the radiologist prior to administering such contrast media. Liver function tests would include information on serum bilirubin level and prothrombin time. Pulmonary function is an evaluation of the exchange of oxygen and carbon dioxide. Coagulation factor is an indicator of clotting time for blood.

960. The answer is D. *(Adler, pp 307, 315. Ballinger, 7/e, vol 3, p 262. Bontrager, 3/e, p 623. Ehrlich, 4/e, pp 243–244.)* For cranial and thoracic CT examinations, water-soluble iodine contrast media are administered intravenously. However, exams of the abdomen and pelvis may require both IV introduction of a water-soluble iodine contrast media and oral administration of barium sulfate. In those patients for whom barium is contraindicated, the use of oral water-soluble iodine contrast media may be substituted. The natural presence of air within the body may act as a contrast agent, but air is not purposefully introduced. Iodized oils are no longer commonly used as contrast agents except for lymphangiograms.

961. The answer is D. *(Ballinger, 7/e, vol 3, pp 292, 308, 365, 368. Bushong, 5/e, pp 477–480, 516–518. Ehrlich, 4/e, pp 246–249.)* Only ultrasound and magnetic resonance imaging (MRI) do not utilize ionizing radiation in the imaging process. Sound waves are a form of mechanical energy that requires a medium through which to be conducted. Reflected sound waves or echoes are then received and used to generate an image. MRI utilizes electromagnetic energy from the radio frequency range to stimulate a tissue sample and generate a return signal, also in the radio frequency range. Although these modalities do not cause biologic effects like those associated with radiation exposure, there are certain biologic and safety issues that must be considered. Fortunately, any biologic effect noted has a threshold level below which no negative effects have been observed. Computed tomography, nuclear medicine, and single photon emission computed tomography (SPECT) all employ ionizing radiation. CT procedures expose patients to a finely collimated beam. All radiation safety practices must be applied to CT exams as for routine radiography. Routine nuclear medicine and the more specialized technique of SPECT require the administration of a radiopharmaceutical to the patient prior to the imaging procedure. Again, all radiation safety practices must be applied.

962. The answer is C. *(Ehrlich, 4/e, p 235. Snopek, 3/e, p 257.)* As part of the myelogram, a lumbar puncture is made and a needle is inserted into the subarachnoid space of the spinal canal. A small amount of CSF is generally removed for laboratory analysis. The contrast medium is then injected and the needle removed before filming. In order to prevent the flow of the contrast medium into the ventricles while the patient is in the Trendelenburg position, the neck and head are extended. Following the exam, the patient is instructed to rest, keep the head slightly elevated (20 to 30°), and increase fluid intake for the next several hours. This action will reduce the incidence of a severe headache while the lost CSF is being replenished.

963. The answer is B. *(Ballinger, 7/e, vol 3, p 103. Bontrager, 3/e, p 676. Ehrlich, 4/e, pp 233–235. Snopek, 3/e, p 257.)* The water-soluble iodinated type of contrast media are currently the agents of choice for myelography, rather than the oily iodinated materials used previously. These current agents are administered via a lumbar puncture, as were the iodized oils. However, since the contrast medium will be absorbed by the body, there is no need to leave the needle in position during the exam for removal of the contrast medium at the end of the exam. This allows for safer positioning of the patient for filming without risk of bumping the needle. The water-soluble agents also provide better opacification of the nerve roots than was possible with the iodized oils. However, the body does begin to absorb the contrast media within 30 min of administration and opacification is good for about an hour, which curtails the amount of time for filming. Following the exam, the patient is instructed to rest in bed with the head elevated 20 to 30° to reduce the occurrence of a headache.

964. The answer is B. *(Snopek, 3/e, pp 277–279.)* The hysterosalpingogram is performed to image the uterus and fallopian tubes. This is achieved by the introduction of water-soluble iodine contrast media directly into the uterus. As the contrast media flows, it fills the fallopian tube (retrograde) and spills out into the peritoneal cavity. As a diagnostic tool, this exam provides an opportunity to evaluate the anatomic structure of the uterus and fallopian tubes, as well as to determine the presence of an abnormality or disease process. However, it is also useful as a therapeutic tool. As a result of the pressure of the contrast media flow, blocked or kinked fallopian tubes may be opened and dilated to a more normal status. This procedure, which is often included as part of a fertility evaluation, often improves infertility problems. The remainder of the radiologic procedures listed as answer options provide diagnostic data only.

965. The answer is D (3). *(Ballinger, 7/e, vol 1, p 42. Snopek, 3/e, pp 309–312.)* Arthrography is the radiographic exam of freely moveable joints, referred to as *diarthrotic* joints, to evaluate the condition of the articular surfaces of the bones and the ligaments supporting the joint. This exam is slowly becoming replaced by MRI procedures. The arthrogram most commonly employs the use of air and water-soluble iodine contrast media to enhance visualization of the joint. The joints most commonly evaluated in this manner include the knee, hip, shoulder, wrist, and TMJ.

966. The answer is B. *(Ballinger, 7/e, vol 1, p 444. Snopek, 3/e, pp 312–313.)* The radiographic exam of the freely moveable joints known as arthrography is slowly being replaced by MRI. The increased quantity of detail visualized as well as continued improvements in the imaging process contribute to this movement. However, in regions where MRI centers are not as available, radiographic arthrography will continue to be performed.

967. The answer is A. *(Ehrlich, 4/e, p 86.)* Cyanotic changes manifest as a bluish tint to the lips or nail beds of the patient. This is in response to a lack of oxygen in the blood for a variety of reasons involving the cardiopulmonary system. For some patients, this may be a fairly normal condition, but if the patient becomes cyanotic during a visit to the radiology department, further observations must be made and a physician consulted to assure proper assistance is provided to the patient.

968–970. The answers are 968-D, 969-A, 970-B. *(Adler, p 348. Ehrlich, 4/e, pp 20–21.)* Radiographers, as any health care professionals, are liable for their actions or lack of action pertaining to any patient in their care. The type of misconduct characterized as battery would be any form of physical contact that is undesirable to a patient. This includes touching patients against their will, even if it is gentle and a part of the procedure, or radiographing the wrong patient. To minimize the chance of committing this type of offense, radiographers must remember to explain their actions as the exam proceeds. Always check patient identification and check the exam request with the patient's history or medical chart.

An invasion of privacy may occur as a breach of patient confidentiality by the radiographer or other health care professional. All information pertaining to a patient is privileged and not to be disclosed inappropriately. This also includes the responsibility of technologists to keep the patient's modesty protected while in their care.

False imprisonment is characterized by any action in which patients feel a procedure is being forced upon them. Patients have the right to refuse to have an exam done at any point. They also have the right to leave the department and not be detained against their wishes. Patient restraints or other immobilization devices should be used prudently and their purpose should be explained to the patient and family members.

971–976. The answers are 971-C, 972-B, 973-C, 974-A, 975-A, 976-B. *(Adler, pp 217, 241, 244–245, 247–249. Ballinger, 7/e, vol 1, p 502; vol 2, p 112; vol 3, p 104. Bontrager, 3/e, pp 429, 462. Ehrlich, 4/e, pp 71–72, 176–177, 184–185, 195.)* The Trendelenburg position requires the placement of the patient's head to be 30 to 45° lower than the body and legs. In radiography, this position is used for evaluation of esophageal reflux during a barium swallow or UGI series. The patient is usually positioned in the right anterior oblique position for this evaluation. The left posterior oblique position may also be used. The prone Trendelenburg position is used during myelography to move the column of contrast media into the upper dorsal and cervical regions of the spinal column. A patient who is in shock or feeling weak and ready to faint should be placed in the Trendelenburg position. These conditions are generally due to a drop in blood pressure and an associated reduction in oxygen to the brain. Since this position places the head lower than the body and legs, it allows for an increased flow of blood to the brain.

The Sims position requires the patient to be positioned on the left side. The right leg is then flexed and placed above and in front of the left leg. This position is used to expose the patient's anus for the insertion of an enema tip. Patients should be informed as to what actions will occur and their modesty protected.

The Fowler position is met by elevating the patient's head about 18 to 20 inches from the flat supine position. Also the knees are bent and raised to a comfortable position. This position is recommended when a patient needs to use a urinal or bed pan. Patients with respiratory illnesses frequently have difficulty breathing when in the supine position. When it is conducive to the radiologic exam being performed, the patient's head should be elevated to assist in the ability to breathe. If the exam requires the patient to be flat, an upright or decubitus alternative may be required.

The ventral decubitus position places the patient prone and employs a horizontal beam to obtain a lateral projection of the area of interest. This position is used to obtain cross-table lateral projections of the spine during myelography.

977–981. The answers are 977-B, 978-A, 979-D, 980-C, 981-B. *(Adler, pp 304–309. Ballinger, 7/e, vol 3, p 173. Bontrager, 3/e, pp 424–425, 464. Ehrlich, 4/e, pp 198–200, 205–206, 215.)* Water-soluble iodine contrast media are the only type that can be administered intravenously due to their ability to be absorbed and excreted by the urinary system. They are used for radiologic procedures of the circulatory system (arterial and venous) and the urinary system primarily. The nonionic types are preferred, especially for angiography where large quantities of contrast media are used, due to the reduced likelihood of an allergic reaction associated with their use. Neither barium nor iodized oils are excreted by the kidneys, and these media are never introduced to the vasculature. Air injected into a blood vessel will act as an embolism, disrupting blood flow and causing a potentially life-threatening situation. Barium sulfate is the standard contrast medium used for opacification of the gastrointestinal tract. It is administered either orally or rectally. The mixture of barium is a suspension and does not react chemically with the body. It is eliminated unchanged through the natural processes of the gastrointestinal tract. A contraindication to the use of barium is the possibility of extravasation of the material from the GI tract into the peritoneum via a perforation. Barium that leaks into the peritoneum will not be absorbed by the body and will most likely have a toxic effect on the patient. A water-soluble iodine-based contrast medium should be used in place of barium. This material will be absorbed by the body if it extravasates out of the alimentary tract. It may be administered orally or rectally. Double-contrast exams of the GI tract are performed using a combination of barium and carbon dioxide crystals for the upper GI and barium and room air for the lower GI series. A thick form of barium is used to coat the gastric or intestinal mucosa, then air is introduced to distend the organ. Double-contrast exams provide enhanced demonstration of the lining of the stomach and intestines. Lymphography is the radiographic study of the lymphatic system, including its vessels and nodes. These structures must be enhanced with contrast media in order to be visualized. Iodized oils are the contrast media of choice for lymphography. Water-soluble iodine contrast media become dilute and are absorbed from the lymph vessels too quickly to be of use.

982–986. The answers are 982-C, 983-A, 984-D, 985-B, 986-C. *(Adler, p 318. Bontrager, 3/e, p 512. Ehrlich, 4/e, p 183.)* Anaphylactic shock is a severe type of reaction to iodine contrast media. This condition is characterized by a drop in blood pressure, dyspnea, and possible respiratory and cardiac arrest. This type of reaction requires immediate response for full emergency treatment in order to prevent death of the patient. Such a response can manifest very suddenly and the radiographer must be aware and ready to respond. For this reason, the patient should not be left alone after receiving iodine-type contrast media. Convulsions are also a severe type of reaction. A physician must be contacted to advise the proper type of medical care.

Moderate reactions include widespread hives, excessive vomiting, and tachycardia (increased or rapid pulse rate). A physician should be notified of these changes in the patient's status so that appropriate treatment will be provided.

The mild reactions include nausea, vomiting, and a possible vasovagal response that includes sweating, dizziness, and weakness. Generally, the radiographer can assist the patient sufficiently and offer comfort in the form of reassurance and a cool cloth on the forehead. These responses will usually pass on their own, but the patient must be observed for progression of symptoms.

987–990. The answers are 987-D, 988-A, 989-C, 990-B. *(Adler, pp 259–264. Ehrlich, 4/e, pp 169–178.)* Medical emergencies require a prompt and appropriate response from any person working in health care. Life-threatening conditions can occur very suddenly. Such emergencies include cardiopulmonary arrest (no respiratory or circulatory actions), shock (another type of failure of the circulatory system), respiratory distress (inability to breathe adequately), and head injury (trauma to the brain affecting its function). Patients who are in cardiac arrest require prompt treatment to reestablish the circulation of oxygenated blood. This can be achieved by mechanical devices, but may need to be initiated through the practice of cardiopulmonary resuscitation. This action provides artificial ventilation through mouth-to-mouth breathing or use of some type of breathing device. CPR also provides circulation of the blood by chest compressions that manually squeeze the heart between the sternum and thoracic spine. The loss of oxygenated blood to the brain for more than 5 min can severely damage the brain. Unresolved respiratory distress can also lead to cardiac arrest. The partial or complete obstruction of the airway results in a decreased supply of oxygen to the brain and may lead to a loss of consciousness or death. Proper training in the technique of CPR and the Heimlich maneuver can prepare the health care worker to provide life-saving measures in these cases. Another type of medical emergency is shock, of which there are various types. The general manifestation of shock is a drastic drop in blood pressure, resulting in an insufficient supply of oxygen to the body. Shock may result from an excessive loss of blood, sudden change in body temperature, or an allergic reaction. Effects of traumatic head injuries may be fairly mild, such as dizziness or a brief loss of consciousness. More severe trauma may cause bruising of the brain and an associated swelling of the brain and increased intracranial pressure. If untreated, the patient may experience seizure activity and become comatose.

991–996. The answers are 991-E, 992-A, 993-D, 994-C, 995-B, 996-E. *(Adler, pp 7–10. Ballinger, 7/e, vol 3, pp 64–65, 204, 292, 318, 362. Bushong, 5/e, pp 336, 407, 450, 500. Ehrlich, 4/e, pp 242–252.)* Numerous specialty imaging modalities are available to optimally image the human body. Some of these techniques employ ionizing radiation in the energy range of that used in traditional diagnostic radiology. These include mammography, CT, and nuclear medicine. Mammography is the specialized technique of imaging the soft tissue structures of the breast. Dedicated equipment and techniques are employed to enhance the naturally low subject contrast of the breast, with an emphasis on maintaining the lowest possible radiation dose. Computed tomography employs very sophisticated equipment to obtain sectional images of the body that are able to be enhanced via computer assistance. Nuclear medicine exams require the patient to be injected with a radiopharmaceutical that concentrates in the organ of interest. A gamma camera is then used to detect and measure the radiation concentration and ultimately an image is produced and may be enhanced through computer manipulation. The two modalities that do not employ ionizing radiation are ultrasound and magnetic resonance imaging (MRI). Ultrasound equipment produces a high-frequency sound wave that is applied to the body and generates a return signal known as an *echo*. These echoes are stored in digital form and reconstructed to yield an image on a computer monitor. Because of its minimal negative effects on biologic tissue, ultrasound is commonly used to image the fetus in utero and is able to provide data to determine gestational age. MRI is a very complex technique that also employs a computer to generate a pulse of electromagnetic energy and then receive a return signal, which is stored and reconstructed into an image. The electromagnetic energies used in MRI are in the radio frequency range, which is the basis for its status as a nonionizing imaging modality. Nuclear medicine, CT, MRI, and ultrasound all employ a computer for the purpose of digitizing the signal generated by the body area imaged. The image is then reconstructed and displayed on a monitor and then recorded onto film from the monitor, using either a multiformat camera or a laser imaging system. Only mammography is still directly recorded on film. However, development of a digital mammography unit is under way and such capabilities are expected to be available in the near future.

997-1000. The answers are 997-D, 998-A, 999-C, 1000-B. *(Ballinger, 7/e, vol 1, pp 444–445; vol 3, pp 102–103, 173. Bontrager, 3/e, pp 669, 676. Snopek, 3/e, pp 257–258, 289–290, 313, 322.)* The radiographic procedures described in these questions are considered to be of a more specialized nature than routine radiography. The frequency of these procedures has been somewhat lessened due to the variety of alternate imaging modalities. However, they are still performed frequently enough to continue to be included in the basic radiography education curriculum. The use of contrast media is required in each of these exams; however, only lymphography also uses a dye to stain the anatomic structures, specifically the small lymphatic vessels, in order to distinguish them for cannulation. The contrast media (iodized oils) are then slowly injected. This is most likely the only radiologic exam for which iodized oils are still the preferred contrast media.

Although iodized oil does have its disadvantages, its high density and long life are advantageous for this procedure.

The need to remove contrast media from an organ was more common when iodized oils were used in myelography, bronchography, and sialography. This was due to the fact that this material was very slowly absorbed by the body and often could be seen years after it was introduced. Currently, bronchography is seldom performed because of bronchoscopy and CT procedures. Myelography and sialography currently use water-soluble contrast media, which are readily absorbed by the body. However, it is still recommended to extract as much contrast material as possible after a sialogram, even though it is water-soluble. This is achieved by having the patient suck on pieces of lemon to stimulate the salivary glands to excrete saliva and the contrast medium.

Of the exams offered as answer options, only arthrography is commonly performed as a double-contrast exam. This is achieved by introducing water-soluble iodine contrast media and air into the joint cavity. The positive contrast agent coats the articular surfaces of the bone and the air acts to distend the cavity and provide for negative contrast.

Current methods of performing myelography often incorporate both routine fluoroscopic/radiographic and CT imaging techniques. Water-soluble iodine contrast media are introduced into the spinal canal via a lumbar puncture and preliminary filming may be obtained. The patient is then transferred to the CT room to obtain enhanced cross-sectional images.

Bibliography

Adler AM, Carlton RR: *Introduction to Radiography and Patient Care,* Philadelphia, Saunders, 1994.

American Registry of Radiologic Technologists: *Handbook for Advanced Level Examinations.* Mendota Heights, MN, The American Registry of Radiologic Technologists, 1991.

Ballinger PW: *Merrill's Atlas of Radiographic Positions and Radiologic Procedures,* 7/e, 3 vols. St. Louis, Mosby-Year Book, 1991.

Bontrager KL: *Textbook of Radiographic Positioning and Related Anatomy,* 3/e. St. Louis, Mosby-Year Book, 1993.

Bushong S: *Radiologic Science for Technologists: Physics, Biology, and Protection,* 5/e. St. Louis, Mosby-Year Book, 1993.

Carlton R, McKenna-Adler A: *Principles of Radiographic Imaging: An Art and a Science.* Albany, Delmar, 1992.

Carroll QB: *Fuch's Radiographic Exposure, Processing and Quality Control,* 5/e. Springfield, IL, Charles C Thomas, 1993.

Cullinan AM: *Producing Quality Radiographs,* 2/e. Philadelphia, Lippincott, 1994.

Curry TS, Dowdey JE, Murry RC: *Christensen's Physics of Diagnostic Radiology,* 4/e. Philadelphia, Lea & Febiger, 1990.

Dowd SB: *Practical Radiation Protection and Applied Radiobiology.* Philadelphia, Saunders, 1994.

Ehrlich RA, McCloskey ED: *Patient Care in Radiography,* 4/e. St. Louis, Mosby, 1993.

Eisenberg RL, Dennis CA: *Comprehensive Radiographic Pathology.* St. Louis, Mosby, 1990.

Ellis DB: *Becoming a Master Student,* 5/e. Rapid City, SD, College Survival, 1985.

Fry RW: *How to Study,* 3/e. Hawthorne, NJ, Career Press, 1994.

Gray JE, Winkler NT, Stears J, Frank ED: *Quality Control in Diagnostic Imaging.* Baltimore, University Park Press, 1983.

Laudicina P: *Applied Pathology for Radiographers.* Philadelphia, Saunders, 1989.

Marieb EN: *Human Anatomy and Physiology,* 2/e. Redwood City, CA, Benjamin-Cummings, 1992.

McKinney WEJ: *Radiographic Processing and Quality Control.* Philadelphia, Lippincott, 1988.

Mosby's Medical, Nursing and Allied Health Dictionary, 3/e. St. Louis, Mosby, 1990.

National Council on Radiation Protection and Measurements (NCRP): *Limitation of Exposure to Ionizing Radiation.* Report No. 116. Bethesda, MD, National Council on Radiation Protection and Measurements, 1993.

NCRP: *Medical X-Ray Electron Beam and Gamma-Ray Protection for Energies up to 50 MeV (Equipment Design, Performance and Use).* Report No. 102. Bethesda, MD, National Council on Radiation Protection and Measurements, 1989.

NCRP: *Quality Assurance for Diagnostic Imaging.* Report No. 99. Bethesda, MD, National Council on Radiation Protection and Measurements, 1988.

NCRP: *Radiation Protection for Medical and Allied Health Personnel.* Report No. 105. Bethesda, MD, National Council on Radiation Protection and Measurements, 1989.

NCRP: *Recommendations on Limits for Exposure to Ionizing Radiation.* Report No. 91. Bethesda, MD, National Council on Radiation Protection and Measurements, 1987.

Pansky B: *Review of Gross Anatomy,* 5/e. New York, McGraw-Hill, 1984.

Selman J: *The Fundamentals of X-Ray and Radium Physics,* 8/e. Springfield, IL, Charles C Thomas, 1994.

Snopek AM: *Fundamentals of Special Radiographic Procedures,* 3/e. Philadelphia, Saunders, 1992.

Statkiewicz-Sherer MA, Visconti PJ, Ritenour ER: *Radiation Protection in Medical Radiography,* 2/e. St. Louis, Mosby, 1993.

Sweeney RJ: *Radiographic Artifacts: Their Cause and Control.* Philadelphia, Lippincott, 1983.

Thompson MA, Hattaway MP, Hall JD, Dowd SB: *Principles of Imaging Science and Protection.* Philadelphia, Saunders, 1994.

Thornborough JR, Schmidt HJ: *How to Prepare for the Step 1 Medical Exam,* 2/e. New York, McGraw-Hill, 1993.

Travis EL: *Primer of Medical Radiobiology,* 2/e. Chicago, Year Book Medical, 1989.

Weir J: *An Imaging Atlas of Human Anatomy.* St. Louis, Mosby-Year Book, 1992.

ISBN 0-07-052078-X